Caring for the
Perioperative Patient

Second Edition

Paul and Joy would like to dedicate this book to:
Our teachers, our students, our colleagues, our friends
Kate, Mairi and Neil Wicker
Barry and Nicola O'Neill
Beth Lynch
Anne Mottram

Caring for the Perioperative Patient

Second Edition

Paul Wicker
Head of Perioperative Studies
Visiting Professor, First Hospital and Medical
School, Nanjing, China
Faculty of Health
Edge Hill University
Ormskirk
Address for correspondence: wickerp@edgehill.ac.uk

AND

Joy O'Neill
Practice Placement Facilitator
Faculty of Health
Edge Hill University
Ormskirk
Address for correspondence: joy.oneill@edgehill.ac.uk

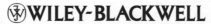

A John Wiley & Sons, Ltd., Publication

This edition first published 2010
First edition published 2006
© 2010 Paul Wicker and Joy O'Neill

Blackwell Publishing was acquired by John Wiley & Sons in February 2007.
Blackwell's publishing programme has been merged with Wiley's global
Scientific, Technical, and Medical business to form Wiley-Blackwell.

Registered office
John Wiley & Sons Ltd, The Atrium, Southern Gate, Chichester, West Sussex,
PO19 8SQ, United Kingdom

Editorial offices
9600 Garsington Road, Oxford, OX4 2DQ, United Kingdom
2121 State Avenue, Ames, Iowa 50014-8300, USA

For details of our global editorial offices, for customer services and for
information about how to apply for permission to reuse the copyright material
in this book please see our website at www.wiley.com/wiley-blackwell.

The right of the author to be identified as the author of this work has been
asserted in accordance with the UK Copyright, Designs and Patents Act 1988.

Library of Congress Cataloging-in-Publication Data
Wicker, Paul.
   Caring for the perioperative patient / Paul Wicker and Joy O'Neill. – 2nd ed.
      p. ; cm.
   Includes bibliographical references and index.
   ISBN 978-1-4051-8850-0 (pbk. : alk. paper)   1. Operating room nursing.
2. Preoperative care.   3. Postoperative care.   I. O'Neill, Joy.   II. Title.
   [DNLM: 1. Perioperative Care–nursing.   2. Perioperative Nursing–
methods.   WY 161 W636c 2010]
   RD32.3.W53 2010
   617'.917–dc22

                                   2009049072

A catalogue record for this book is available from the British Library.
Set in 9 on 11 pt Palatino by Toppan Best-set Premedia Limited

Printed and bound in Malaysia by Vivar Printng Sdn Bhd

1 2010

Contents

Foreword by Mary Moore *Associate Director, National Orthopaedic Project, Department of Health, London*   vi
Preface   viii
Acknowledgements   xii

Section 1   Core Issues   1
 1   Perioperative homeostasis   2
     Paul Wicker
 2   Managing perioperative equipment   51
     Joy O'Neill
 3   Perioperative pharmacology   101
     Paul Wicker and Africa Bocos
 4   Perioperative communication   134
     Joy O'Neill
 5   Managing perioperative risks   179
     Joy O'Neill

Section 2   Perioperative Practice   229
 6   A route to enhanced competence in perioperative care   230
     Paul Wicker and Jill Ferbrache
 7   Preoperative preparation of perioperative patients   247
     Paul Wicker
 8   Patient care during anaesthesia   271
     Joy O'Neill
 9   Patient care during surgery   339
     Paul Wicker and Adele Nightingale
 10   Patient care during recovery   379
     Paul Wicker and Felicia Cox

Index   413

Foreword

In recent years the NHS has seen unprecedented change, resulting in significant healthcare improvement for patients and
increased career opportunities within the NHS and its partners.
These developments in innovative and advancing levels of
practice are also reflected across Europe and many parts of the
world.

The dynamic pace of this change has presented significant
challenges for clinicians as they endeavour to acquire high-level
clinical skills and deliver care while adapting to many new
ways of working.

The UK NHS has had to respond dramatically to the changing
demographics of its workforce and to high-level policy to drive
down waiting times for patients and to increase the capacity for
surgery. The perioperative workforce has been at the forefront
of such changes and has had to undergo significant transforma-
tion in the way it works, crossing traditional healthcare boundaries. The aspirations of health professionals, structured NHS
career frameworks, pay modernisation, working practice legislation, advancing levels of practice and the skills escalator
concept of skills progression all contribute to the complexity of
delivering care to patients.

The provision of education to health professionals giving
perioperative care has also undergone significant change, with
much more cross-profession delivery of core skills, increased
e-learning opportunities and the development of nationally led
Advanced Practitioner programmes. This education and exposure to hands-on learning is against a backdrop of increasing
workload and advances in technology that now support clinical
intervention.

Clinical input for trainees is a vital component in the education of our perioperative workforce, but both students and
teachers within the many specialisms that encompass peri-

operative practice need access to a knowledge base that is modern, comprehensive and fit for purpose. The publication of such a clinically based and up-to-date resource is well overdue, and this book promises to fill that gap.

This text is well structured for easy reference and lends itself to detailed underpinning of knowledge, while at the same time being suitable for use as a quick reference guide. I am confident that it will fulfill a need for both learners and teachers within perioperative care.

Mary Moore
Associate Director, National Orthopaedic Project
Department of Health, London

Preface

Perioperative care has been through a number of changes and has now developed into a truly patient-centred, holistic, evidence-based speciality that offers practitioners challenges and opportunities that are rarely seen outside the perioperative environment. Perioperative practitioners are defined in this book as nurses or operating department practitioners (ODPs) who perform scrub, circulating, anaesthetic and recovery roles whilst caring for perioperative patients.

The pressures brought about by initiatives such as the NHS Plan, Clinical Governance and Agenda for Change mean that the care of the patient undergoing surgery is now carried out by many different professionals. Old technique-centred practice has given way to a patient-centred, evidence-based approach. A diverse and challenging perioperative environment has therefore developed with subsequent challenges for the practitioners who work there.

The purpose of this book is to identify and discuss the essential core skills and knowledge required by perioperative practitioners to care for their patients. It is primarily aimed at the period following registration but before the development of advanced perioperative skills, such as those displayed by advanced practitioners. As such it is also a source of information for nursing and ODP students working in perioperative care.

This evidence-based and innovative book has been written to embrace the changes in the perioperative role. It is skills-orientated and uses examples of techniques or procedures to illustrate how those skills can be applied in perioperative practice. It refers to practitioners rather than nurses or ODPs to ensure the inclusion of all practitioners working in the perioperative environment.

This book is arranged in two sections: Core Issues and more specific Perioperative Practice.

CORE ISSUES
Chapter 1 describes the practitioner's role in the delivery of therapeutic interventions required because of the anatomical and physiological influences of anaesthesia and surgery. The chapter reviews the concept of homeostasis in the context of holistic perioperative care and identifies the impact of anaesthesia and surgery on the systems of the body. Topics include principles of perioperative homeostasis, fluid balance, cardiovascular homeostasis, the respiratory system, wound healing and trauma.

Chapter 2 discusses the overall management of perioperative equipment with specific reference to the most common types currently in use in the perioperative environment. There is an emphasis on the safe use and maintenance of anaesthetic and surgical equipment.

Chapter 3 discusses the implications of the use of various drugs on perioperative care. There is a discussion on the metabolism of drugs, and the uses, administration and side effects of common perioperative drugs. Drugs included in this chapter include opiates, muscle relaxants, analgesics, local anaesthetic agents, general anaesthetic agents and antiemetics.

Chapter 4 considers ways to enhance communication in the perioperative environment. There is an exploration of important aspects of communication in relation to perioperative patients to ensure safe and effective care. There is also reference to the different roles of the perioperative practitioner within the perioperative team. Topics include perioperative patient checklists, patient advocacy, consent, clinical governance, change management, principles of record keeping and NHS and patient agencies.

Chapter 5 looks at risk management in the perioperative environment. It explores the main principles of risk management and identifies some of the common perioperative risks to patients. Topics include discussion on specific perioperative risks, such as infection control, pressure area care, deep vein thrombosis prophylaxis, inadvertent hypothermia, latex allergy and smoke inhalation.

The following chapters explore the indicators further and discuss some of the important skills and knowledge displayed by practitioners in anaesthesia, surgery and recovery.

PERIOPERATIVE PRACTICE

Chapter 6 presents the competencies associated with the role of the perioperative practitioner. It is based on the work carried out by NHS Education Scotland (NES) working parties in 2001–2002 and 2006–2008. This chapter presents a discussion of perioperative competencies and their associated indicators for perioperative practitioners and also specifically anaesthetic assistants. The indicators are measurable markers of the achievement of the competencies and are provided as examples of the competencies that practitioners develop in specific clinical areas.

Chapter 7 considers the role of the practitioner in the preoperative preparation of perioperative patients. It explores the techniques and methods of perioperative assessment and the role of the perioperative practitioner in preoperative visiting and care planning. Topics include selection of patients for surgery, assessment of patient's condition, common concurrent diseases, illnesses and conditions, and preoperative planning to prevent intraoperative and postoperative complications.

Chapter 8 explores the skills and knowledge required by anaesthetic practitioners in the assistance of the establishment and maintenance of anaesthesia. It discusses the different types of anaesthesia, many of the clinical techniques used in anaesthesia and the role of the anaesthetic practitioner in the anaesthetic team. Topics include patient care during different types of anaesthesia, airway management and patient monitoring.

Chapter 9 discusses the roles of the scrub and circulating practitioners. It explores some of the clinical techniques that practitioners use during surgery and the part that the practitioner plays within the surgical team. Content includes discussion on surgical scrubbing, haemostasis, wound closure, positioning the patient and wound care.

Finally, Chapter 10 considers unique aspects of the role of the recovery practitioner and the main clinical techniques used in recovery. Content includes discussion on the principles of patient care after clinical intervention, patient assessment, airway maintenance, pain management and discharge criteria in postoperative patients. Topics also include common postoperative complications such as nausea and vomiting, shock, hypothermia and airway complications.

We hope that you enjoy using this book to enhance your practice and that it helps you to provide optimum patient care.

Joy O'Neill and Paul Wicker

Readers' note: Every effort has been made to check the accuracy of drug and product information, and clinical content. However, readers should check the manufacturer's product information and local workplace policies and protocols before undertaking any intervention.

Acknowledgements

We would like to say thank you to several people for helping us to produce this book. For help with the first edition, we would like to say thank you to Caroline MacDonald, Joanne Wildman and Linda Faulkener for their help reviewing the book proposal. We also thank all the people who have read, reviewed, edited and commented on our work as it has developed, including Rachel Astle, Janet Bidwell, Samantha Mills, Caroline Macdonald, Amanda Clarke, Andrew Clancy, Robert Hughes, Jonathon Kenworthy, Shahid Mirza, Mujahid Zaheer, Janet Barrie, Brian Allsop for the photographs, Beth Lynch for help with the illustrations, and all our colleagues at work. Finally thank you to Beth Knight for her confidence in us and for the role she has played in helping us to achieve our goal.

For help with the second edition, we would also like to thank Adele Nightingale, Jill Ferbrache, Felicia Cox, Africa Bocos, Teresa Hardcastle, Chris Wiles, Victoria Mason and Bernard Pennington.

Section 1

Core Issues

1 | Perioperative Homeostasis

Paul Wicker

LEARNING OUTCOMES
- ❑ Understand *homeostasis*.
- ❑ Discuss *fluid and electrolyte balance* in the perioperative patient.
- ❑ Describe the *structure, function and regulation of the cardiovascular and respiratory system.*
- ❑ Describe *blood pressure regulation*.
- ❑ Discuss the implications of the *metabolic response* and the *stages of wound healing*.

INTRODUCTION
Teamwork is the focus of good perioperative practice. Nowhere is teamwork more obvious than within the human body itself, where the close and efficient functioning of all the individual parts is essential for survival.

The purpose of this introductory chapter is to set the context of perioperative care and to identify links between the patient's anatomy and physiology, and perioperative care. Everything that happens to the perioperative patient during surgery and anaesthesia has an effect on his or her anatomy and physiology. This makes it important to understand the internal maintenance and control of the body's systems, and the external control through medical interventions.

The human body is a complex system of parts which can protect itself against major changes to its own internal environment. It does this by preserving a fine balance between all its major organs and systems, by maintaining fluids and electrolytes, blood pressure and oxygenation between particular limits to ensure efficient functioning. Every part of the system is related: for example, the lungs absorb oxygen which is transported by the blood to muscles such as the heart, allowing it to beat and maintain blood pressure. The blood pressure in turn pushes the oxygenated blood around the body to the tissue cells. The blood then progresses back to the lungs where it supplies the lung tissue itself, as well as going on to provide a further source of oxygenated blood to all the cells of the body.

The term homeostasis is often used to refer to the maintenance of a constant environment. In perioperative care; however, it is better to see homeostasis as a dynamic process that results in a peak state for the body under existing circumstances (Clancy *et al*. 2002). Hence, for example, blood pressure may or may not be maintained at preoperative levels during the perioperative experience, and during surgery a low blood pressure may be helpful to reduce bleeding, ensuring a bloodless field. However, the main principles of control still hold true – maintaining an ideal environment for body processes to take place under current circumstances. The aim of medical interventions, as external homeostatic controllers, is to support the body's natural ability to maintain this dynamic homeostatic environment.

The topics associated with homeostasis are huge and this chapter will highlight selected areas of interest and relate them to clinical issues raised later in the book. This chapter therefore, describes some of the ways in which the human body maintains equilibrium, how anaesthesia and surgery affect this balance and how medical interventions support the return to normal homeostasis. Finally, this chapter will look at the human body's response to stress and the process of wound healing.

PRINCIPLES OF HOMEOSTASIS

To maintain homeostasis naturally, the body needs to:

- detect and analyse changes;
- take measures to address the changes;
- evaluate the effect of measures taken.

Control mechanisms carry out these processes, acting as receptors (detecting the changes), analysers (interpreting the changes) and effectors (acting on the changes to minimise, maximise or regulate them). These mechanisms detect changes in normal values and try to bring them back to within the normal homeostatic range. An example of this system is the acid–base balance, where the buffer systems (described later in this chapter) act in unison to maintain the pH of body fluids within a normal range of around 7.35–7.45. Under normal circumstances, the body's buffer systems are able to maintain this balance; however, during illness, disease or because of trauma such as surgery or anaesthesia, the body may need support from external controls (medical interventions) to regain equilibrium.

Most of the body's own control mechanisms work through negative feedback – a change occurs to the body's environment and then mechanisms to cancel the changes are activated. Blood glucose regulation, for example, involves either the release of insulin to lower blood glucose or the release of glucagon to raise it. In either case, blood sugar levels are brought back to within the normal range.

Occasionally the control mechanisms work through positive feedback and a control mechanism to promote changes is activated – for example, blood clotting, where the blood undergoes changes that allow it to clot and therefore reduce blood loss. Once the need has passed, the blood then returns to its normal state.

Internally, the organs act as both independent and interactive homeostatic controllers. This topic goes beyond the scope of this book. However, in the perioperative patient, several systems are specifically important because they are critical to the patient's immediate survival and are also the target of many perioperative interventions. Fluid and electrolyte balances are important perioperative considerations because of the potential for blood loss and possible hypovolaemia. Medical interventions that support the effects of blood and fluid loss, and help maintain electrolyte balance, therefore, merit consideration. The regulation of the respiratory and cardiovascular systems is also crucial in both the long and the short term. The aim of many anaesthetic functions is to control these systems to provide the optimum physiological environment during surgery.

Table 1.1 Terminology associated with fluid compartments.

Fluid compartment	Description
Extracellular (extracellular fluid = ECF)	Outside cells
Intracellular (intracellular fluid = ICF)	Inside cells
Interstitial	Between cells
Intravascular	Inside blood vessels (this is also extracellular)
Extravascular	Outside blood vessels (this may be intracellular, interstitial or transcellular)
Transcellular	Within hollow spaces, such as cerebrospinal fluid, the joints, the gastrointestinal tract, the urinary tract and the ducts of glands. Also called the 'third space'

WATER AND ELECTROLYTE HOMEOSTASIS

Table 1.1 describes the fluid compartments of the body. Total body water is distributed among all the fluid compartments of the body. Of the 40 litres present in a 68 kg (150 lb) male, 65% is intracellular and 35% is extracellular. Extracellular fluid is composed of 25% tissue fluid, 8% blood plasma and lymph, and 2% transcellular fluid such as cerebrospinal fluid (CSF) and synovial fluid.

Osmosis is the main process that distributes fluid throughout these compartments (Watson & Fawcett 2003). The term 'osmolarity' refers to the concentration of solutes (such as potassium) in the solution (such as water). Osmosis is a special form of diffusion which involves the passage of water across a selectively permeable cell membrane that is freely permeable to water but not freely permeable to solutes. This process aims to equalise the concentrations of the solution on each side of the membrane. In osmosis, water will flow across a membrane toward the solution that has the higher concentration of solutes, because that is where the concentration of water is lowest (Figure 1.1). A solution with a high osmolarity has high osmotic pressure.

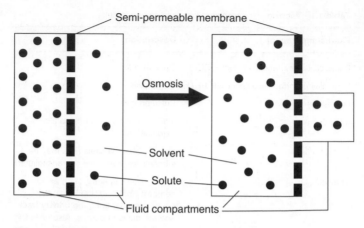

Fig. 1.1 Osmosis.

An important effect of the movement of ions and water across cell membranes is the development of an electrical charge across the membrane. The resting potential is the charge across the membrane of an undisturbed cell. When the cell is stimulated, the electrical charge may be increased, causing an 'action potential'. In nerves, for example, this represents the movement of information away from the cell body and down the nerve. In muscles, the action potential causes the contraction of muscle fibres.

Other methods which the cell uses to transport water and electrolytes include:

- filtration, which is a passive process where hydrostatic pressure (blood pressure) forces fluid and solutes across a membrane barrier;
- carrier-mediated transport, which involves specialised cell proteins binding to ions or organic substances, facilitating their entry to or exit from the cell;
- vesicular transport, which involves the movement of materials within small membranous sacs or vesicles.

Fluid balance

A person is in a state of fluid balance when water gain equals water loss; for example, a water intake of 2.5 litres a day, taken in by food and drink, is balanced by water loss via routes such as faeces, expired air, sweat and urine.

Fluid intake is mainly controlled by the thirst centre in the hypothalamus which generates the sensation of thirst. Water output is regulated by varying urine volume. This system is mainly controlled by the antidiuretic hormone (ADH), but also to a lesser extent by aldosterone and atrial natriuretic factor (ANF). Blood osmolarity is maintained because both sodium and water are either retained or excreted.

Changes in the osmotic pressure exerted by plasma influence the release of ADH. High osmotic pressure (i.e. dehydration) leads to release of ADH; low osmotic pressure (i.e. hydration) reduces excretion of ADH. This system is so efficient that under normal conditions water balance is maintained to within 2% of the normal homeostatic range (Clancy *et al*. 2002).

ANF is a peptide released by walls of the cardiac atrium in response to high sodium chloride (NaCl) concentration, high extracellular fluid volume or high blood volume. ANF inhibits NaCl reabsorption in the distal convoluted tubule and cortical collecting duct of the kidneys. It also dilates the afferent glomerular arteriole and constricts the efferent glomerular arteriole. This increases the glomerular filtration rate, which increases NaCl excretion, raises urinary filtration rate and therefore increases the rate of urine production.

Volume depletion (hypovolaemia) is a loss of total body water volume when osmolarity remains normal. Vomiting, diarrhoea, burns, haemorrhage or renal failure can cause this. Addison's disease results in dehydration leading to loss of total body water volume with an associated rise in osmolarity. This condition can also be caused by lack of drinking water, diabetes, profuse sweating or diuretics. Infants are more vulnerable to this condition.

Electrolyte balance

The balance of major electrolytes such as sodium (Na^+), potassium (K^+), calcium (Ca^{2+}), hydrogen (H^+) and bicarbonate (HCO_3^-

) is essential to ensure homeostasis and the proper functioning of the body's processes (Saladin 2009).

Maintaining electrolyte and water balance are three major hormones: ADH, which promotes water retention independently of Na^+ and K^+ concentration; aldosterone, which promotes retention of water and Na^+, and secretion of K^+; and ANF which increases NaCl secretion.

Electrolyte metabolism

Sodium and potassium

Sodium and potassium levels are critical to homeostasis because of their many roles. These two electrolytes contribute to maintaining membrane potentials, a major role of the sodium–potassium pump. Sodium is also responsible for 90–95% of osmolarity of extracellular fluid (ECF) and potassium is the primary cation in intracellular fluid (ICF).

The normal sodium intake of around 3–7 g/day exceeds the 0.5 g/day needed for survival. Normal blood level ranges are:

- Na^+, 130–145 mmol/litre;
- K^+, 3.5–5.5 mmol/litre.

The homeostasis of water, sodium and potassium levels occurs by various linked systems:

- aldosterone/ANF;
- ADH;
- oestrogen/progesterone;
- salt craving.

Intercalated cells in the collecting duct of the kidneys also control potassium levels (Saladin 2009).

Calcium

ECF contains a low concentration of calcium; however calcium exerts great influence on the body systems. Low calcium concentration increases the excitability of cells and in muscle cells this may lead to tetany. High concentrations of calcium ions make the cells less excitable and may lead to symptoms such as muscle weakness and bowel stasis. Other roles of calcium include skeletal mineralisation, muscle contraction, exocytosis (release of substances such as hormones from the vesicles of certain tissue cells) and blood clotting. Blood levels of 2.25–2.9 mmol/litre are normal.

Calcitonin is a hormone that takes part in calcium and phosphorus metabolism and affects bone deposition and resorption. Low intracellular Ca^{2+} levels influences calcitonin. The thyroid gland produces most calcitonin.

Phosphate

Phosphate is concentrated in ICF and variations in levels are well tolerated. Roles include being an ingredient of nucleic acids, phospholipids and some enzymes and coenzymes such as adenosine triphosphate. Phosphate also activates enzymes in metabolic pathways and buffers pH. Maintenance and control of phosphate homeostasis is by tubular reabsorption in the kidneys.

Chloride

Sodium and chloride homeostasis are linked. Chloride preserves osmolarity of ECF and plays a part in stomach acid production. The so-called 'chloride shift' (influx of chloride ions into cells) helps to maintain pH and electrical neutrality within cells. Chloride has a strong attraction to Na^+, K^+ and Ca^{2+}, and is retained or secreted with Na^+ by the kidneys.

Acid–base balance

The acid–base balance is a critical part of homeostasis – the normal pH range of ECF (including blood) is 7.35–7.45. Several processes within the body affect acid–base balance maintenance. For example, normal metabolism produces substances such as lactic acids, phosphoric acids, fatty acids, ketones and carbonic acids, which all affect pH. Even absorption of acidic foods may alter blood pH (Saladin 2009). Maintenance of acid–base balance is through buffer systems in the blood, respiration and renal systems.

Blood-based buffers

The blood itself contains three buffering systems that help to stabilise pH – the bicarbonate buffer, the phosphate buffer and the protein buffer. The bicarbonate buffering system works through the association and disassociation of carbon dioxide, water, hydrogen, carbonic acid and bicarbonate, according to the following formula:

$$CO_2 + H_2O \leftrightarrow H_2CO_3 \leftrightarrow HCO_3 + H^+$$

One molecule of carbon dioxide (CO_2) combines with one molecule of water (H_2O) to become one molecule of carbonic acid (H_2CO_3). The release of hydrogen ions from the carbonic acid increases the acidity of blood.

The carbonic acid molecule is not especially stable and will break down in one of two ways. The carbonic acid molecule may break down back to carbon dioxide and water; the equation moves to the left, resulting in alkalosis. Alternatively it could break down into one molecule of bicarbonate and one hydrogen ion and the equation moves to the right, resulting in acidosis. The chemical reactions have the effect of equalising the levels of bicarbonate/hydrogen and carbon dioxide/water – so regulating the balance between alkalinity and acidity.

The phosphate buffer system works as follows:

$$H_2PO_4 \leftrightarrow HPO_4^{2-} + H^+$$

Again, an increase in hydrogen ions increases acidity.

The protein buffer system works because the acidic side groups of protein molecules release hydrogen ions (increasing acidity) and amino side groups bind hydrogen ions (increasing alkalinity).

Respiratory buffer

The second main buffering system is a bicarbonate buffer within the respiratory system. This system is nearly three times more powerful as a buffer system than blood. The process is the same as the bicarbonate system in blood.

Renal buffer

The third and most powerful buffer system to adjust pH is renal control. The renal tubules secrete H^+ into urine and this secretion involves chemical processes using ammonium chloride and phosphate. The pH of urine affects the pH of blood by the diffusion of hydrogen ions through the membranes of the renal tubules into the kidney's capillaries (Saladin 2009).

Acidosis and alkalosis

Increasing acid or a significant loss of bicarbonate results in acidosis. H^+ ions diffuse into cells where they are buffered by the protein buffer system, and simultaneously K^+ ions are driven into the ECF. The result is membrane hyperpolarisation, which affects, for example, muscle and nerve cells function. Alkalosis is essentially the opposite of this: H^+ ions diffuse out of the cells, K^+ ions diffuse in and the membrane becomes hypopolarised.

Acidosis has several possible causes, for example carbon dioxide retention (leading to increased carbonic acid); ketone or organic acid production (such as ketoacidosis or lactic acidosis); the use of acidic drugs; or renal failure resulting in the inadequate excretion of H^+ ions. The patient may suffer symptoms of headache, blurred vision, fatigue and weakness.

Metabolic alkalosis may be the result of various conditions including, for example, inadequate generation of metabolic acids, overuse of antacids or severe vomiting. Symptoms may include weakness, muscle cramps and dizziness.

Perioperative implications of fluid and electrolyte balance

Various factors present during anaesthesia and surgery can lead to water imbalances which must either be controlled by the body systems or supported through medical interventions (Heitz & Horne 2004).

Preoperative fasting, while necessary to reduce the risk of aspiration of stomach contents during induction or recovery from anaesthesia, may also result in dehydration in elderly, young or sick patients.

Surgery may have a significant effect on water balance because of rapid changes in water level and distribution. High blood loss, for example, and resulting hypovolaemia can be quickly fatal. Hypovolaemia can also develop because of acute renal failure following disruption of perfusion of the kidneys, respiratory losses during ventilation or insensible losses through sweating because of postoperative pyrexia or disturbances in temperature. Other reasons include blood loss from wound drains, loss of peritoneal fluid and loss by vomiting, diarrhoea and evaporation by exposed moist tissues.

Surgery also has an effect on other systems of the body, especially the endocrine system, which can lead to changes in the homeostasis of water and electrolytes. For example, ADH is released because of hypotension, blood loss or dehydration, leading to water retention. Adrenaline (epinephrine) is released because of surgical stress and can lead to sodium and water retention by the kidneys (Clancy *et al.* 2002).

Management of the water balance is necessary because of these perioperative challenges. Fluid balance charts are the most common means of recording and estimating the fluid needs of patients. Consumed or infused fluids are matched against fluid losses such as urine output, exudates from wounds or blood loss. Weighing swabs during surgery gives an estimate of the volume of blood loss. The continuing assessment of patients to guard against dehydration or overhydration is therefore essential during all phases of their care (Hatfield & Tronson 2008).

Conditions such as renal depression, blood loss, vomiting or diarrhoea are likely to affect the perioperative electrolyte balance. Vomiting in particular leads to the loss of Na^+, Cl^- and K^+ ions, and gastric acids, leading to metabolic alkalosis. Anaesthetic drugs, such as morphine can stimulate vomiting, and so antiemetics (such as metoclopramide, cyclizine or ondansetron) are often administered concurrently. The problems of unproven efficacy and sometimes serious side effects of antiemetics have led to alternatives such as acupressure and acupuncture being evaluated in some areas (Abraham 2008).

Diarrhoea is common following abdominal surgery for various reasons, such as the use of enemas, use of antiemetic drugs, and following trauma or excision of the large or small bowel. When there is diarrhoea the bowel secretes several litres of fluid a day, which is high in bicarbonate, and may therefore lead to metabolic acidosis and overall electrolyte loss (Waugh & Grant 2004).

Intravenous replacement

The perioperative infusion of fluid and blood products supports homeostasis. Using fluid replacement therapies it is possible to influence the water and electrolyte content of the fluid compartments to achieve the desired result. It is important to realise that surgery and anaesthesia may have altered the body's needs either permanently, because of anatomical and physiological changes, or temporarily during the recovery phase and period of return to normality. The continuing assessment of the patient's needs is part of the science of anaesthesia and is beyond the scope of this book. However, following diagnosis and establishment of the patient's requirements, fluid and electrolyte replacement therapy will involve the practitioner in the use of colloids, crystalloids and blood products.

Colloids are plasma expanders – they selectively increase fluid in plasma while having a small effect on the intracellular compartments. Colloids include the protein-based gelatin (Gelofusine) and the carbohydrate-based dextran. They work by increasing or restoring the colloid pressure of plasma, resulting in increased fluid movement into the intravascular space. Infusion provides a short-term increase in plasma volume and their effects reduce as they are excreted.

Crystalloid infusions provide electrolytes and water, and support both intracellular and extracellular compartments. Crystalloids can be hypertonic, hypotonic or isotonic. Hypertonic solutions draw water out of cells, causing them to shrink. Mannitol is an example of such an infusate that shrinks brain cells and reduces pressure inside the cranium. Hypotonic solutions draw water into cells causing them to swell. There is a potential danger of lysis, where the cell membranes burst, and therefore it is rare to use hypotonic solutions. Cells suspended in an isotonic solution would neither increase nor decrease in size because the osmotic pressure of the fluid inside the cells is equal to that outside the cells. Isotonic solutions are widely used because they support both the intracellular and extracellular compartments.

Isotonic solutions, such as saline 0.9%, dextrose 5% and Hartmann's solution, have an osmotic pressure similar to that of plasma and therefore move between the compartments in a similar way to normal body fluids. In hypovolaemia, isotonic crystalloids, the most common of which is sodium chloride 0.9% (normal saline), replace fluid in the intravascular compartment and will slowly diffuse into the intracellular space.

Dextrose 5% is a solution of glucose in water. At a concentration of 5% it has an equal osmolarity to body fluids and so on infusion it remains largely in the intravascular compartment since it cannot diffuse rapidly into the cells. However, the body's normal metabolic processes use up the glucose, leaving behind water, which is hypotonic. Intracellular volume increases as this water is drawn into the cells. Dextrose 5% is therefore effective at increasing both extracellular and intracellular fluid. The 25 g of glucose in 0.5% solution also provides a little energy – roughly equivalent to two chocolate biscuits per 500 ml!

Hartmann's solution provides a more complex mix of electrolytes, which closely resembles that of extracellular fluid, except for the presence of lactate rather than the bicarbonate normally found in blood. Other less common infusates include potassium chloride infusion, combinations such as dextrose/saline infusions and hyper/hypotonic variations of these solutions, such as 2.5% sodium chloride (Hatfield & Tronson 2008).

THE CARDIOVASCULAR SYSTEM

For the body to stay alive, each of its cells must receive a continuous supply of nutrition and oxygen. Simultaneously, the body removes carbon dioxide and other materials produced by the cells. The body's circulatory system – the heart and blood vessels – continuously support this process of nutrition delivery and waste removal. The circulatory system pumps blood from the heart to the lungs to receive oxygen. Blood then returns to the heart to be pumped throughout the body and then returns to the heart to begin again. The lymphatic system, which is an important constituent of the circulatory system, collects interstitial fluid and returns it to the blood. The cardiovascular system and the respiratory system are linked and could be seen as interlocking and interdependent systems. They are jointly

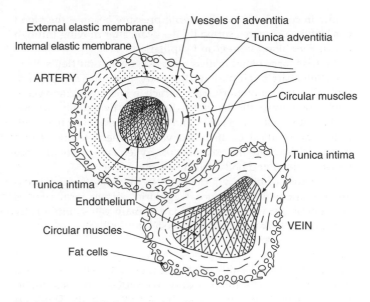

Fig. 1.2 Anatomy of an artery and a vein.

responsible for carrying oxygen from the air to the bloodstream and tissues, and expelling the waste product of carbon dioxide.

Arteries and veins

Both arteries and veins consist of three major layers called 'tunica' (Figure 1.2). Endothelium lines the inner layer of the vessel, the tunica intima. The tunica media is the middle layer, which is much thicker in arteries and contains an extra thick layer of smooth muscle that can constrict to reduce the diameter of the vessel. Blood vessels have an outer layer called the tunica adventitia. Arteries use smooth muscle contractions to alter their internal diameter, which increases or decreases the resistance to the flow of blood provided by pressure from the heart. Smooth muscle in veins can only contract weakly and so there are one-way valves that aid the flow of blood. Squeezing veins, by contracting muscles (such as calf muscles in the leg), produces blood flow through the one-way valves. Venous pressure is low in comparison with arterial pressure because the blood has lost the pressure exerted by the heart after moving through the smaller blood vessels and capillaries.

Arteries carry blood loaded with oxygen and nutrients away from the heart to all parts of the body. The only exception to this rule is the pulmonary artery which in fact carries deoxygenated blood from the heart to the lungs. Eventually arteries divide into smaller arterioles and then into even smaller capillaries, the smallest of all blood vessels. The network of tiny capillaries is where the exchange of oxygen and carbon dioxide between blood and body cells takes place.

The return of blood via the heart to the lungs for reoxygenation is of equal importance. Capillaries join to form venules and then veins, which flow into larger main veins, until finally they deliver deoxygenated blood back to the heart.

The heart
The heart consists mainly of cardiac muscle which works like a pump and contracts automatically (without conscious thought) to send blood to the lungs and the rest of the body. The heart consists of four chambers: each half of the heart consists of an upper chamber (called the atrium) and a larger lower chamber (called the ventricle). The major blood vessels entering and leaving the heart are shown in Figure 1.3.

The aorta is the largest artery in the body. It extends upward from the left ventricle of the heart, arches over the heart to the left, and descends just in front of the spinal column. The first portion of the aorta is the ascending aorta, which curves into the arch of the aorta. Three major arteries originate from the aortic arch: the brachiocephalic artery (which then branches into the right common carotid artery and the right subclavian artery), the left common carotid artery and the left subclavian artery.

The cardiac cycle
Each heartbeat consists of a 'cardiac cycle'. As the heart relaxes, both atrium chambers fill with blood: deoxygenated blood comes into the right side from the superior and inferior vena cava, and oxygenated blood returns to the left side from the lungs via the pulmonary veins. The heart valves open and the

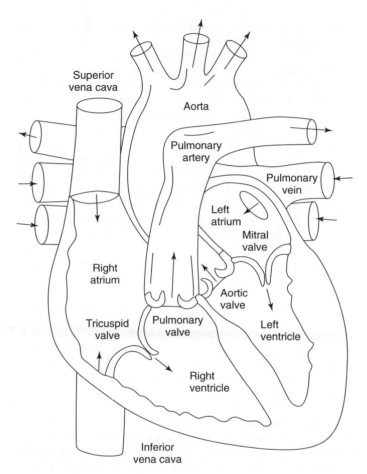

Fig. 1.3 The heart.

atria contract (systole) and force the blood into the ventricles. The ventricles then contract to pump the deoxygenated blood through the pulmonary valve into the lungs and the oxygenated blood through the aortic valve into the body's main circulatory system. The atria relax once more (diastole) and fill with blood to restart the cycle. As the valves slap shut to prevent the blood's backflow, they make a noise described as the 'lub–dub' sound of a heartbeat (Tortora 2008).

Conduction of impulses within specialised muscle tissue in the heart itself largely controls this process. The sinuatrial node, found in the right atrium, starts an impulse which spreads throughout the atrium, causing atrial contraction. It then arrives at the atrioventricular (AV) node which 'forwards' it to the bundles of His and the Purkinje fibres, spreading the signal throughout the ventricles, which cause these parts to contract. The intrinsic properties of these nodes normally control the rate of heartbeat; however, the autonomic nervous system (producing emotions such as anxiety or fear) and hormones such as thyroxine and adrenaline (epinephrine) also influence the rate of the heartbeat. The electrical activity of the heart produces the signals that can be picked up by electrocardiographs.

This outline of the cardiovascular system serves only to show the complexity of the system. Reference to texts on anatomy and physiology are essential for a full understanding of this system (e.g. Tortora 2008).

The cardiovascular system delivers oxygen and nutrients to the cells of the body, and removes waste products. This system is inextricably linked to the survival of the patient and is thus vitally important in perioperative care (Clancy *et al.* 2002). Two important areas for the perioperative patient will now be considered – interpreting cardiac rhythms and the homeostasis of blood pressure.

The electrocardiogram

The electrocardiogram (ECG) measures the electrical changes of the heart as it goes through the cardiac cycle. It is therefore useful for diagnosis of abnormal cardiac rhythms and other cardiac pathology. Therefore, ECG machines provide early warning of cardiac problems during anaesthesia and surgery.

Normal sinus rhythm (NSR)

The sinus node produces an electrical impulse that launches a normal heart rhythm. This signal radiates through the right and left atrial muscles, producing electrical changes represented by the P-wave on the ECG. The electrical impulse stimulates the

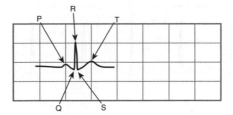

Fig. 1.4 ECG of a single cardiac cycle.

atria causing them to contract. This contraction of cardiac muscle is known as systole. The electrical impulse then continues to travel into and through specialised cardiac tissue known as the AV node, which conducts electricity at a slower pace, and forwards the impulse into the ventricles causing ventricular systole. The slower conduction rate will create a pause (PR interval) before stimulation of the ventricles. The pause between atrial and ventricular systole allows blood to empty into the ventricles from the atria before ventricular contraction, which propels blood out towards the aorta and the pulmonary artery. The QRS complex of waves on the ECG represents ventricular contraction. The T-wave follows, representing the electrical changes in the ventricles as they are relaxing. The QRS complex hides the electrical changes produced by atrial relaxation. The cardiac cycle then repeats itself after a short pause (Jevon & Ewens 2002).

Therefore, a cardiac cycle is represented on an ECG by P-waves which are followed after a brief pause by a QRS complex, then a T-wave (Figure 1.4).

Normal sinus rhythm (Figure 1.5) suggests that the rhythm produced by the sinus node is travelling through the tissues of the heart in a normal fashion and rate. The normal range of heart rate varies by individual and is influenced by factors such as age, health, body mass index, fitness and emotional state. An adult's heart rate is around 60–80 beats per minute at rest. A newborn infant may have a heart rate up to 150 beats per minute, while a child of 5 years old may have a heart rate of 100 beats per minute.

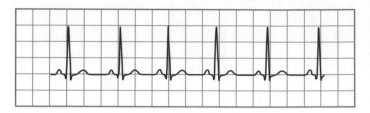

Fig. 1.5 Normal sinus rhythm.

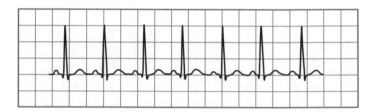

Fig. 1.6 Tachycardia.

Tachycardia

Sinus tachycardia is a fast heart rate which occurs with a normal heart rhythm (Figure 1.6). This means that although the impulses producing the heartbeats are normal, they are occurring at a faster pace. This occurs because of conditions such as shock and drug actions, as well as exercise, excitement, anxiety or as a reaction to stress.

Supraventricular tachycardia (SVT)

This is an abnormal heart rhythm because the sinus node does not produce the impulse stimulating the heart, which instead comes from tissues around the AV node. Rapid generation of these abnormal electrical impulses leads to a heartbeat that may reach up to 280 beats per minute (Figure 1.7).

Ventricular tachycardia is similar; however, it results from abnormal tissues in the ventricles producing a rapid and irregular heart rhythm. Poor cardiac output usually accompanies this rapid heart rhythm and can therefore be significant during surgery.

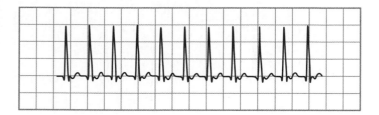

Fig. 1.7 Supraventricular tachycardia.

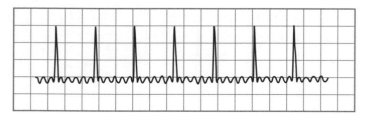

Fig. 1.8 Atrial flutter.

Atrial flutter

This abnormal rapid heart rhythm arises because the impulse which arises from the abnormal tissue in the atria bypasses the AV node. Without the dampening effect of the AV node, the impulse is repeated rapidly, resulting in the faster abnormal rhythm (Figure 1.8).

Sinus bradycardia

Sinus bradycardia presents as a slow heart rate with a normal sinus rhythm (Figure 1.9). It is usually benign, although in some circumstances it may need treatment, for example when caused by stimulation of the vagus nerve during surgery. It is also a result of using medications such as beta-blockers (see Chapter 3).

Atrioventricular block (AVB)

This abnormal rhythm occurs because of a block in conduction between the sinus node and the AV node. There are various types of AV block depending upon the mechanism of block. For

21

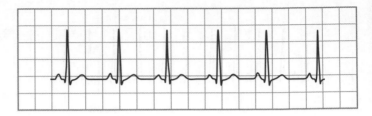

Fig. 1.9 Sinus bradycardia.

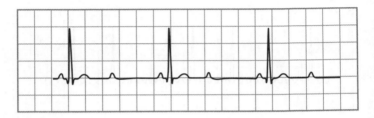

Fig. 1.10 Atrioventricular block.

example, second-degree heart block occurs when some signals from the atria do not reach the ventricles, resulting in 'dropped beats' (Figure 1.10). Third-degree or complete AV block results in a total lack of atrial impulses passing through the AV node and the ventricles therefore create their own rhythm. This rhythm is usually extremely slow and so the heartbeat must be raised to within the normal range with a pacemaker.

Premature atrial contraction (PAC)
The sinoatrial node fires early, causing the atria to contract early in the cycle, resulting in an irregular rhythm (Figure 1.11).

Premature ventricular contraction (PVC)
The AV node fires early, causing the ventricles to contract early in the cycle, resulting in an irregular rhythm (Figure 1.12).

Atrial fibrillation
This is a result of many sites within the atria firing electrical impulses in an irregular fashion, causing irregular heart rhythm

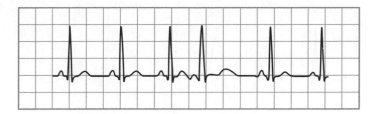

Fig. 1.11 Premature atrial contractions.

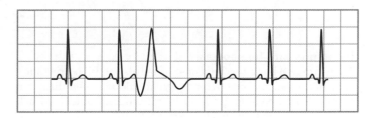

Fig. 1.12 Premature ventricular contractions.

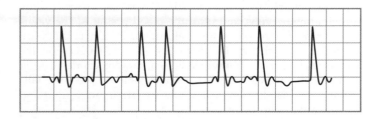

Fig. 1.13 Atrial fibrillation.

(Figure 1.13). This abnormal heart rhythm is unusual in children.

Asystole
Asystole represents the lack of electrical activity of the heart and therefore the ending of heartbeats. Note the absence of a completely straight line which signals continuing residual electrical activity (Figure 1.14).

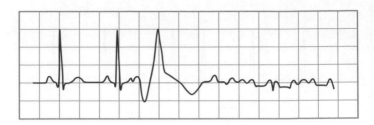

Fig. 1.14 Asystole.

Blood pressure homeostasis

There are two basic mechanisms for regulating blood pressure: short-term mechanisms, which regulate blood vessel diameter, heart rate and contractility; and long-term mechanisms, which regulate blood volume (Clancey *et al.* 2002).

Nervous control of blood pressure

The sympathetic and parasympathetic nervous systems mainly provide the nervous control of the blood pressure. The vagus nerve provides the parasympathetic nerve supply to the heart. Stimulation of the vagus nerve (e.g. during surgery on the vagus such as a vagotomy) leads to a paradoxical decrease in sympathetic nervous system activity. Blood pressure falls because of vasodilation, a lower heart rate (bradycardia) and lower cardiac output.

Sympathetic nerve fibres stimulate vasomotor fibres within the smooth muscle of arteries, resulting in vasoconstriction; this causes blood pressure to rise. Lack of sympathetic stimulation results in relaxation of the arteries, an increased arterial diameter, and therefore reduces blood pressure.

In the heart, sympathetic activity stimulates the sympathetic cardiac nerves, which results in increased heart rate and contractility, higher cardiac output and increased blood pressure. Simultaneously the vagus (parasympathetic) nerve displays decreased activity.

Hormonal control of blood pressure
Increased sympathetic impulses to the adrenal glands lead to the release of adrenaline (epinephrine) and noradrenaline (norepinephrine) into the bloodstream. These hormones act on chemoreceptors to increase heart rate, contractility and vasoconstriction. The effect is slower acting and more prolonged than nervous system control.

Short-term regulation of rising blood pressure
Baroreceptors, specialised areas of tissue which are sensitive to pressure, provide short-term control of rising blood pressure. Rising blood pressure leads to stretching of arterial walls and stimulation of baroreceptors in the carotid sinus, aortic arch and other large arteries of the neck and thorax. The baroreceptors send an increased frequency of impulses to the brain, which leads to increased parasympathetic activity and decreased sympathetic activity. This results in a decreased heart rate and an increase in arterial diameter, which aim to reverse the increasing blood pressure (Jevon & Ewens 2002).

Short-term regulation of falling blood pressure
Falling blood pressure inhibits the baroreceptors, leading to a decrease in impulses sent to the brain. This causes a paradoxical increase in sympathetic activity leading to three effects:

- increased heart rate and increased contractility;
- increased vasoconstriction;
- release of adrenaline (epinephrine) and noradrenaline (norepinephrine) from the adrenal glands, which increases heart rate, contractility and vasoconstriction.

The combined effect helps to increase blood pressure.

Long-term regulation of blood pressure
Long-term control of blood pressure is primarily accomplished by altering blood volume. The loss of blood through haemorrhage, accident or donating a pint of blood will lower blood pressure and trigger processes to restore blood volume and therefore blood pressure back to normal. Long-term regulatory

processes conserve body fluids by renal mechanisms and stimulate intake of water to normalise blood volume and blood pressures. (See section on water/electrolyte balance pages 5–14.)

Haemorrhage (loss of blood)

When there is loss of blood, blood pressure and blood volume decrease. Juxtaglomerular cells (a small endocrine organ associated with individual nephrons within the kidneys) monitor changes in the blood pressure. If blood pressure falls too low, these specialised cells release the enzyme renin into the bloodstream and launch the renin/angiotensin mechanism. This process consists of a series of steps aimed at increasing blood volume and blood pressure.

The first step of this process is angiotensin I formation. As renin travels through the bloodstream, it binds to an inactive plasma protein, angiotensinogen, activating it to become angiotensin I.

The second step is the conversion of angiotensin I to angiotensin II as it passes through the lung capillaries. Angiotensin II is a vasoconstrictor and therefore raises blood pressure in the body's arterioles, however, its main effect is on the adrenal gland. Here, in the third step, it stimulates the cells of the adrenal cortex to release the hormone aldosterone.

Aldosterone stimulates increased sodium reabsorption from the tubule cells. The increased sodium levels in the tubules make sodium move into the bloodstream, closely followed by water.

Increase in osmolarity

Dehydration resulting from sweating, diarrhoea or excessive urine flow will cause an increase in osmolarity of the blood and result in a decrease in blood volume and blood pressure. As osmolarity increases there is both a short- and long-term effect. In the long term, the hypothalamus sends a signal to the posterior pituitary to release ADH, which increases water reabsorption in the distal convoluted tubules and collecting tubules of the kidney. Water moves back into the capillaries, decreasing the osmolarity of the blood, increasing the blood volume, and therefore increasing the blood pressure.

A short-term effect of increased osmolarity is the activation of the thirst centre in the hypothalamus. The thirst centre stimulates the individual to drink more water and thus rehydrates the blood and the extracellular fluid, restoring blood volume and therefore blood pressure.

Pharmacology and blood pressure homeostasis

There are many chemicals that influence blood flow and blood vessel diameter and therefore have a direct action on blood pressure. Table 1.2 gives some examples of drugs that act on the cardiovascular system. See Chapter 3 on pharmacology for further discussion of such drugs.

Shock

Shock is a condition that arises from a failure of the circulatory system to deliver oxygen and nutrients to the tissues of the body, and to remove waste products. Before going into shock in detail it is important to understand the relationship between cardiac output, peripheral resistance and blood pressure. Control of blood circulation is through the interaction of blood volume (provided via cardiac output), blood vessel diameter (vasoconstriction – especially peripherally) and the pressure gradient that 'pushes' blood through the tissues (blood pressure).

Cardiac output is the volume of blood per minute ejected from the heart. The volume of blood ejected every beat is the stroke volume.

$$\text{Cardiac output} = \text{stroke volume} \times \text{heart rate}$$
$$= 140 \text{ ml} \times 60 \text{ beats per minute}$$
$$= 8400 \text{ ml per minute}$$

This is the cardiac output for an average heart beating 60 times per minute with a stroke volume per ventricle of 70 ml (so 140 ml total).

Various factors affect stroke volume. For example, low venous return reduces the volume of blood refilling the heart between beats (end-diastolic volume) and therefore reduces stroke volume. Cardiac contractility affects the percentage of blood ejected from the heart on every beat – a strong contraction will empty the heart more efficiently than a weak contraction. A

Table 1.2 Examples of drugs acting on the cardiovascular system.

Drug	Action	Uses
Adrenaline (epinephrine)	α agonist – coronary and peripheral vasoconstriction β agonist – increased heart rate and myocardial contractility	Used in cardiac arrest to stimulate the heart muscles
Isoprenaline, dopamine	β agonist – increased rate and force of heart beat, vasodilation	Cardiogenic shock in infarction or cardiac surgery
Ephedrine	Increases heart rate and myocardial activity. Increases peripheral vasoconstriction	Reversal of hypotension, e.g. from spinal or epidural anaesthesia
Phentolamine	α antagonist – vasodilation and myocardial stimulant. Overall effect of reducing blood pressure	Used as a vasodilator in cardiobypass surgery and in cardiogenic shock
Atenolol	Slows the heart beat and reduces myocardial oxygen demand	Prophylaxis of angina, treatment of dysrhythmias and hypertension
Propranolol (also oxprenolol and atenolol)	β antagonist – reduces heart rate and output, reduces myocardial oxygen demand	Control of ectopic heartbeats and tachycardia. Reduces incidence of angina
Digoxin	Cardiac glycoside – increases the force of myocardial contraction and reduces conductivity within the atrioventricular (AV) node	Most useful in the treatment of supraventricular tachycardias, especially for controlling ventricular response in persistent atrial fibrillation
Atropine	An antimuscarinic drug which blocks acetylcholine	Prevention and reversal of excessive bradycardia

huge variety of factors such as autonomic nervous stimulation, hormones and drugs affect the heart rate.

Peripheral resistance refers to the tissue's resistance to blood flow. The diameter of blood vessels directly influences the resistance to blood flow – narrow vessels conduct blood at a slower rate than wide vessels. Control of blood vessel diameter occurs at a local tissue level through the release of lactic acid and other metabolites of normal cellular function. These metabolites cause local vasodilatation and therefore reduce peripheral vasoconstriction. Control of peripheral resistance occurs centrally through neural and hormonal activity, in particular the sympathetic nervous system.

Blood pressure is also subject to many controls. The higher the pressure gradient the faster blood will flow. The difference between the heart contractions (systole) and the relaxation phase (diastole) produces a pressure gradient. In humans, systolic pressure is normally around 120 mmHg and diastolic pressure is around 80 mmHg. The difference between these two measurements is the pulse pressure and it is this pressure that represents the pressure gradient. Pulse pressure is influenced by a combination of the contractility of the heart, the circulating volume and the peripheral resistance.

Shock, therefore, can be defined as acute circulatory failure leading to inadequate tissue perfusion, resulting in generalised cellular hypoxia and end-organ injury. It is caused by a disruption to the cardiovascular system and inadequate compensation to maintain tissue perfusion (Jevon & Ewens 2002).

Shock can be classified according to its three known causes:

- a fault of the heart, which is cardiogenic shock;
- a fault of the vascular system, which is distributive shock;
- a fault of fluid regulation, which is hypovolaemic shock.

Keeping in mind the previous discussion on blood pressure regulation, it can be seen that hypotension and shock are therefore caused by a problem with heart rate, stroke volume or peripheral resistance.

A clinical approach to shock (Table 1.3) identifies the main clinical problems associated with shock that can be treated by medical interventions such as drugs or surgery:

Table 1.3 A clinical approach to shock.

Overall effect		Physiological problem	Clinical focus
Failure of cardiac output	Heart rate	Inappropriate heart rate	• Heart block/pacemaker • Hypotension • Bradycardia
	Stroke volume	Inadequate filling time	• Tachycardia • Arrhythmias
		Failure to receive blood	• Haemorrhage • Hypovolaemia • Dehydration • Inadequate fluid intake • Excessive fluid loss • Interstitial fluid loss (e.g. bowel surgery, pancreatitis) • Inflow obstruction • Mitral stenosis • Tamponade
		Failure to eject blood	• Muscle dysfunction • Myocardial ischaemia or fibrosis • Valvular/septal damage • Ventricular damage • Aortic regurgitation • Septal defects • Outflow obstruction • Pulmonary obstruction • Aortic/pulmonary stenosis
Failure of peripheral resistance		Inappropriate vasodilation	• Anaphylaxis • Shock • Sepsis

- low blood pressure, because of inadequate cardiac output or low peripheral resistance;
- low cardiac output, caused by a problem with heart rate or stroke volume;
- heart rate abnormalities – too fast (tachycardia) or too slow (bradycardia);

- stroke volume abnormalities, caused by failure to receive blood, failure to eject blood or inadequate volume;
- low peripheral vascular resistance, because of inappropriate vasodilation.

Hypovolaemic shock

During shock, the body protects itself from hypovolaemia by a series of reflex mechanisms involving the cardiovascular and neurohormonal systems as described previously. The result is a decrease in cardiac output and increased peripheral resistance. The selective shunting of blood occurs to essential organs such as the brain, heart and kidneys, which are further protected by autoregulatory reflexes. This state is 'compensated shock' and may occur with up to 20% of blood loss (approximately 1 litre) (University of Pennsylvania 2006).

The clinical signs of compensated shock may be subtle: blood pressure may be normal; there is tachycardia, cold and clammy peripheries, decreased capillary refill; and a widened gap between core and peripheral temperature (Astiz *et al.* 1993).

As circulating volume decreases (1–2 litres blood loss) blood pressure begins to fall, resulting in increased peripheral vasoconstriction and tachycardia. Blood pressure may become unrecordable and there are signs of end-organ failure (oliguria and confusion) following the loss of more than 40% (2 litres) of circulating volume. The drop in urinary output is a reliable way of identifying progressive loss of circulating volume.

Treatment of hypovolaemic shock

Treatment of shock addresses the cause by replacing lost fluids and supporting the body's essential systems against the effects of hypovolaemia. Techniques and protocols are constantly being reviewed as new research evidence becomes available.

Replacement of lost fluids by colloids and crystalloids is normally a priority for treating shock. Progressively worsening shock necessitates monitoring of arterial and central venous pressure (CVP) to assess the effects of fluid replacement. The end point of fluid replacement will be: blood pressure within normal limits; urinary output of greater than 1 ml/kg; CVP of over 12 mmHg; and lactate readings of less than 2 mmol/litre

(University of Pennsylvania 2006). If the patient remains hypotensive after the volume replacement, then the problem lies with the cardiovascular system which must be supported through medical interventions. Noradrenaline (norepinephrine) and low dosage vasopressin may increase stroke volume, which can be measured with a pulmonary artery catheter or oesophageal Doppler. Dobutamine may be useful at this point to increase the efficiency of the heart pump.

The stroke volume, CVP, pulmonary capillary wedge pressure (PCWP) and venous oxygen saturation may guide fluid resuscitation. Since over-transfusion of patients rarely occurs during shock, non-invasive monitors such as the oesophageal Doppler may provide more rapid and less dangerous measurement of stroke volume. Close monitoring is essential since the patient's fluid status may change as the body recovers from shock or as the effects of medical interventions progress (Pinsky & Payen 2004)).

THE RESPIRATORY SYSTEM

The respiratory system transports gases between the bloodstream and the outside air. Blood delivers oxygen to the tissues of the body, while carbon dioxide from tissue activity is returned to the lungs. The carbon dioxide waste leaves the body during exhalation.

Breathing is the process of moving air into and out of the lungs. An adult normally breathes from 14 to 20 times per minute, rising to 80 breaths per minute on effort and dropping to 8 or 10 breaths per minute at rest. A child's rate of breathing at rest is faster than an adult's at rest, and a newborn baby has a rate of about 40 breaths per minute. In adults the tidal volume (amount of air taken in a normal breath) is about 0.5 litres. The vital capacity (the maximum amount) is about 4.8 litres in an adult male.

The process of breathing comprises two phases, inspiration and expiration. The lungs themselves have no muscle tissue so the ribcage and the diaphragm control their movements.

The diaphragm is a large, dome-shaped muscle that lies just under the lungs, which flattens when stimulated. This expands the volume of the thoracic cavity. The rib muscles also contract on stimulation, pulling the ribcage up and out, also expanding the thoracic cavity. The increased volume of the thoracic cavity creates a partial vacuum which sucks air into the lungs. The diaphragm and rib muscles relax when the nervous stimulation ends, the thoracic cavity shrinks and exhalation occurs.

Conscious control and overriding of the respiratory centre alter the rhythm, for example when singing or whistling, or when holding the breath.

Structure

The respiratory system extends from the nose to the lungs and is divided into the upper and lower respiratory tracts. The upper respiratory tract consists of the nose and the pharynx, or throat. The lower respiratory tract includes the larynx, or voice box; the trachea, or windpipe, which splits into two main branches called bronchi; tiny branches of the bronchi called bronchioles; and finally the lungs. The nose, pharynx, larynx, trachea, bronchi and bronchioles conduct air to and from the lungs. The lungs interact with the cardiovascular system to deliver oxygen and remove carbon dioxide.

Nose and nasal cavity

Capillaries in the nose and nasal cavity warm and humidify the air. Hairs and mucus inside the nasal cavity help to trap dust and other particles to protect the lungs. Stimulation of chemo-receptors inside the nose activates the olfactory nerve which eventually leads to the sensation of smell.

Pharynx

The pharynx is a short, funnel-shaped tube about 13 cm long that links the nose and the larynx. The pharynx transports air to the larynx and is lined with a protective mucous membrane and ciliated cells to remove impurities. The pharynx also houses the tonsils, which are lymphatic tissues that contain white blood cells. The tonsils help to protect against upper respiratory tract infections. High in the rear wall of the pharynx are the adenoids. Located at the back of the pharynx on either side of the tongue are the palatine tonsils. The lingual tonsils are found at the base of the tongue. The tonsils can become swollen with infection (tonsillitis), causing various symptoms associated with airway blockage and sepsis.

Viral infections such as the common cold, influenza, German measles (rubella), herpes and infectious mononucleosis cause pharyngitis, giving symptoms of a sore throat. Infection can also be caused by diphtherial, chlamydial, streptococcal and staphylococcal bacteria.

Larynx

Air moves from the pharynx to the larynx and on to the trachea. The larynx is about 5 cm long and consists of several layers of cartilage. The Adam's apple is a prominent bulge visible on the neck formed by a projection in the cartilage.

The larynx also produces sound, prevents food and fluid from entering the trachea, and helps filter air. The presence of food or fluid in the larynx produces a cough reflex. If the cough reflex does not work, a person can choke.

The larynx houses two pairs of vocal cords made of elastic connective tissue covered by folds of mucous membrane. One pair, the false vocal cords, narrows the glottis (the pharyngeal opening of the larynx) during swallowing. Below this and extending as far as the thyroid cartilage are the true vocal cords. Sound is created when this pair of cords vibrates as air passes through them.

Laryngitis, which often accompanies colds, is the larynx's most common affliction and can lead to voice loss. Other diseases include croup, diphtheria and cancer. Cancer is often treated by radiotherapy and surgery – partial or total laryngectomy.

Trachea

The trachea extends from the larynx to the right and left primary bronchi in the lungs (Tortora 2008). The trachea is lined by ciliated mucous membrane; the mucus traps tiny particles and the cilia move the mucus up and out of the respiratory tract. Rings of cartilage reinforce the trachea and prevent it from collapsing. If the airway blocks above the larynx, a tracheostomy may be performed to bypass the blockage and ease breathing.

Alternatively, the patient may need intubation using an endotracheal tube.

Bronchial tree and lungs

The trachea divides into the right and left primary bronchi which transport air to and from the right and left lungs respectively. Inside the lungs, each bronchus divides into smaller bronchi, bronchioles, terminal bronchioles and finally the respiratory bronchioles.

The lungs, two pink and spongy sacs, occupy the chest cavity from the collarbone down to the diaphragm, which separates the contents of the abdominal cavity from the chest cavity. At birth the lungs are pink but as a person ages they become grey and mottled from tiny particles breathed in with the air.

The visceral pleura lines the outside of lungs and the parietal pleura lines the inside walls of the chest. The narrow space between the visceral and parietal pleurae is called the pleural cavity. A thin layer of pleural fluid in this cavity causes the visceral pleura to stick to the parietal pleura so the lungs stick to the chest wall. This causes them to expand and contract with the chest during breathing, drawing air in on inspiration and forcing it out on expiration.

Air entering the lungs contains about 21% oxygen and 0.04% carbon dioxide. Air leaving the lungs contains about 14% oxygen and about 4.4% carbon dioxide.

Alveoli

The bronchioles divide many more times in the lungs to end in tiny air sacs called alveoli. Each lung is composed mostly of about 150 million alveoli. Alveoli resembling tiny, collapsed balloons are arranged in grape-like clusters surrounded by tiny capillaries. The air in the wall of the alveoli is only about 0.1–0.2 µm from the capillary blood. The alveoli are where gaseous exchange occurs between the air in the alveoli and the blood in the capillaries in their walls (Figure 1.15). In the capillary beds of the lungs, carbon dioxide diffuses down its concentration gradient into the air inside the alveoli and is exhaled from the body during the next breath. Oxygen in the alveoli diffuses down its own concentration gradient into the blood.

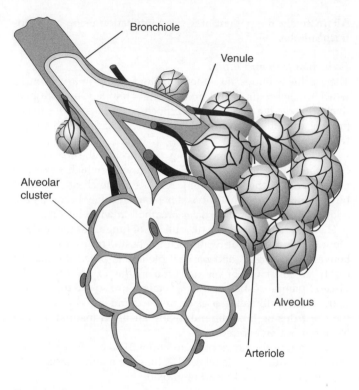

Fig. 1.15 Terminal bronchiole and alveoli.

The oxygenated blood leaves the lungs, returns to the heart by the pulmonary arteries and then continues out of the heart into the body to restart the process (Figure 1.16).

The role of surfactant

Some of the cells forming the alveoli secrete a chemical called surfactant, which decreases surface tension of the fluid in the alveoli. This reduces the attraction between water molecules and prevents the walls of the alveolus from collapsing.

Infant respiratory distress syndrome (IRDS) is caused by a deficiency in surfactant. This syndrome is often seen in prema-

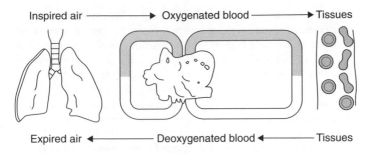

Inspired air ⟶ Oxygenated blood ⟶ Tissues

Expired air ⟵ Deoxygenated blood ⟵ Tissues

Fig. 1.16 Exchange of oxygen and carbon dioxide between the blood and lungs.

ture babies who may be unable to produce adequate amounts of surfactant. The alveoli collapse on exhalation making reinflation difficult. Giving surfactant and hormones can stimulate the surfactant-producing cells.

Regulation of breathing

Aerobic respiration is the process within cells in which nutrients and oxygen build the energy molecule adenosine triphosphate (ATP) through a process known as the Krebs' cycle. The overall effect of aerobic respiration is that body cells use oxygen to metabolise glucose, forming carbon dioxide as a waste product.

The oxygen and carbon dioxide concentrations in various parts of the body are measured as partial pressures – the pressure exerted by any one gas absorbed within a fluid. For example, pO_2 is the partial pressure of oxygen in the blood – the pressure exerted by oxygen which contributes to the entire pressure of all the absorbed gases.

The rate and pattern of breathing is controlled by a cluster of nerve cells in the brain stem called the respiratory centre – a circuit of neurons in the base of the brain (the medulla oblongata and pons). Motor neurons from the respiratory control centre innervate the diaphragm and chest muscles. When stimulated, they contract and change the volume of the thoracic cavity. The respiratory control centre also receives input from many other neurons.

Nerves from the higher brain centres controlling emotion stimulate or depress the respiratory control centre and cause changes in the rate and depth of breathing when the person is excited or relaxed. Sensory neurons such as proprioceptors from the joints and chemoreceptors from the arteries also interact with the respiratory control centre. On exercising, action potentials from proprioceptors in joints stimulate the respiratory control centre and increase the rate of breathing.

However, the levels of carbon dioxide in the blood and cerebrospinal fluid (CSF) are the major factors regulating both the rate and depth of breathing (Figure 1.17). If carbon dioxide levels in the blood increase, the carbon dioxide will diffuse into the CSF. Central chemoreceptors in the medulla oblongata of the brain stimulate the respiratory control centre, increasing the rate and depth of breathing and so reducing pCO_2.

Hypercapnia is caused by high carbon dioxide concentration in blood. The carbonic acid equation moves to the right and the hydrogen ion concentration increases (see page 10). The increase in hydrogen ion concentration increases the acidity of blood and CSF, and can cause respiratory acidosis. The respiratory control centre will respond by increasing the speed and depth of breathing, causing carbon dioxide to diffuse from blood to the lungs more rapidly.

Hypocapnia is caused by low partial pressure of carbon dioxide in blood. In this case, the carbonic acid equation moves to the left, and hydrogen ion concentration will decrease as a new equilibrium is reached (see page 10). The decrease in blood hydrogen ion concentration causes respiratory alkalosis. The respiratory control centre reacts by decreasing the respiratory rate, causing carbon dioxide from cellular respiration to build up in the bloodstream. The carbonic acid equation moves to the right again, reversing the respiratory alkalosis. The respiratory control centre constantly adjusts the depth and rate of breathing to maintain the proper balance. Although some degree of conscious control can be exerted over the amount of air inhaled, the most important factors controlling breathing are the carbon dioxide and hydrogen ion concentrations of the blood and CSF (Jardins 2007).

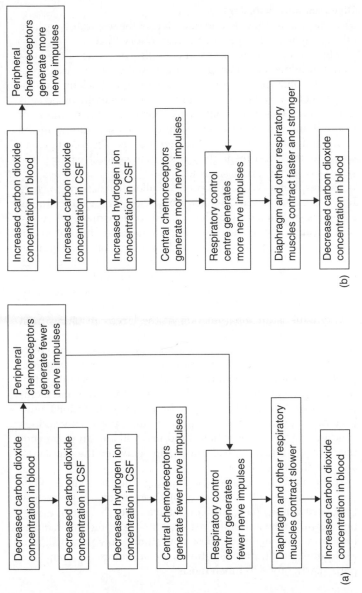

Fig. 1.17 Regulation of breathing and respiration by carbon dioxide concentration in the blood: (a) decreased; (b) increased.

Diseases and disorders

There are many diseases and disorders of the respiratory system which can affect any part of the respiratory tract.

Infection by a huge variety of cold viruses is one of the most common ailments affecting the membranes of the nasal passages and pharynx. The immune system fights back by increasing blood flow to the area, bringing numerous white blood cells to the scene. This inflammatory reaction causes the membranes to swell and increase the secretion of mucus, resulting in the stuffy and runny nose associated with colds. The infection can spread to the lower respiratory tract, to the middle ear or to the sinuses where it causes sinusitis.

The respiratory system is prone to allergic reactions, such as hay fever and asthma, which are caused when the immune system is stimulated by pollen, dust or other irritants. A runny nose, watery eyes and sneezing characterise hay fever. In asthma, temporary constriction and inflammation of the bronchi and bronchioles causes difficulty in breathing. An asthma attack is typically mild in otherwise healthy patients, but can be severe enough to be life-threatening when anaesthesia and surgery, or other concurrent conditions compromise the patient.

Laryngitis is an inflammation of the larynx resulting from causes such as viral infections, trauma caused by endotracheal tubes, irritants such as cigarette smoke or overuse of the voice. Laryngitis may result in hoarseness or whispering until the swelling subsides. Bronchitis, caused by viral or bacterial infection or by irritating chemicals, is an inflammation of the membranes that line the bronchi or bronchioles. Infections with bacteria or viruses can lead to pneumonia, a potentially serious condition of the lungs where fluid and inflammation prevent the flow of oxygen and carbon dioxide between the capillaries and the air in the alveoli.

Tuberculosis bacteria attack the lungs and sometimes other body tissues as well. Untreated infections in the lungs destroy lung tissue. In the past, antibiotics have controlled tuberculosis, but recently, new antibiotic-resistant strains of the tuberculosis bacterium have evolved. These new strains now pose a significant public health problem. Immunocompromised patients are particularly prone to tuberculosis.

In emphysema the alveolar bundles coalesce, resulting in an overall smaller surface area for the exchange of gases. Weakened bronchioles collapse on exhalation, trapping air in the alveoli. This eventually hinders the exchange of oxygen and carbon dioxide with the circulatory system, leading to hypoxia and difficulty in breathing. Emphysema is a non-contiguous disease that can result from various causes including a genetic tendency to the condition, smog, cigarette smoke or infection.

Exposure to cancer-causing agents, such as tobacco smoke, asbestos or radiation, can lead to lung cancer in individuals with a genetic inclination to the disease. Cancerous tumours can start in the bronchi, bronchioles or in the alveolar lung tissue. Treatments are more effective on early detection of lung cancer, before it has spread to other parts of the body, and provide a good prognosis for full recovery. The prognosis is poor if the cancer has had the opportunity to spread.

Respiratory distress syndrome (RDS) is the name for a cluster of symptoms that suggest severe failure of the lungs. In infants, RDS is termed infant respiratory distress syndrome (IRDS). As mentioned above, IRDS is commonly found in premature infants when the alveoli fail to expand fully during inhalation. Expansion of the alveoli requires surfactant, but in many premature infants the alveoli cannot produce this substance. Treatment of IRDS is by artificial ventilation and giving surfactant until the alveoli begin producing surfactant on their own. Severe damage to the lungs caused by, for example, trauma, poisonous gases or as a response to inflammation in the lungs, causes acute (adult) respiratory distress syndrome (ARDS). ARDS is a life-threatening condition with a survival rate of about 50%.

TRAUMA AND WOUND HEALING

Anaesthesia and surgery cause stress to the body, so it comes as no surprise that the perioperative patient presents many of the responses found with naturally occurring stressors. This section describes the body's metabolic response to anaesthesia and surgery and then, the process of wound healing.

Stressors such as surgery and anaesthesia, as well as others such as injury, burns, vascular occlusion, dehydration, starvation, sepsis, acute medical illness or psychological stress, may launch the metabolic response to trauma. The body responds locally by an inflammatory response designed to protect tissues from further damage and to encourage repair. The purpose of the somatic response is to conserve fluid and provide energy for tissue repair.

Two phases characterise the somatic response. Initially the body produces an *acute catabolic reaction* where the patient is in shock, characterised by:

- depression of enzymatic activity;
- decreased oxygen consumption;
- low cardiac output;
- low core temperature;
- lactic acidosis.

An *anabolic phase* follows where fat and protein stores are regained and weight increases, characterised by:

- increased cardiac output;
- increased oxygen consumption;
- increased glucose production;
- lactic acid may be normal.

The state of normal homeostasis returns as the triggers resolve and the body returns to its normal metabolic balance (Tortora 2008)).

The form of the metabolic response depends chiefly on the degree of trauma suffered. Other contributing factors include the influence of drugs, sepsis, underlying systemic disease, underlying nutritional state and efficacy of the medical interventions. Although the metabolic response is protective, it can become harmful if excessive or prolonged. The aim of medical interventions is to revive body systems, control pain and temperature, and provide acceptable fluid and nutrition.

Factors starting the metabolic response
The factors that start the metabolic response include hypovolaemia, factors exuded by the wound, hormonal responses, sepsis and the inflammatory response.

Hypovolaemia is common in major surgery but the body's own response and the early use of fluid replacement therapy may significantly reduce the metabolic response. Pain and anxiety can also initiate a hormonal response, but this can be adjusted by analgesia so that a metabolic response is not stimulated.

Tissue injury activates two specific responses, inflammatory (humoral) and cellular. Products of these responses play a role in organ dysfunction. For example, the inflammatory mediators of injury have been implicated in membrane dysfunction, leading to various conditions affecting every organ of the body.

The inflammatory response is a complex collection of reactions involving macrophages, polymorphonuclear leucocytes and phagocytic cells, such as neutrophils and eosinophils. Normal phagocytosis (engulfing of foreign bodies by phagocytes) is one of the primary activations of the metabolic response. This results in responses such as neutrophil aggregation, and secretion of histamine and serotonin, which may increase vascular permeability and vasodilation. A combination of these reactions results in the inflammatory response.

The action and release of adrenaline (epinephrine), noradrenaline (norepinephrine), cortisol and glucagon are increased, while other hormones are decreased during trauma. The hypothalamus has a major role in coordinating the stress response through endocrine actions by the pituitary and the sympathetic and parasympathetic nervous systems. The pituitary gland responds to trauma by increasing adrenocorticotrophic hormone (ACTH), prolactin and growth hormone levels.

Pain receptors, osmoreceptors, baroreceptors and chemoreceptors stimulate the hypothalamus to induce sympathetic nerve activity. Stimulation of the pain receptors results in the secretion of endogenous opiates, which adapt the response to pain.

Hypotension, hypovolaemia and hyponatraemia stimulate the anterior pituitary to secrete ACTH. ACTH stimulates the secretion of antidiuretic hormone (ADH) from the anterior hypothalamus, aldosterone from the adrenal cortex and renin from the juxtaglomerular apparatus of the kidney. This has the overall effect of increasing water reabsorbtion and thereby increasing blood volume.

Reactions to changes in glucose concentration include the release of insulin from the cells of the pancreas, while high amino acid levels stimulate the release of glucagon from the pancreatic cells.

Result of the metabolic response

The stress of major surgery can lead to the initiation of the metabolic response. Many of the interventions carried out on the perioperative patient are aimed at moderating the metabolic response, which if untreated may rapidly prove fatal.

As can be seen from the above, the metabolic response results in systemic inflammatory responses which increase the activity of the cardiovascular system, reflected as tachycardia, widened pulse pressure and a greater cardiac output. As metabolic rate increases, there is an increase in oxygen consumption, increased protein catabolism and hyperglycaemia.

The resting energy expenditure can rise to more than 20% above normal, if the patient is well enough to respond. In an inadequate response, oxygen consumption may fall and endotoxins and anoxia may injure cells and limit their ability to utilise oxygen. Cellular injury, impaired hepatic gluconeogenesis and lack of oxygen may result in rapid deterioration of processes requiring energy. As a result of the inefficient energy-making process, lactate is produced, causing a severe metabolic acidosis.

The oliguria, which often follows major surgery, is a consequence of the release of ADH and aldosterone. As well as promoting the reabsorption of water, aldosterone also releases large quantities of intracellular potassium into the extracellular fluid, possibly causing a significant rise in serum potassium, especially if renal function is impaired. Retention of sodium and bicarbonate may contribute to metabolic alkalosis with impairment of the delivery of oxygen to the tissues.

Critically ill postoperative patients may develop a glucose intolerance which resembles that found in pregnancy and in diabetic patients. This is as a result of both increased mobilisation and decreased uptake of glucose by the tissues. The turnover of glucose is increased and the serum glucose is higher than normal.

The glucose level following surgery should therefore be carefully monitored since hyperglycaemia may exacerbate ventilatory insufficiency and may provoke an osmotic diuresis. The optimum blood glucose level is between 4 and 10 mmol/litre. Control of blood glucose is best achieved by titration with intravenous insulin, based on a sliding scale. However, because of the degree of insulin resistance associated with trauma, the quantities required may be considerably higher than normal.

The principal source of energy following trauma is adipose tissue and as much as 200–500 g of fat may be broken down daily after major surgery. High levels of ketones are produced as free fatty acids are broken down to provide energy. Because of the possible problems with glucose metabolism, nutritional support of traumatised patients requires a mixture of fat and carbohydrate.

The intake of protein by a healthy adult is between 80 and 120 g of protein, or around 1–2 g protein/kg/day. Lack of protein intake leads to the breakdown of skeletal muscle in order to produce essential amino acids. After major surgery, or with sepsis, as much as 20 g/day of urea nitrogen from protein breakdown may be excreted in the urine. A severely ill patient may lose over 600 g of muscle mass per day, leading to marked muscle wasting. Depletion of amino acids also results in atrophy of the intestinal mucosa and failure of the mucosal antibacterial barrier. This may lead to systemic infection and multisystem failure after severe trauma. This is normally fatal in patients who lose more than 40% of body protein because of failing immunocompetence. The protein intake can be improved dramatically by parenteral or enteral feeding, as long as adequate liver function is present.

Survival after trauma such as surgery depends on a balance between the extent of cellular damage, the efficacy of the metabolic response and the effectiveness of supporting treatment. Hypovolaemia is a major initiating trigger for the metabolic sequence; therefore, adequate fluid resuscitation to shut off the hypovolaemic stimulus is important during and following

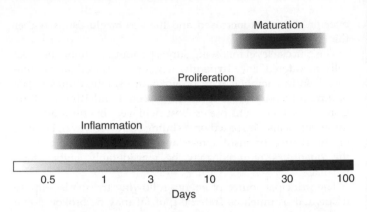

Fig. 1.18 Phases of wound repair: inflammation, proliferation and maturation.

surgery. Fear and pain, tissue injury, hypoxia and toxins from infection add to the initiating factor of hypovolaemia and so it is important that these are also moderated by perioperative interventions in order to reduce the metabolic response.

Patient support during perioperative care should be aimed at reducing the factors triggering the metabolic response. During surgery, important aspects of patient care include adequate fluid volume, maintenance of oxygen delivery to the tissues, careful handling of tissues and removal of pus or devitalised tissue, combined with control of infection, respiratory and nutritional support to aid defence mechanisms.

Wound healing

Wound healing is the process of tissue repair. It involves the interaction of epithelial, endothelial and inflammatory cells, platelets and fibroblasts which are activated and act together in order to repair the damaged tissue. The overall process can be divided into the three overlapping phases of inflammation, proliferation and maturation (Figure 1.18) (Dealey 2005).

Inflammatory phase (day 0–5)

Tissue healing follows essentially the same process regardless of the tissue involved or the type of injury sustained, although healing times and the duration of each phase depend on a variety of factors, such as health of the individual, nutritional status, mode of injury, tissue type, blood supply, moisturisation and so on.

The healing response is initiated from the moment that the surgical incision is made. Blood filling the wound interacts with collagen and leads to platelet degranulation and activation of Hageman factor (factor XII). This factor in turn sets into motion the clotting cascade, which serves to bind the wound and also alerts the systemic system to a local injury.

Kinins and prostaglandins produced by the process cause local vasodilatation and oedema, and are responsible for the pain and swelling which occurs after injury. Leucocytes enter the wound site shortly after injury and their numbers increase steadily, peaking at 24–48 hours. Their main function appears to be phagocytosis of the bacteria that have been introduced into the wound during injury.

The next cells to enter the wound are macrophages, which are derived from circulating monocytes. They first appear within 48–96 hours post-injury and persist in the wound until healing is complete. T lymphocytes appear around the fifth day post-injury, peaking about 7 days after injury. The presence and activation of both macrophages and lymphocytes in the wound is critical to the progress of the normal healing process because they phagocytose and digest pathological organisms and tissue debris. Macrophages, platelets and lymphocytes also release growth hormone and other biologically active substances known collectively as cytokines. Cytokines are small proteins released by cells that communicate with, and affect the behaviour of, other cells. In the context of wound repair, they initiate and support granulation tissue formation.

Proliferative phase (day 3–14)
The proliferative phase of healing commences once the wound has been successfully cleared of devitalised and unwanted material. This phase is characterised by the formation of granulation tissue in the wound. Granulation tissue consists of a combination of cellular elements, including fibroblasts and

inflammatory cells, along with new capillaries embedded in a loose extracellular matrix of collagen, fibronectin and hyaluronic acid. In a process of fibroblast proliferation and synthetic activity known as fibroplasia, fibroblasts are induced to proliferate and are attracted into the wound by cytokines. Fibroblasts are responsible for tissue reconstruction through the production of structural proteins, in particular the glycoprotein collagen, which forms the main constituent of the wound matrix and which imparts tensile strength to the scar. The collagen forms into an organised matrix along the wound's stress lines.

Wound revascularisation also occurs at this time. In response to a variety of local mediators, capillary buds sprout from venules, form capillary loops, connect to the bloodstream and then join together to form a capillary plexus.

Re-epithelialisation of the wound surface begins within a couple of hours of the injury. Epithelial cells from the periphery of the wound begin to migrate under the scab and over the underlying viable connective tissue, filling the wound. Once the defect is bridged the migrating epithelial cells proliferate through mitosis and the surface layer eventually becomes keratinised. Re-epithelialisation is normally complete in less than 48 hours in approximated surgical wounds, but will take longer in larger wounds where there is tissue loss. Epithelialisation can also take place in the absence of fibroplasia and granulation tissue formation in wounds (such as skin graft donor sites) where only the epithelium is damaged. Again, the mediators for re-epithelialisation include a variety of cytokines and other local cellular products.

Maturation phase (day 7 to 1 year)
Almost as soon as the extracellular matrix is laid down it becomes cross-linked and aggregated into fibrillar bundles, which gradually provide the healing tissue with increasing stiffness and tensile strength through collagen fibrogenesis. The wound develops 20% of its final strength after 3 weeks, with the maximum breaking strength of the scar reaching 70% of that of the intact skin.

This gradual gain in tensile strength is due not only to continuing collagen deposition, but also to collagen remodelling. Collagen synthesis and catabolism leads to the formation of larger collagen bundles and increased crosslinking. As this occurs, a thin pale scar is formed from collagen which is relatively avascular and acellular.

Wounds healed by primary intention are those which require minimal granulisation tissue and minimal loss of wound volume. Large and complex wounds, associated with significant tissue loss, heal by secondary intention. Granulation tissue gradually fills the defect and epithelialisation proceeds slowly from the wound edges. The wound area starts to contract rapidly through the inward movement of the uninjured skin edges caused by an interaction between fibroblast locomotion and collagen reorganisation. The result of the healing process is a scar that helps to restore tissue continuity, strength and function.

REFERENCES

Abraham, J. (2008) Acupressure and acupuncture in preventing and managing postoperative nausea and vomiting in adults. *Journal of Perioperative Practice* **18** (12), 543–551.

Astiz, M.E., Rackow, E.C. & Weil, M.H. (1993) Pathophysiology and treatment of circulatory shock. *Critical Care Clinics* **9** (2), 183–203.

Clancy, J., McVicar, A.J. & Baird, N. (2002) *Perioperative Practice: Fundamentals of Homeostasis*. Routledge, London.

Dealey, C. (2005) *The Care of Wounds: A Guide for Nurses*. Blackwell, Oxford.

Hatfield, A. & Tronson, M. (2008) *The Complete Recovery Book*, 4th edn. Oxford University Press, Oxford.

Heitz, U. & Horne, M. (2004) *Pocket Guide to Fluid, Electrolyte, and Acid-Base Balance*. Mosby, St Louis.

Jardins, T. (2007) *Cardiopulmonary Anatomy & Physiology*, 4th edn. Delmar, New York.

Jevon, P. & Ewens, B. (eds) (2002) *Monitoring the Critically Ill Patient*. Blackwell Science, Oxford.

Pinsky, M. & Payen, D. (2004) *Functional Hemodynamic Monitoring*. Springer-Verlag, New York.

Saladin, K.S. (2009) *Anatomy and Physiology: The Unity of Form and Function*, 3rd edn. William C Brown, New York.

Tortora, G.J. (2008) *Principles of Anatomy and Physiology*, 12th edn. Wiley, Oxford.

University of Pennsylvania (2006) *Critical Care Medicine Tutorials: Cardiovascular System.* www.ccmtutorials.com/cvs/index.htm (accessed 25 January 2009).

Watson, R. & Fawcett, T.N. (2003) *Pathophysiology, Homeostasis and Nursing.* Routledge, London.

Waugh, A. & Grant, A. (2004) *Ross and Wilson Anatomy and Physiology in Health and Illness*, 9th edn. Churchill Livingstone, New York.

Managing Perioperative Equipment

2

Joy O'Neill

LEARNING OUTCOMES

❑ Understand the principles underlying the *safe use of equipment* in the operating room.

❑ Understand the principles of the *efficient checking of perioperative equipment* before and after use.

❑ Understand the *use and preparation of anaesthetic and surgical equipment*.

❑ Describe the *measures to be taken if equipment is faulty*.

❑ Discuss the *need for infection control* and the implications of not undertaking such measures.

INTRODUCTION

Surgical equipment is expensive and represents a major investment for the NHS. Surgical procedures have become more complicated and intricate and, as a result, equipment has become more technical, more precise in design and more delicate in structure. Misuse, inadequate cleaning and rough handling can cause damage, reduce life expectancy and produce safety risks due to malfunction.

Perioperative practitioners need to keep up-to-date with the continually changing technology and legislation to ensure their professional competence and accountability in their perioperative practice. It is essential that they have the knowledge and an understanding of the use of operating room equipment. It is the responsibility of the perioperative team to ensure the availability of all relevant equipment, to check it before use and to ensure that it is in full working order for the surgical procedures.

Competent use of equipment is an important part of risk management. Practitioners should continuously monitor the operating room for potential hazards to patients during surgical procedures.

DUTIES OF THE EMPLOYER

It is important that practitioners are aware of the Health and Safety at Work Act 1974 and the implications for perioperative practice. The basic duty of every employer is set out in Section 2 of the Health and Safety at Work Act (HMSO 1974): 'it shall be the duty of every employer to ensure, so far as is reasonably practicable, the health, safety and welfare at work of all its employees'. According to the law, the employer has to do only what is reasonably practicable. The law however requires the employer to be able to prove, on a balance of probabilities, that it did all that was reasonably practicable to carry out its statutory duty (AfPP 2007, p 42).

The management of Health and Safety at Work Regulations (HMSO 1992, 1994, 1999) introduced more specific requirements to manage health and safety, and required employers to carry out a risk assessment and implement changes as necessary.

In addition, hospitals also develop their own policies and procedures for equipment use, safety and training, which are reviewed and revised as necessary. Perioperative practitioners need to know the location of the local policies in their department so they have easy access to them for reference.

The operating department manager has a responsibility to set up a planned maintenance programme agreed between the operating room department and the electrical and biomedical department (EBME). Training and regular updates on equipment use are essential and the operating room manager must keep documentation of attendance as proof in case of an inquiry following an incident. The EBME marks all operating room equipment and it undertakes annual equipment audits in liaison with the operating manager.

DUTIES OF THE EMPLOYEE

Local policies govern the use and safety of the operating department equipment for the perioperative practitioners. Practitioners should be familiar with all operating department equipment, its use and potential hazards, to ensure a safe environment for patients and members of the perioperative team. Practitioners check all equipment before an operating list, identify any faults and follow the proper local procedures to ensure effective maintenance and/or repair of the faulty item.

All equipment to be used for patient care is regularly maintained according to manufacturer's instructions. It is checked before use and records are kept. The staff have been trained especially to ensure it is fit for purpose and safe for use (EORNA & IFPN 2005).

To minimise the risk of equipment failure, all equipment should be assembled and tested in advance of its use. All practitioners who work in theatres should read the safety alerts issued from time to time by the Medicines and Healthcare Products Regulatory Agency (MHRA) and also feedback their experience of incidents to the agency (Edozien 2005).

Practitioners should not operate any item of equipment without instruction or knowledge of its use, as this could be dangerous for the practitioner, other perioperative personnel and especially the patient.

Before an operating list

Before an operating list it is vital that the perioperative team checks all the equipment and formalises this check by signing a checklist as illustrated in Box 2.1.

The provision and use of electrical equipment within the perioperative setting should comply within the recommendations

---

Box 2.1 Procedure before an operating list

- Select the correct equipment and accessories according to the needs of the operating list and the patients' individual needs.
- Identify promptly any faults or malfunctioning equipment, take it out of use and report the fault to the relevant personnel or the EBME department. Do not return it to the operating department until it is repaired and ready for use.
- Calibrate equipment in line with the manufacturer's instructions.
- Monitor equipment while in use according to the manufacturer's instructions.

---

of the Provision and Work Equipment Regulations (HMSO 1998) and therefore should:

- be checked by authorised designated personnel on delivery and before use;
- be used in accordance with the manufacturer's recommendations;
- only be used by employees who have been instructed in its use;
- have a planned preventative maintenance programme, including a regular maintenance contract;
- ensure all loan or trial electrical equipment has a current certificate of indemnity and that checks are carried out prior to use (AfPP 2007).

ANAESTHETIC EQUIPMENT

The anaesthetic machine

All anaesthetic equipment must be checked, prepared and demonstrated as functional before induction of anaesthesia is commenced. A major cause of anaesthetic critical incidents has been when anaesthetic machines and breathing systems have not been adequately checked by an anaesthetists before the commencement of the operating list (AfPP 2007).

The anaesthetic machine is checked before use by the anaesthetic practitioner to maintain patient safety. He or she should follow the local protocol using the guidelines described by the Association of Anaesthetists of Great Britain and Ireland (AAGBI 2007), and the manufacturer. The misuse and failure of the machine can have serious consequences for the patient.

A typical anaesthetic machine is illustrated in Figure 2.1. The components of an anaesthetic machine are:

- gas supply: via pipeline or cylinder supply;
- pressure regulators;
- oxygen pressure failure devices;
- flow control valves and flowmeters;
- scavenger systems;
- vaporisers;
- ventilators;

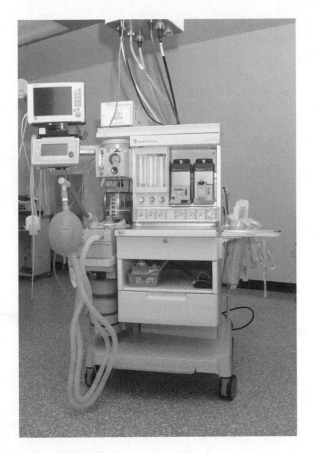

Fig. 2.1 Anaesthetic machine.

- oxygen analysers;
- suction.

Gas supply

The gas supply of an anaesthetic machine consists of a pipeline or cylinder source. The anaesthetic practitioner checks both types of gas supply before each operating session.

The common units of pressure used in the operating room environment are:

- bar pressure (bar);
- kilopascals (kPa);
- pounds per square inch (psi);
- pounds per square inch gauge (psig) (this is the pressure above atmospheric pressure).

Their relationship is:

- 1 bar = 14.5 pounds per square inch (psi);
- 1 bar = 100 kilopascals (kPa) (SI unit).

As a rule of thumb 1000 psi approximately equals 70 bar and 100 bar equals 1450 psi (Meyer 1998).

Pipeline
Hospital stores supply medical gases from a central store via pipelines or by large cylinders or tanks. The gases are delivered to specific ports located in the wall or from the ceiling, via a boom in the operating and anaesthetic rooms (Figure 2.2). Non-interchangeable spring-loaded valves are inserted into the wall ports and connect to the anaesthetic machine via flexible non-crushable tubing. The pipes are colour coded and are bonded to the valve. The pressure in the anaesthetic gas pipeline is 4 bar (400 kPa) and is the same as the working pressure of the anaesthetic machine.

While the nitrous oxide and medical air lines directly connect with the flowmeters, the oxygen line passes via pressure-failure devices, the oxygen flush valve and the ventilator power outlet. If oxygen pressure falls below 25 psig (roughly 50% of normal), a fail-safe valve automatically closes the nitrous oxide flow and other gas lines to prevent accidental delivery of an hypoxic mixture to the patient. In this event an audible alarm to warn of failure of oxygen is activated (Gwinnutt 2008).

The majority of anaesthetic machines possess a mechanical linkage between the nitrous oxide and oxygen flowmeters. This causes the nitrous flow to decrease if the oxygen flowmeter is adjusted to give less than 25–30% of oxygen. The use of an

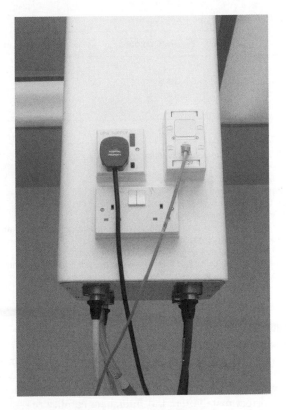

Fig. 2.2 Gas pipelines attached to an anaesthetic boom.

oxygen analyser with an audible alarm is mandatory for all patients breathing anaesthetic gases. The sampling port must be placed so that the gas mixture delivered to the patient is monitored continuously. The analyser should provide a clearly visible readout of the concentration of oxygen in the inspired gas and sound an alarm if an hypoxic mixture is delivered.

Safety checks are illustrated in Box 2.2 and pipeline details are summarised in Table 2.1.

Table 2.1 Pipeline colours and gas pressures.

Gas	Pipe colour	Gas pressure (kPa)
Oxygen	White	400
Nitrous oxide	Blue	400
Medical air	Black	400
Suction vacuum	Yellow	53

Box 2.2 Safety checks for pipeline gas supply

- Check all pipeline connections.
- Perform the Westminster tug test to ensure connections are secure. Take care because the high pressure of the gas from the boom can cause the pipeline to disconnect at speed.
- Check the pressure of gas (400 kPa) on the front of the anaesthetic machine.
- Check the individual gas bobbins rotate on the anaesthetic machine with gas flow and they do not stick throughout the range.
- Check the nitrous oxide flow falls before the oxygen flow (on disconnection of the oxygen pipe) to prevent an hypoxic mixture occurring.
- Check the oxygen alarm sounds to identify no flow of oxygen gas.

Cylinders

Cylinders are made from molybdenum steel, are colour coded (same as pipelines) and consist of a body and a shoulder which contains threads into which are fitted a pin-index valve block, a bull-nosed valve or a hand-wheel valve. The pin index is to ensure correct installation and interchangeability of gas cylinders. The washer at the pin index is called a Bodok seal and its function is to prevent leakage. The anaesthetic practitioner or operating department support worker should change the seal if it shows signs of wear or damage.

Full cylinders are supplied with dust covers and they should be stored separately from empty cylinders in the relevant store cupboard. Anaesthetic practitioners or operating room support workers should take care when they change any gas cylinder. They should ensure that they close the cylinder valve before disconnection from the machine. Safety checks are outlined in Box 2.3 and cylinder details are summarised in Table 2.2. Figure 2.3 shows anaesthetic gas cylinders.

Table 2.2 Cylinder colours and gas pressures.

Gas	Body	Shoulder	Pressure (bar)
Oxygen	Black	White	137
Nitrous oxide	Blue	Blue	44
Medical air	Grey	White and black	137

Box 2.3 Safety checks for cylinder gas supply

- Ensure correct installation of the cylinders. Open and close the cylinders slowly to prevent a surge of gas pressure and damage to the machine.
- Check for any leaks from the cylinders, check the Bodok seal and change it if necessary.
- If the gas cylinder registers as empty or almost empty, change it before the beginning of the operating list.
- Turn off cylinders when not in use.
- Check that individual bobbins are rotating with gas flow, will rotate throughout the range and do not stick.
- Check that the nitrous oxide flow falls before the oxygen flow to prevent an hypoxic mixture being delivered to the patient.
- Check the oxygen alarm sounds to identify no flow of oxygen gas.
- To prevent slippage or accidents such as burns, do not use hand cream before handling cylinders.

Pressure regulators

Pressure regulators have two important functions:

- they reduce high pressures of compressed gases to manageable levels, acting thus as pressure-reducing valves;
- they minimise fluctuations in the pressure within an anaesthetic machine, which would otherwise necessitate frequent manipulations of flowmeter controls (Mushambi & Smith 2007).

Piped gases are delivered to the anaesthetic machine at pressures of between 45 and 50 psig through the pin-index system. The high pressure in the gas cylinder makes the flow difficult and dangerous, and the pressure regulator ensures a safe delivery of gas to the patient at a pressure of less than 50 psig.

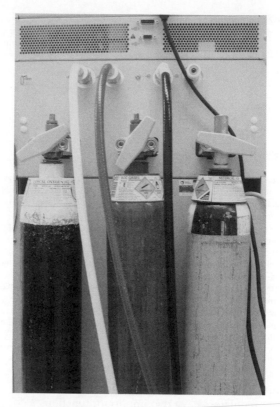

Fig. 2.3 Anaesthetic gas cylinders. Left to right: oxygen (black), nitrous oxide (blue), medical air (grey).

Oxygen pressure failure devices

The nitrous oxide and medical air gas flows connect directly with the flowmeters, but the oxygen gas flow passes via the pressure-failure devices, the oxygen flush device and the ventilator power outlet.

If oxygen gas (piped or cylinder) fails, a fail-safe valve automatically closes off the nitrous oxide flow and prevents the patient receiving an hypoxic mixture of gas. An alarm should sound to alert the anaesthetist or anaesthetic practitioner of this event. Anaesthetic practitioners should check the alarm works before the operating list begins. The anaesthetist can give emergency oxygen by pressing or pushing the oxygen flush valve. The oxygen flush provides a high flow of oxygen to the patient direct from the common gas outlet.

Flow control valves and flowmeters

Gas flows from the anaesthetic machine to the patient through a breathing system. When the anaesthetist switches on the gas flow controls (e.g. oxygen, nitrous oxide, medical air) by turning them anti-clockwise, the gas flows through the valve and the bobbin turns, indicating that the gas is on. The ball or bobbin rises or falls depending on the level of gas delivered to the patient.

Scavenging systems

The scavenging system removes waste gases from the operating room environment by a system of valves and tubing and a pump. This is essential for the well-being of the members of the operating room team. Anaesthetic practitioners should check that they have connected all attachments into the boom in the operating room and into the fitting in the wall of the anaesthetic room. The valve attaches to the expiratory valve of the breathing system or the ventilator (in the anaesthetic room or operating room). Safety checks to be carried out are summarised in Box 2.4.

Vaporisers

Anaesthetic vaporisers are used to administer anaesthetic agents such as halothane, enflurane, isoflurane and sevoflurane by means of the anaesthetic circuit, and are used to maintain

---

Box 2.4   Safety checks for the scavenging system

- Check the security and fitting of attachments.
- Check the tubing is not too long or the resistance to gas flow will rise, leading to possible backing up of scavenged gases and leakage into the operating room atmosphere.

anaesthesia. They should be checked every time the anaesthetic machine is checked. This includes ensuring that they are working, are correctly attached to the anaesthetic machine and are full of the volatile agent (Oakley & Van Limburgh 2005).

A vaporiser is designed to add a controlled amount of an inhalational agent, after changing it from liquid to vapour, to the fresh gas flow. This is normally expressed as a percentage of saturated vapour added to the gas flow.

Characteristics of an ideal vaporiser are (Al-Shaikh & Stacey 2007):

- its performance is not affected by changes in fresh gas flow, volume of the liquid agent, ambient temperature and pressure, decrease in temperature due to vaporisation and pressure fluctuation due to the mode of respiration;
- low resistance to flow;
- light weight with small liquid requirement;
- economy and safety in use with minimal servicing requirements;
- corrosion and solvent-resistant construction

There are two types of vaporiser. In one type (drawover) the anaesthetic agent is vaporised by the negative pressure generated by the patient's respiratory effort and in the other type (plenum), the positive pressure of the gas supply is used to vaporise the anaesthetic agent.

In a drawover vaporiser, the gas is pulled through the vaporiser when the patient inspires, creating a sub-atmospheric pressure. In a plenum vaporiser, the gas is forced through the vaporiser by the pressure of the gas supply (Mushambi & Smith 2007).

There are different types of vaporising agent and each type has its own vaporiser and filling outlet to prevent incorrect filling with the wrong agent. The vaporising agents (coloured bottles) are stored away from the light to prevent breakdown of the consistency of the agent. There may be one, two, three or more vaporisers on the anaesthetic machine, but the anaesthetist will only use one vaporiser at a time. Each vaporiser fits onto the back bar of the anaesthetic machine and will not lock onto this bar if not fitted properly.

Box 2.5   Checklist for vaporisers

- Check the security and fitting of individual vaporisers. Remove and refit if the vaporiser is not seated properly.
- Ensure there is sufficient anaesthetic agent within each vaporiser (up to the indicated line for full).
- Check only one vaporiser will turn on at a time.
- Check that gas flowmeter moves when the vaporiser is switched on.
- Check for leaks within the breathing circuit.

Most anaesthetic machines allow more than one vaporiser to be fitted at any time. To prevent more than one vapour being given, an interlock device is fitted. This is usually a mechanical device that prevents more than one vaporiser being turned on simultaneously (Gwinnutt 2008). A checklist for vaporisers is given in Box 2.5.

Properties and side effects of vaporising agents are discussed in Chapter 3. A vaporiser is illustrated in Figure 2.4.

Ventilators

The principles of effective practice for maintenance of anaesthesia by controlled ventilation are to maintain a safe environment for the patient and staff, to perform careful patient management and effective patient physiological monitoring, and to provide efficient documentation of the patient care record.

The most commonly used type of ventilation is intermittent positive pressure ventilation (IPPV). The lungs are intermittently inflated by positive pressure generated by a ventilator and gas flow is delivered through an endotracheal tube (O'Higgins 2003).

Ventilators may be integrated with the anaesthetic machine or configured later. They are often electronically controlled and pneumatically powered. The autoclave bellows are often suitable for adult and paediatric use. Traditionally, anaesthetic machine ventilators have had a minimal number of controls. The anaesthetist can vary minute volume by setting tidal volume and ventilatory frequency directly or by adjusting inspiratory time, inspiratory flow rate and the rate of inspiratory or expiratory time. They may perform self-test start-up

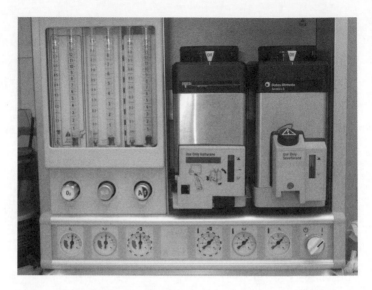

Fig. 2.4 Anaesthetic gas vaporiser.

(usual dual processor technology), volume- or pressure-controlled ventilation modes, assisted spontaneous ventilation and electronically adjustable positive end-expiratory pressure (PEEP).

Sophisticated spirometry compensates for changes in fresh gas flow, small leaks or patient compliance (Sinclair *et al.* 2006).

In volume-controlled ventilators, the flow delivered is constant and the tidal volume is targeted, with a variable pressure delivered relative to compliance of the lung.

In pressure-controlled ventilators, the flow decelerates through the breath to maintain the targeted pressure at the peak inspired pressure. The tidal volume delivered is determined by the compliance of the ventilated lung (UK Anaesthesia 2003).

The goals of ventilation are to deliver oxygen to the alveoli and to remove carbon dioxide. Ventilators collect gas and the vaporising agent into a bag or bellows, and deliver these to the patient's lungs. They create a pressure gradient between the proximal airway and the alveoli, and there are four phases during the ventilation cycle:

* inspiration;
* the transition from inspiration and expiration;
* expiration;
* the transition from expiration to inspiration.

Anaesthetists may use different ventilators in conjunction with the insertion of an endotracheal (ET) tube and the rapid sequence induction procedure. These are described in Chapter 8. Ventilators can be of two types – mechanical and power driven. Anaesthetic practitioners should familiarise themselves with the different types of ventilator and their checking procedures.

When IPPV ventilation is used during anaesthesia, airway pressure alarms must be used to detect excessive pressure within the airway and also to give warning of disconnection or leaks. The upper and lower alarms must be reviewed and set appropriately before anaesthesia commences (AAGBI 2007). The gases are pneumatically driven into a bag or bellows and are compressed. The bellows take the place of the breathing bag used in spontaneous breathing.

The power source of power driven ventilators can be either compressed gas, electricity or both.

The possible hazards with ventilators are:

* no available alarm;
* disconnection of electricity or tubing can occur;
* failure of oxygen gas supply and delivery of ventilation.

Before anaesthesia, and at any appropriate time during anaesthesia, the anaesthetic practitioner must check all aspects of the ventilator to prevent occurrence of these hazards. These checks are outlined in Box 2.6.

Total intravenous anaesthesia (TIVA)

TIVA techniques for induction and maintenance of anaesthesia are widely used. The pharmacokinetic and pharmacodynamic prolife of agents such as propofol, alfentanil and remifentanil permit rapid titration of drug dose to the required effect in

---

Box 2.6 Checklist for ventilators

• Check the efficient working of the ventilator before the operating list.
• Check the correct configuration as per the local anaesthetic checklist.
• Check the attachment of the breathing bag to the ventilator tubing and check that the ventilator works efficiently on the set configuration.
• Check all connections, leak test and ventilator alarm.
• During ventilation of the patient:
  — observe the colour of the patient, chest movements and bellow movements or sound of the ventilator;
  — observe the waveform of end-tidal carbon dioxide on the monitor.

---

individual patients. Target controlled infusion (TCI) devices enable the theoretical drug concentration in the plasma of propofol to be controlled continuously and administered without the need for complex calculation by the anaesthetist. The computer program in the TCI device continuously calculates the distribution and elimination of propofol, and automatically adjusts the infusion rate to maintain a predicted plasma drug concentration.

Advantages of TIVA include the avoidance of some of the complications of inhalational anaesthesia, such as distension of gas-filled spaces, diffusion hypoxia and production of fluoride ions. It may be used safely in patients susceptible to malignant hyperpyrexia. There is also a reduced incidence of postoperative nausea and vomiting (Fell & Kirkbride 2007).

TIVA equipment is illustrated in Figure 2.5.

Syringe pumps use a driver that pushes the preferred drug out of the syringe (50 ml) by advancing its plunger while the barrel is kept stationary. The important features of the syringe pump are:

• a bolus facility which gives the ability to increase quickly the plasma concentration;
• flow rate – the pump should be able to function accurately on small flows of gas (oxygen or oxygen and medical air);
• battery – there should be an indication of the status of the battery;
• tight syringe fitting – the syringe plunger must fit securely in the clamp.

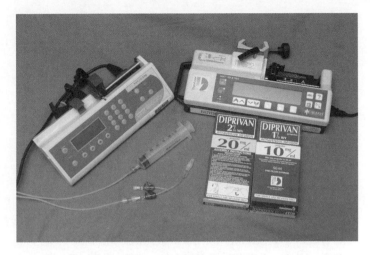

Fig. 2.5 TIVA equipment.

The role of the anaesthetic practitioner in TIVA is illustrated in Box 2.7.

Oxygen analyser

The anaesthetist uses an oxygen analyser to ensure that the patient receives a correct concentration of oxygen. There is 21% of oxygen in the air and the anaesthetic practitioner checks and calibrates the oxygen analyser before each operating list to ensure it has the correct setting. For instructions on how to calibrate the analyser for 21% and 100% see Box 2.8b, page 70.

Suction

A pipeline vacuum suction is available with the anaesthetic machine. It is controlled by an on and off switch and it usually has a medium and a high setting. Operating support workers or anaesthetic practitioners insert new disposable linings into the suction machine for each patient. Relevant suction catheters are used for the patients.

Box 2.7 TIVA checklist

• Locate the appropriate syringe pumps, drug infusion set (propofol) and accessories (connecting tubing and a Y-connector) to deliver the induction agent and opiate through the venous cannula.
• Attach the syringe pumps to a drip stand and plug them in.
• Give the anaesthetist the opiate and record it in the controlled drugs book.
• Have other propofol infusion sets available for a long surgical procedure.
• Ensure that vaporisers are filled in case the anaesthetist changes from TIVA to an inhalational anaesthesia technique.
• After use, syringe pumps should be plugged in to ensure that they are charged up and ready to use again.

Checking the anaesthetic machine

The checking procedure for the anaesthetic machine covers all aspects of the anaesthetic delivery system, including the gas supply pipelines, machine, breathing systems (filters, connectors and airway devices), ventilators, suction monitoring and ancillary equipment (AAGBI 2004). This is outlined in Box 2.8a and b.

ANAESTHETIC MONITORING EQUIPMENT

During anaesthesia the anaesthetic team observes the patient and monitors his or her physiological status throughout the perioperative stage and throughout transfer to the intensive care ward or to another hospital. They document the recordings on the patient's anaesthetic record and the care plan. See Chapter 8 (page 315) for an example of the anaesthetic record of the care plan. Anaesthetic practitioners should attach all monitoring devices before the commencement of anaesthesia and record the first physiological readings on the patient's care plan.

During the establishment and maintenance of anaesthesia, the patient's physiological state, depth of anaesthesia and functioning of the equipment need continual assessment. To achieve this, monitoring devices are used to supplement clinical observation.

Box 2.8
(a) Anaesthetist's check list for the anaesthetic machine (AAGBI guidelines) (AAGBI 2004)

- The anaesthetic machine is connected to the electricity supply and switched on.
- All monitoring devices, oxygen analyser, pulse oximeter and capnograph are functioning and have appropriate alarm limits.
- Gas sampling lines are attached and free from obstructions.
- An appropriate frequency of recording of blood pressure is selected.
- Correct insertion of pipeline gases and perform Westminster tug test for all gases.
- The anaesthetic machine is connected to a supply of oxygen and there is an oxygen cylinder with an adequate supply fitted to the back of the machine.
- All pipeline gas pressure gauges indicate 400–500 kPa.
- Operation of flowmeters.
- Each flow operates smoothly and bobbins move freely throughout the range.
- The antihypoxic device is working correctly.
- The emergency oxygen bypass control.
- Vaporisers are fitted correctly, filled and leak tested.
- Breathing circuit, leak test and patency of flow of gas.
- Face mask, filter and catheter mount are available.
- Ventilator tubing is securely attached, leak tested and works efficiently on set configuration, and alarms are set.
- Alternative ventilation means is available (breathing circuit and oxygen cylinder).
- Scavenging tubing is attached to appropriate exhaust port of the breathing system, ventilator or workstation and is in set limits.
- Ancillary equipment is available (intubation equipment as described in Chapter 8, page 282).
- Recording of the anaesthetic machine check by anaesthetic team.

(b) Anaesthetic practitioner's check list for the anaesthetic machine (Pennine Acute NHS Hospitals Trust guidelines)

- Observe the machine for damage and that the mains cable is plugged in.
- Check that all accessories are present.
- Press the drain button if appropriate.
- Disconnect all pipeline supplies and turns off any fitted gas cylinders.
- Ensure all flow controls are off (fully clockwise).
- Open slowly the oxygen cylinder valve. Check amount of oxygen in the cylinder.
- Close the oxygen cylinder valve and observe the gauge. The gauge must not fall by more than 690 kPa (100 psi) in 1 minute.
- Repeat for air and nitrous oxide cylinders.

Cont.

Box 2.8 *Continued*

- Drain all cylinders.
- Check there is a 'No oxygen pressure' audible alarm.
- Change cylinders if necessary.
- Full cylinders:

  oxygen – 2175 psi, nitrous oxide – 725 psi, medical air – 1450 psi.

- Plug in all pipeline gases.
- Ensure each gauge registers approximately 400 kPa.
- Perform the Westminster tug test.
- Ensure the scavenging system is connected and efficient.
- Remove the oxygen sensor from the circuit.
- Calibrate the cell to 21%. This will take up to 3 minutes.
- Once calibrated, refit the oxygen cell to the circuit.
- Once a month calibrate the cell to 100%.
- After fitting the cell, flow 5 litres of oxygen through the system.
- Calibrate to 100%.

Negative leak test
- Switch off the machine.
- Turn all controls to 1.5 turns anti-clockwise.
- Switch on auxiliary common gas outlet (ACGO).
- Test the leak device to the ACGO by squeezing the bulb and blocking the end off (the bulb should stay collapsed).
- Fit the test device to the ACGO and squeeze the hand bulb several times until the bulb collapses.
- If the bulb reinflates within 30 seconds there is a leak on the anaesthetic machine.
- Initially the gas flow bobbins will rise.
- The bulb should not inflate within 30 seconds.
- Turn one vaporiser on initially to 0%.
- Re-squeeze the bulb several times until the bulb collapses. Ensure the bulb does not reinflate.
- Repeat this with any other vaporiser.
- Ensure that only one vaporiser can be turned on at one time.
- Remove the hand bulb from the ACGO and turn the flow controls off.
- Return the ACGO to the off position.

Breathing system leak tests
- Occlude the patient breathing circuit at the end, remembering to remove any filters or gas sampling lines.
- Switch the bag/vent switch on the absorber to vent mode.
- Use the oxygen flush to fill the bellows.
- Turn on the machine and switch the vent to bag mode.
- The bellows should not fall by more than 100 ml in 30 seconds.

Box 2.8 *Continued*

- While in bag mode, turn the adjustable pressure limiting (APL) valve to 30 cmH$_2$O.
- Ensure a 2-litre bag is connected to the side arm.
- While pressing the flush button, observe the pressure guage dial to ensure that it reads approximately 30 cmH$_2$O (±5%, i.e 28.5–31.5 cmH$_2$O).
- Release the flush button.
- Following an initial drop in pressure, ensure the dial stabilises at a pressure of approximately 30 cmH$_2$O (±5%, i.e 28.5–31.5 cmH$_2$O).
- Check the 2-litre bag for any leaks.
- Open the APL valve to ensure that it is not sticking.

Hypoxic guard test
- Use the oxygen analyser for this test.
- Turn all controls fully clockwise and observe the flows:
  oxygen – 25–75 ml, nitrous oxide – zero, medical air – zero.
- Adjust the nitrous oxide flow from 900 ml, 1.5 litres, 3 litres, 6 litres and 9 litres and the oxygen flow from 300 ml, 500 ml, 1 litre, 2 litres and 3 litres.
  The oxygen analyser percentage should stay within 21–30% to ensure there is no hypoxic flow.

Oxygen failure test
- Turn all the gas flows to mid range. Disconnect the oxygen pipeline and ensure the following:
  — an oxygen failure alarm appears on the ventilator;
  — nitrous oxide and oxygen flows stop. The small oxygen bobbin must reach the bottom of the flow tube after the nitrous oxide bobbin. The medical air will still flow.
- Reconnect the oxygen and all flows should reinstate themselves.
- Turn off the medical air and nitrous oxide controls (fully clockwise).

Vaporiser back pressure test
- Turn the oxygen flow to 6 litres.
- Slowly turn the first vaporiser to 1%.
- The oxygen flow should not drop by more than 1 litre.
- Repeat for each vaporiser fitted.

Ventilator operation
- Connect a re-breathe bag to the patient circuit.
- Set the ventilator to the required settings.
- Switch to mechanical ventilation.
- Press the oxygen flush button to completely fill the bellows.
- The ventilator should reach within 10% of the set readings within seven cycles.

Cont.

Box 2.8 *Continued*

- Check the absorber valves are working.
- Turn off the ventilator flow controls.

Suction
- Ensure the suction is connected and working efficiently.

Auxiliary oxygen meter
- Check the bobbin flows throughout the range.

The anaesthetist observes:

- mucosal colour;
- pupil size;
- response to surgical stimuli;
- movement of the chest wall.

The anaesthetist can also undertake palpation of the pulse, auscultation of breath sounds and, if appropriate, measurement of urine and blood loss.

The anaesthetist observes physiological monitoring (AAGBI 2004):

- pulse oximetry;
- non-invasive blood pressure;
- electrocardiography;
- capnography;
- vapour analyser;
- temperature.

Monitoring devices
For all monitoring devices the anaesthetic team set appropriate parameters before use and these include:

- cycling times;
- frequency of recordings;
- alarm settings.

Pulse oximetry

The pulse oximeter measures the oxygen saturation of the patient's blood. The pulse oximeter probe is attached to the patient's finger, toe or ear. The probe contains a light source and, when it is attached to a monitor, the patient's oxygen saturation percentage is displayed as a light absorption trace and a reading on the monitoring machine. It is non-invasive and easy to apply.

Pulse oximeters provide rapid, non-invasive measurement of pulse rate and haemoglobin saturation by measuring changes in light absorbed by an extremity. One side of the probe contains an array of light-emitting diodes and the other contains a light sensor. The method relies on the principle that the amount of light absorbed by a solution is proportional to the concentration. Therefore if the absorption can be measured, the concentration can be calculated. As both oxyhaemoglobin and deoxyhaemoglobin are present within a sample of blood, the oxygen saturation may be calculated by measuring the absorption at two different wavelengths (Byrne 2007).

The anaesthetic practitioner should check the probe, during a long anaesthetic or with patients who have impaired circulation, to identify any pressure on the probe site, and should change the probe site if necessary. Details of any pressure should be documented on the patient's care plan and the appropriate operating personnel informed.

Non-invasive blood pressure measurement

The anaesthetic practitioner attaches the appropriate size of blood pressure cuff to the patient. The cuff is usually fitted to the dominant arm of the patient, unless the identified surgery is on that arm. In this circumstance the anaesthetist should be asked for his or her preference and the cuff may be positioned on the leg instead.

The tubing is attached to the monitor and the blood pressure reading will be displayed on the monitor. The cuff inflates and deflates, and the machine detects arterial wall motion and calculates systolic, mean and diastolic pressures. Most machines have a trend setting where the anaesthetic team can read blood pressure readings from the first reading until disconnection from the monitor machine.

Electrocardiograph (ECG)

The anaesthetic practitioner attaches the ECG electrodes to the patient before the induction of anaesthesia. The leads are attached to the monitor and the ECG reading is displayed on the monitoring machine. See Chapter 1 (pages 20–24) for discussion of these physiological readings.

Capnography

A capnograph measures end-tidal carbon dioxide and this helps the anaesthetist to confirm correct placement of the ET tube and ventilation. The anaesthetic practitioner should check correct attachment of the gas sampling lines and that they are free from obstruction or kinks before the start of the operating list and between surgical procedures if necessary. The carbon dioxide gas sampling line connects to the distal end of the breathing circuit or ventilator tubing and the other end attaches to the monitoring machine. Carbon dioxide absorbs infra-red light. The amount of carbon dioxide present is given by the absorption reading on the monitor as a waveform. The shape of this waveform determines the level of expired carbon dioxide.

Capnography provides indications of:

• correct placement of the laryngeal mask airway (LMA) or ET tube if the patient is breathing and has a circulation.
  Fall in end-tidal carbon dioxide indicates:

• disconnection of the breathing circuit or ventilator tubing;
• leaks from the breathing circuit during spontaneous ventilation;
• hypotension (fall in end-tidal carbon dioxide).

  Rise in end-tidal carbon dioxide indicates:

• re-breathing of the patient during ventilation;
• malignant hyperthermia.

Vapour analyser

The anaesthetist monitors the amounts of vaporising agent during anaesthesia. The vapour analyser measures the concentration of vapour over a range of gas flows and identifies the type of vaporising agent and displays the percentage on the monitoring machine.

Temperature

Monitoring devices must be attached before induction of anaesthesia and their use continued until the patient has recovered from the effects of anaesthesia. Accurate records of these measurements provided by monitors must be kept (AAGBI 2007).

Healthcare professionals should measure and document the patient's temperature prior to induction of anaesthesia and every 30 minutes until the end of surgery. They should not commence induction of anaesthesia unless the patient's temperature is above $36.0°C$ (NICE 2007).

It is important to monitor the patient's temperature during long surgical procedures, where warming devices are being used and if the patient has a low temperature before surgery. During the first 30–40 minutes of anaesthesia, a patient's core temperature can drop to less than $35°C$. Reasons for this include the loss of the behavioural response to cold and the impairment of thermoregulatory heat-preserving mechanisms under general or regional anaesthesia, anaesthetic-induced peripheral vasodilation (with associated heat loss) and the patient getting cold while waiting for surgery on the ward or in the emergency department (NICE 2007).

Heat production is decreased during anaesthesia. Anaesthetic agents alter hypothalamic function, reduce metabolic rate, abolish behavioural responses to heat loss and abolish shivering. Heat loss increases during anaesthesia and surgery because of heat redistribution to the peripheries by vasodilatation and increased radiation by exposure of large moist surfaces. Evaporative heat loss is increased by ventilation of the lungs with cold, dry gas, the use of wet packs and operations on open body cavities (Hardman 2007).

The patient's temperature can alter with:

- a lengthy surgical procedure;
- exposure of abdominal contents during surgery;
- use of wet packs or washout during the surgical procedure.

The perioperative team has a responsibility to ensure that the temperature of the operating room is optimal for the surgical procedure. The anaesthetic practitioners prepare an intravenous infusion by attaching a blood coil to the warming machine and attaching one end to the infusion and the other to an extension tube and three-way tap; if relevant for the anaesthetic and patient's medical condition.

A warming blanket can be used to warm the patient during the surgical procedure. These come in various designs including:

- upper body;
- surgical access;
- dual-port torso;
- full body surgical.

The anaesthetic practitioner hands a nasopharynx temperature probe to the anaesthetist to measure the patient's temperature during the surgical procedure. The end of the probe is attached to the monitor and a reading of the patient's temperature will be displayed on the monitor.

Neuromuscular block

If the patient has been given a muscle relaxant, the anaesthetic practitioner should have a nerve stimulator available for the anaesthetist to identify muscle relaxation and paralysis. A nerve stimulator can identify the depth of the neuromuscular blockade and the amount of reversal drug required.

The role of the anaesthetic practitioner during the monitoring of the patient is summarised in Box 2.9. Monitoring equipment is illustrated in Figure 2.6.

SURGICAL EQUIPMENT

Electrosurgery (diathermy)

One of the most commonly used items of equipment within the operating room is the electrosurgery machine. Electrosurgery is a technique providing both coagulation and cutting effects by application of a high frequency alternating electric

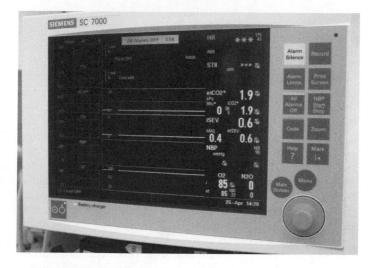

Fig. 2.6 Monitoring equipment.

Box 2.9 Monitoring the patient

- Be aware of the patient's base readings of the physiological observations from the ward.
- Be familiar with all equipment.
- Check monitoring machine and accessories before the commencement of anaesthesia.
- Set parameters to correct settings.
- Ensure all alarms work efficiently.
- Report any faults to appropriate personnel, locate and check replacements if necessary.
- Obtain printouts from the machine for the anaesthetist if necessary.
- Clean devices and accessories following local policies.
- Document recordings of physiological readings on the patient's care plan.
- Have all available monitoring for transfers.

---

current to the tissue. Two methods of electrosurgery are commonly used in the operating room environment: these are monopolar and bipolar electrosurgery. The method of completion of the electrical circuit is the fundamental difference between them.

Monopolar electrosurgery

Monopolar circuitry current originates in the generator, flows through the active electrode and into the patient. It is then recaptured by the return electrode attached to the patient's body, and finally channelled back into the generator. The patient forms the major part of the electrical circuit. An active cable from the electrical surgical unit carries current to the monopolar electrode.

Monopolar electrosurgery is the passage of a high frequency current through the patient from the active electrode (electrosurgical forceps or pencil) to the return electrode (sometimes called the patient plate, dispersive electrode or indifferent electrode). The flow of the current is resisted in body tissue, producing a rise in temperature. The small tip of the active electrode produces 'high current density', which in turn results in the greatest heating effect as current is concentrated in this area. The large area of the return electrode produces 'low current density', which results in a low heating effect since the current is dissipated over a large area. It is important to note that both electrodes are capable of producing the same heating effect since they both carry the same current. It is the difference in size which makes the small active electrode concentrate the heating effect to a small area of tissue, leading to the desired electrosurgical effects.

The greater the current density, the greater the heating effect, leading to the three known electrosurgical effects of cutting, coagulation and fulguration (AfPP 2007).

The surgeon has two foot pedals to control the electrosurgical machine and these are colour-coded as follows:

- blue for coagulation and fulguration. Coagulation is caused by relatively low power, low voltage current heating cells to produce a soft coagulation. Fulguration is caused by non-contact high power, high voltage current to spray sparks over a wide area, leading to superficial destruction of tissues;
- yellow for cutting. Cutting is the use of non contact high power, low voltage current to disrupt cells causing a split in the tissues.

Box 2.10   Checklist for monopolar electrosurgery use

- Check equipment for any damage or loose connections (including of electric plugs and wiring). The alarm sounds if the theatre support worker does not attach all connections into the machine or patient.
- Use the correct position of the electrosurgical patient pad for the surgical procedure.
- The patient's skin should be dry, clean and free of excess hair before applying the return electrode.
- Do not place patient return electrode over bony or scarred tissue or near metal implants. It should be as close to the operative site as is practical and should remain dry throughout surgery.
- Ensure the patient's skin is not in contact with any metal (e.g. operating table or supports).
- Adjust electrosurgical settings according to local policy or surgeon's preference. Alter if necessary.

The circulating practitioner will:

- Inform the scrub practitioner of the electrosurgical settings.
- Place the correct electrosurgical foot pedal or pedals in position (next to the surgeon's feet) before commencement of the surgery.
- Record pad position and state of skin after removal.

The scrub practitioner will:

- Ensure the surgeon is aware of the electrosurgical settings before they begin the surgery.
- Place the active electrosurgical handle in an insulated quiver when it is not in use to avoid any burns to the patient.

The safety checklist for monopolar electrosurgery use is summarised in Box 2.10. The electrosurgical machine and accessories are illustrated in Figure 2.7.

Patient return electrode positions
The preferred return electrode positions are buttock, posterior thigh, anterior thigh, mid back, lower back, upper calf and abdomen. These are illustrated in Figure 2.8.

Bipolar electrosurgery
A bipolar machine has both the active and return electrodes in the one instrument. The current originates in the generator and flows down one tine of the forceps through the tissue between the forceps and back to the generator through the other tine of

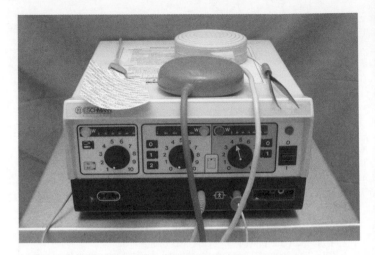

Fig. 2.7 Monopolar machine.

the forceps. Current does not flow through the patient, since it is contained within the wound, travelling between the tines of the forceps. Therefore a return electrode attached to the patient is not necessary. The machine and accessories are illustrated in Figure 2.9 and the safety checks are summarised in Box 2.11.

Considerations before the use of electrosurgery

- Ask surgeons which type of electrosurgery they will use during the surgical procedure, but have all appropriate choices available.
- Communication between the scrub practitioner, the surgeon and the anaesthetist needs to be at its optimum to avoid any hazards.
- Always check the machine and attachments and identify any faulty equipment. If necessary remove it from the operating room and ask the EBME department to check it before reuse.
- Never switch on the machine before attaching all relevant leads and accessories.
- During laparoscopic surgery be aware of other laparoscopic instruments (clamps or clip applicator) during electrosurgery.

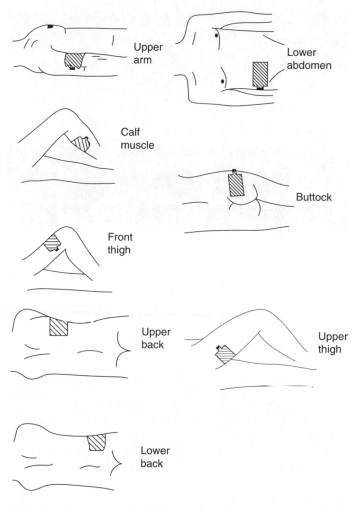

Fig. 2.8 Positions for the return electrode.

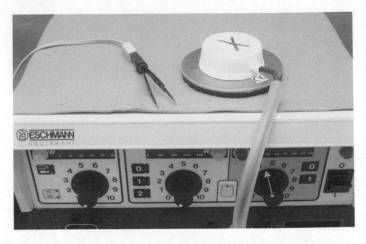

Fig. 2.9 Bipolar machine and accessories.

Box 2.11 Checklist for bipolar electrosugery use

• Check equipment for any damage or loose connections (inclusive of electric plugs and wiring). An alarm sounds if the connections are not correctly attached.

• Use a scratch card to clean off any debris during the surgical procedure to ensure efficiency of the electrosurgery electrode.
• Wash pedals, machine and accessories if relevant at the end of each surgical procedure and at the end of the operating list following local policy.
• Inform the anaesthetist and surgeon if the patient has a pacemaker.

Hazards of electrosurgery

Burns
Accidental burns still occur despite the advances in technology which have produced safe and efficient electrosurgical equipment (MHRA 2005, Cunnington 2006). The practitioner should

be aware of and follow the operating department policy and undertake safety checks to ensure patient safety.

Burns may occur with:

- poor contact of electrosurgical pad;
- pooling of fluids (e.g. when the surgeon prepares the patient's skin);
- breakage of the electrical circuit (e.g. disconnection of the leads or pad);
- patient contact with metal (e.g. operating table).

Electrocution

Undertake regular safety checks of wiring and plugs, according to health and safety requirements, to avoid electrocution of staff or patient.

Interference with medical equipment

- Cardiac pacemakers can interfere with monitors and video equipment.
- The anaesthetic practitioner should always inform the anaesthetist and surgeon if the patient has a pacemaker. The surgeon can use bipolar electrosurgery in this case.

Smoke inhalation of electrosurgical plume

Surgical plume is the smoke which is released when an electrosurgery, laser or ultrasonic device is used on body tissue. Surgical plume contains toxins such as chemicals, carbonised tissue, blood particles, viral DNA particles and bacteria that can have a chemical and biological impact on those exposed (Association of Operating Room Nurses [AORN] 2006, Scott *et al*. 2004). These hazards and implications for perioperative staff are discussed in Chapter 5 (page 210).

Exposure to smoke plume generated during electrosurgery should be minimised. Inhalation of smoke generated by electrosurgery should be minimised by implementing control measures that include, but are not limited to, the use of:

- smoke evacuation systems;
- wall suction with in-line filters, which is only appropriate for a minimal amount of plume.

Box 2.12   Issues the practitioner should consider in the use of suction

- Use suction tubing that has an acceptable circumference to avoid blockage or collapse.
- Select the correct pressure during suction. Advise surgeons, if relevant, of the pressure and let them see the gauge and suction pressure during surgery (gynaecological surgery).
- Use a relevant filter with the suction unit.
- Use a disposable suction lining and the operating room support worker will dispose of it following local policy and standard precautions.

Smoke evacuation systems and accessories should be used according to manufacturers' written instructions. When a smoke evacuation system is used, the suction wand should be placed as close to the source of the smoke as possible. This will maximise smoke capture and enhance visibility at the surgical site (AORN 2005).

Suction

Suction equipment is used during surgical procedures for removal of blood or tissue fluids from the surgical field to improve visibility (Figure 2.10). This can be achieved either by use of a portable machine or via piped access.

A suitable style tip and suction tubing are used dependent on the surgery and the surgeon's preference. A Yankauer attachment is most commonly used in anaesthetics (adult and paediatric) and a Wheeler or Yankauer suction for surgery. Suction use in the recovery area is discussed in Chapter 10 (page 394).

The issues to consider in suction use are summarised in Box 2.12.

Pulse lavage

Surgeons can use pulse lavage which is a powered suction irrigation system. It can be used simultaneously to irrigate the wound and to remove blood and tissue fluids. The pulse switch can be used intermittently or continuously according to preference.

The surgeon can regulate the flow of irrigation and suction by controls on the disposable tip assembly. Members of the

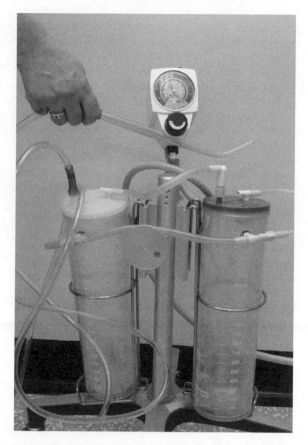

Fig. 2.10 Suction equipment.

surgical team should wear masks with visors for their own safety. The machine and accessories are illustrated in Figure 2.11.

Laser

The use of laser technology in different surgical specialities and techniques decreases blood loss, reduces operative time,

85

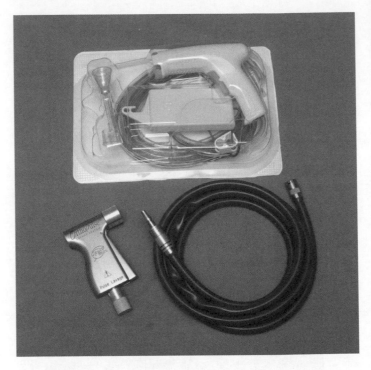

Fig. 2.11 Pulse lavage.

postoperative complications and pain, and aids wound healing. The development of medical lasers has revolutionised surgery.

There are many types of laser and the members of the perioperative team have to consider each laser as they require different operational techniques. They will need consideration of their various features and associated hazards.

It is essential that perioperative practitioners adhere to local policies and recommendations at all times.

Any staff member who will be involved in surgical procedures involving a laser must have undertaken a training programme and have been assessed as having the knowledge and skills to participate in the use of the equipment. The individual practitioner must acknowledge his or her competence to participate and this should be recorded in his or her personal portfolio/personal file. For each specific laser in an operating theatre, authorised operators and safety officers must be clearly identified within the local policy. These individuals will carry total responsibility for security of the laser keys and safe practice for that area of care (AfPP 2007). This management development and initiative has enhanced the safety of perioperative care of the patient.

The term laser is an acronym for light amplification by simulated emission of radiation. The laser focuses light on atoms to stimulate them to a high point of excitation. The resulting radiation is then amplified and metamorphosed into the wavelengths of laser light. The light beam is monochromatic (one colour) because all of the electromagnetic waves are the same length and collimated, or parallel to each other. The light is totally concentrated and easily focused. Unlike conventional light waves, which spread and dissipate electromagnetic radiation by many wavelengths, the coherence of the laser beam is sustained over space and time with wavelengths in the same frequency and energy place.

Lasers use argon, carbon dioxide, holmium, krypton, neodymium, phosphate, ruby or xenon as their active medium. When delivered to tissues, laser light can be absorbed, reflected, transmitted or scattered depending on the characteristics of the laser and the type of tissue. Only absorbed light produces thermal effects in tissue. Thermal penetration varies according to the ratio of absorption versus scattering. Energy absorbed at the surface will destroy superficial cells, further penetration extends cell destruction in surrounding tissues. The wavelength of the laser light, power density rate of delivery of energy and exposure time will vary the effects on tissue (Phillips 2004).

A laser beam is created by stimulating photons inside a resonating chamber. As the photons bounce back and forth, they gain energy, which is emitted through the delivery system, producing a laser beam that can be used to cut or coagulate tissue.

The components of a laser include:

- a medium to produce a laser effect of the stimulated emission. Gases, solid rods or crystals, liquid dyes and free electrons are used. Each produces a different wavelength, colour and effect;
- a power source to create population inversion by pumping energy into the lasing medium. This may be electrical, radio-frequency or an optical power;
- an amplification mechanism to change random directional movement of stimulated emissions to a parallel direction. The power density of the beam determines the laser's capacity to cut, coagulate or vaporise tissue;
- wave guides to aim and control the direction of the laser beam;
- backstops to stop the laser beam from penetrating beyond the expected impact site and affecting non-targeted tissue (Phillips 2004).

There are two different types of system:

- pulsed laser – emits its energy in short, repeating emissions that have a short duration;
- continuous wave – produces continuous light when activated by the perioperative practitioner.

The parts of the each laser system are the same and have a combination of length, level and output of radiation emitted when operated. Power density, the irradiance, is the amount of power per unit surface area during use. Power density is defined as watts per centimetre squared. The most commonly used lasers in the operating room are the carbon dioxide laser and the ND:YAG laser.

Carbon dioxide laser
The carbon dioxide laser uses molecules of carbon dioxide as the medium and may be used in many surgical specialities such as gynaecology, neurosurgery, plastic, general, and ear, nose and throat surgery. It has the ability to cut and coagulate tissues and it is used with the pulsed or continuous systems.

Different wavelengths and frequencies of the laser beam are used for cutting or coagulation of the tissue. The laser is operated through an endoscope or directly onto the tissue, and different sized pieces of tissue can be removed. The beam of this laser is precise and therefore only diseased tissue is selected, which allows for decreased postoperative pain and a faster recovery.

The carbon dioxide wavelength is readily absorbed by water and, as the body's cells are 75–90% water, the carbon dioxide beam is absorbed rapidly at the surface of the tissues. The surface temperature increases and as the water temperature increases it vaporises tissue. Vaporisation is the conversion of solid tissue to smoke and gas – the plume produced should be evacuated or suctioned through a filter device for safety reasons. As the beam is so accurate, the thermal effect on the surrounding tissue is minimal.

Holmium:neodymium-doped yttrium aluminium garnet (ND:YAG) laser

The laser light comes from a crystal containing the metal holmium. The surgeon can use the laser to cut tissue or coagulate blood vessels. The laser beam delivery can be through a hollow needle or through an optical fibre via an endoscope, either continuously (steady beam) or on pulse mode (emits short emissions of light), and it can be used in urological, orthopaedic, or ear, nose and throat surgery. Vaporisation occurs, resulting in the removal of the tissue in a plume of vapour. The surgeon selects the laser wavelength, pulse mode and power for the procedure, and the laser operator controls these.

Developments in the use of laser within the operating room have introduced extra responsibilities for the perioperative practitioner. Perioperative practitioners need to address these responsibilities, in conjunction with the EBME and risk management department, when preparing local policies, and consider the potential hazards associated with lasers and the general standards to protect patients and staff. The general rules for laser use are summarised in Box 2.13.

Box 2.13   General rules for laser use

- One or more operating rooms are designated for the use of the laser.
- Store laser equipment in a locked cupboard and only allow designated personnel to have access.
- Laser warning signs or lights indicate that the laser is in use in the operating room environment (operating room and anaesthetic room doors).
- Windows in operating room door covers have opaque glass to avoid inadvertent eye injuries.
- All perioperative personnel are aware of the fire and safety procedures to be adopted during laser use.
- Keep perioperative team to a minimum during use of the laser.
- All members of the perioperative team should be aware of the fire and safety procedures during laser use.
- Ensure all perioperative personnel and the patient wear eye protection.
- In head and neck surgery, the anaesthetic practitioner will cover the patient's eyes and face with saline or water swabs before surgery.
- Prevent plume inhalation by wearing relevant face masks.
- Use portable or piped suction to evacuate plume.

The laser operator undertakes the following safety checks:

- Tests the laser machine and accessories before use.
- Ensures that the laser is always on stand-by mode until required.
- Does not enable the laser unless it is directed towards the treatment site or a beam stop.
- Switches the machine off and withdraws the key from the machine if laser is not in use.
- The laser foot pedal should be placed in a position convenient to the operator therefore reducing easy access and avoidance of unintended activation of the laser beam and potential injury to the operator, patient or theatre staff.
- Completes all relevant documentation:
  — the name of the laser operator;
  — type of laser used, the use of wattage and the number of joules.
- Reports any incident to the appropriate personnel.
- The surgeon uses instruments with diffuse reflecting surfaces rather than those that give secular reflection.

Hazards of laser use

Eye injuries

Eye injuries can occur with accidental eye exposure during alignment of the laser beam as part of the checking procedure or during use; because of lack of eye protection or because of problems with equipment. Improper handling owing to unfamiliarity with equipment and improper restoration of equipment following service can also cause possible eye injuries.

Laser light can strike the cornea of the eye causing vaporisation and possible destruction of the outer layer, and it can destroy the retina. Laser light may also pass through the cornea, be focused by the lens and destroy the retina (AfPP 2007). The eye is most vulnerable to injury from the laser beam. The injury depends on the power and wavelength of the beam. It can be caused by a break in the laser fibre or the reflection of energy from the beam. The approved laser operator ensures all members of the perioperative team wear eye protection throughout the surgical procedure when the laser machine is in use. Practitioners should check their specific laser glasses before use to ensure that they are not faulty. These glasses are of the appropriate optical density and wavelength. Glasses or moistened eye pads can protect the patient's eyes. It is the operator's responsibility to ensure that all staff and the patient's eyes are protected before operating the laser.

Skin preparation solutions

Surgeons should use aqueous prepping solutions and avoid pooling of these fluids in the prepping procedure of the patient. Alcoholic solutions are not used because of the fire hazards associated with them. The laser beam could possibly heat the volatile fluid and ignite it.

Burns

Burns can be caused by direct or indirect emission of the laser beam. Eye and skin burns are caused by the laser beam shining on the body. The laser operator, scrub practitioner, surgeon and anaesthetists should be vigilant and aware of the risks, and check the surgical instruments and patient for any incidents.

Surgical instruments should have a non-reflective surface and should be blackened to reduce the potential risk of reflection of the laser beam. Such instruments should be inspected regularly to ensure the integrity of the coating (AfPP 2007).

Fire hazard

All members of the perioperative team must observe their local fire policy if the laser beam accidentally causes a burn and ultimately a fire. Specialised laser ETs should be used during intubation.

Laser plume
Chemical hazards from lasers include infective agents in laser plume (smoke). All thermal instruments used in surgery produce smoke and it is possible the infective agents can be present in the laser plume. These may be a potential risk to staff (AfPP 2007).

Non-beam hazards are associated with laser equipment. The hazardous substances are released from the equipment and are emitted from materials exposed to laser plumes produced during surgical procedures. The same hazards as with electrosurgery use apply to the laser machine. The use of smoke evacuators and efficient face masks can minimise these hazards.

Electrical hazards
All laser equipment should adhere to the British Safety Standard BS EN 60825-1 (British Standards Institute [BSI] 1994) and where relevant BS EN 60601-2-22 (BSI 1993). If manufactured after June 1996, the equipment should have the European manufacturing standard CE mark on it.

Specialised laser electrical outlets are used within identified operating rooms for laser machines. The practitioner checks the machine and all attachments before their use. Suitable action should be taken if any faults are identified in the pre-use check.

The legislation identified in the Health and Safety Etc. Act 1974 places a duty on the employers to maintain a working environment for employees that is as safe as is reasonably practicable. This duty extends to incorporate the environment, safe equipment, safe systems of work, as well as providing necessary education, training and supervision to ensure safe working practices (AfPP 2007).

The Association of Laser Safety Professionals (ALSP) is a professional society of laser safety experts actively engaged in providing advice, support and training in laser safety, and it covers all applications of laser technology. The primary aims of the Association are to (Association of Laser Safety Professionals 2008):

- provide a forum in the UK for laser safety expertise;
- establish, promote and maintain high standards in the provision of laser safety services;
- award the qualification of certified Laser Protection Advisor (LPA) to those who are sufficiently competent and knowledgeable in matters of laser safety;
- Organise meetings, events and other appropriate activities relating to laser safety.

The LPA is someone having sufficient skill in, and knowledge and experience of, relevant matters of laser safety, and is able to provide appropriate professional assistance in determining hazards, assessing risks and proposing any necessary protective controls and procedures. Many LPAs also provide training in laser safety.

TV and camera

A visual display unit (VDU) is used to monitor and provide the primary source for information on the surgical procedure. The surgeon gathers anatomical information (state of the organs, position of blood vessels) visually by inspecting the surgical operative site via a camera which is attached to the end of a laparoscope. Surgeons are dependent on this technology for accurate visualisations of the operative field and need an efficient system that will provide the information.

A laparoscopic camera is a special lightweight attachment that fixes to the eyepiece of the laparoscope and it is able to pick up a video image of whatever the surgeon can see through the laparoscope. A cable sends the video signal to a video processing unit – an electronic box that converts the signals into a picture that the surgeon sees on a VDU. A halogen or a high performance xenon light with a fibre-optic cable transmits the light source to the telescope, which has a special attachment point for the light cable.

How to get the best from your camera system (Olympus 2009)

Laparoscopes are precision optical instruments – to ensure clear images, always check the lenses at either end of the laparoscope are clean prior to use. Also, check the optics are in good working order by viewing down the eyepiece, looking for foggy/misty/ fractured or discoloured images, all tell tale signs of a damaged scope. The camera can magnify any deterioration in image quality, especially high-definition (HD) systems.

Most cases of poor image quality will be caused by insufficient illumination from broken light guide fibres. Therefore, examine the light guide cables and telescopes prior to use by directing one end towards (ambient) room light and then checking the opposite end or scope light post to verify the end of the fibre bundle is bright and clear. Always consider the light cable and scope as being an integral part of the camera 'system'. The quality of the image is only as good as the weakest link in the chain!

White balance

This is one of the most important functions on the camera. White balancing calibrates the camera to the colour white and it is from this baseline that it reproduces all other colours. The check for the white balance test is summarised in Box 2.14.

Laparoscopy

Minimal invasive or laparoscopic surgery is performed by inflating the abdomen with gas, (carbon dioxide), which creates a space between the wall of the abdomen and the organs inside. Using short incisions in the skin, trocars are inserted through the abdominal wall so laparoscopic instruments can be passed through them to perform the surgery This is observed directly

---

Box 2.14   White balance test (Olympus 2009)

- With the system fully functional, wrap a clean swab around the distal end of the laparoscope, ensure it forms a cone or funnel, or use the 'white balance cap' that accompanies the system.
- When the laparoscope is 'looking' into the funnel of white, activate the white balance function. Do not remove the swab until the white balancing process is complete.
- A message will appear on the monitor to tell you the procedure is successful.

---

on a monitor which receives its picture from a video camera attached to the laparoscope.

The laparoscope has a light source at the end and a camera that allows the surgical team to observe the contents of the abdomen under magnification and in great detail on VDUs. Video laparoscopy was introduced in the late 1970s and early 1980s.

To improve visualisation of the peritoneal cavity and ease instrument manipulation during laparoscopy, the abdominal cavity is filled with an insufflating gas, producing a pneumo-peritoneum. This gas helps to keep the walls of the abdomen and the organs separated from each other, and allows excellent exposure.

The scrub practitioner attaches gas tubing to the laparoscope and the other end is attached to an insufflator machine. The gas inflates and distends the abdominal cavity (belly) through a trocar and gas tubing.

An insufflator is a machine for inflating the body cavity with the gas of choice. It delivers gas at a desired rate and measures the absolute pressure generated within the body cavity being filled. Laparoscopic insufflators are pressure-limiting gas flow regulators that make it easy to establish and maintain a pneu-moperitoneum. The source of gas is a high-pressure cylinder and the pressure is stepped down by the insufflator.

Electronic insufflators are programmable and maintain an accurate intra-abdominal pressure and have warning signs and alarms. The insufflator maintains the intra-abdominal pressure at a constant pre-set level. Thus the surgeon will normally perform the procedure without having to monitor constantly the pressures and volumes.

If the gas pressure drops below the pre-set level needed to keep the body cavity inflated, then extra gas flow is necessary to re-inflate the body cavity. This requires direct operation of the insufflator by the operating room support worker on the surgeon's instructions.

An added problem is that loss of pressure often occurs slowly (e.g. via a slow leak in the skin incision). The surgeon may only realise the problem when there is a loss of vision or a loss of space, restricting instrument manipulation. The scrub practitioner or surgeon will ask the operating room support worker to increase the gas flow and surgery will restart when the pressure in the abdominal cavity is re-established.

Carbon dioxide is readily absorbed, non-toxic and does not support combustion. The only serious risk is that of hypercarbia, which only develops at an absorption rate of greater than 100 ml a minute. Therefore the anaesthetist usually ventilates the patient during surgery.

The surgeon can make one to three additional incisions, 5–10 mm in length, close to the pubic bone to insert long thin instruments. These instruments are essentially extensions of the surgeon's hands and allow the surgeon to use these instruments from outside the body and perform surgery inside the abdominal cavity. Throughout the surgical procedure the surgical team needs to regulate the flow of gas from the insufflator.

The perioperative team should use filters for the foreign gases going into the body. The filters will stop bodily fluids accidentally flowing back through the tube and into the insufflator. Insufflators are expensive units and they are difficult to clean and recondition if they become contaminated.

Some surgeons prefer to use a gasless method for displacing and extending the abdomen during laparoscopy. A device referred to as an 'abdominal lift' can be used to elevate the abdominal wall for minimal access procedures without the use of carbon dioxide. Shorter instrumentation can be used, because the internal organs are closer to the surface (Phillips 2004).

Using these techniques, elective and emergency surgical procedures of the gastrointestinal, gynaecological and urological surgical specialities can be performed.

There is a possibility that the surgeon may have to abandon the laparoscopic procedure and revert to open surgery. The practitioner should have the appropriate instrument sets for this occurrence. A swab, needle and instrument check should be undertaken when possible to ensure that all these are accounted for.

Advantages of laparoscopic surgery are the minimisation of:

- trauma of access to the internal organs;
- incisions;

- postoperative pain;
- respiratory problems;
- convalescence period.

Possible complications are:

- haemorrhage;
- leakage of carbon dioxide inside the abdominal wall tissues, this may cause crepitus (cracking sensation), which will resolve after a few days;
- absorption of carbon dioxide (embolus);
- injury to other organs within the abdomen;
- shoulder tip pain due to insertion of carbon dioxide and surgical positioning during the procedure;
- reduced urine output; during exit – bleeding;
- postoperative infection;
- deep vein thrombosis.

Laparoscopic surgery is not complication-free. The top four complications resulting in a claim following laparoscopic procedures are (MPS 2007):

- 47% of claims feature damage to adjacent structures such as the common bile duct, ureters, bladder or uterus;
- perforated bowel;
- vascular damage;
- failed procedure or problem occurred.

Perioperative practitioners should (Girard 2009):

- be aware of all that is happening within the room at all times;
- anticipate additional needed instruments, supplies, blood products, or medication;
- understand potential intraoperative complications;
- foster team communication before, during and after surgery;
- document accurately at all times.

An orthopaedic scrub practitioner and the operating room support worker will prepare for an arthroscopy procedure in a similar way to that described for a laparoscopy procedure (Box 2.15).

Box 2.15   Role of the scrub practitioner and operating room support worker during a laparoscopy procedure

Scrub practitioner
- Check and prepare all laparoscopy instruments.
- Ensure all trocar ports are closed before procedure commences.
- Pass gas tubing, light cable, suction tubing and electrosurgical cable to the operating room support worker to attach to relevant machines.
- Monitor gas flow settings during surgery and amount used.
- Ensure a filter is used with the suction machine.
- Prepare irrigation fluid and check it is flowing efficiently.
- Undertake white balance test.
- Prepare clips for clip applicator for surgeon.
- Have a bag available for gall bladder retrieval.

Operating room support worker
- Check insufflator, electrosurgery machine and TV monitors.
- Check gas pressures of insufflator machine.
- Check carbon dioxide flow and replace cylinder if empty.
- Check TV monitors for clarity of picture.
- Attach all connections from scrub practitioner and ensure all settings are correct.
- Alter settings if required by surgeon.

Infection control

Efficient cleaning of equipment should be undertaken by anaesthetic practitioners to maximise high levels of infection control. Standard precautions need to be undertaken to ensure patient and staff safety. Hand washing is very important in this process and in the prevention of methicillin-resistant *Staphylococcus aureus* (MRSA). Infection control and MRSA are discussed in further detail in Chapter 5.

REFERENCES

Al-Shaikh, B. & Stacey, S. (2007) *Anaesthetic Equipment*, 3rd edn. Churchill Livingstone, Edinburgh.

Association of Anaesthetists of Great Britain and Ireland (AAGBI) (2004) *Checking for Anaesthetic Equipment*. AAGBI, London.

Association of Anaesthetists of Great Britain and Ireland (AAGBI) (2007) *Recommendations for Standards of Monitoring During Anaesthesia and Recovery*. AAGBI, London.

Association of Laser Safety Professionals (ALSP) (2008) www.laserprotectionadviser.com

Association for Perioperatice Practice (AfPP) (2007) *Standards and Recommendations for Safe Perioperative Practice*. AfPP, Harrogate.

Association of Operating Room Nurses (AORN) (2005) AORN Recommended Practices Committee *Journal* **3** (81), 616–631.

British Standards Institute (BSI) (1993) *Medical Electrical Equipment Part 2: Particular Requirements for the Safety of Diagnostic Therapeutic Laser Equipment*. BS EN 60601-2-22 (IEC 601-2-22 1922:BS724: Section 2.122:1993. BSI, London.

British Standards Institute (BSI) (1994) *Radiation Safety of Laser Products; Equipment Classification, Requirements and User's Guide*. BS EN 60825-1. BSI, London.

Byrne, A.J. (2007) Monitoring. In: Aitkenhead, A.R., Smith G. & Rowbotham, D.J. (eds) *Textbook of Anaesthesia*, 5th edn. Churchill Livingstone, Edinburgh, pp 345–366.

Cunnington, J. (2006) Facilitating benefit, minimising risk: responsibilities of the surgical practitioner during electrosurgery. *Journal of Perioperative Practice* **6** (4), 195–202.

Edozien, L. C. (2005) Risk management in gynaecology: principles and practice. *Clinical Risk* **11** (5), 177–184.

Fell, D. & Kirkbride, D. (2007) The practical conduct of anaesthesia. In: Aitkenhead, A.R., Smith G. & Rowbotham, D.J. (eds) *Textbook of Anaesthesia*, 5th edn. Churchill Livingstone, Edinburgh, pp 297–314.

Girard, N.J. (2009) Perioperative grand rounds. Procedural mishap: learning curve? *AORN Journal* **89** (2), 468–469.

Gwinnutt, C. (2008) *Clinical Anesthesia*, 3rd edn. Wiley-Blackwell, Chichester.

Hardman, J.G. (2007) Complications during anaesthesia. In: Aitkenhead, A.R., Smith G. & Rowbotham, D.J. (eds) *Textbook of Anaesthesia*, 5th edn. Churchill Livingstone, Edinburgh, pp 367–399.

Her Majesty's Stationery Office (HMSO) (1974) *Health and Safety at Work Etc. Act*. HMSO, London.

Her Majesty's Stationery Office (HMSO) (1992) *Management of Health and Safety at Work Regulations*. HMSO, Norwich.

Her Majesty's Stationery Office (HMSO) (1994) *Management of Health and Safety at Work (Amendment) Regulations*. HMSO, Norwich.

Her Majesty's Stationery Office (HMSO) (1998) *The Provision and Use of Work Equipment Regulations*. The Stationery Office, Norwich.

Her Majesty's Stationery Office (HMSO) (1999) *Management of Health and Safety at Work Regulations*. HMSO, Norwich.

Medicines and Healthcare Products Regulatory Agency (MHRA) (2005) *High Power Electrosurgery Review Update*. MHRA, London.

Meyer, V.R. (1998) *Practical High Performance Liquid Chromatography*, 3rd edn. Wiley, Chichester.

Medical Protection Society (MPS) (2007) www.medicalprotection.org/Default.aspx

Mushambi, M.C. & Smith, G. (2007) Common complications in keyhole surgery result in higher number of claims. In: Aitkenhead, A.R., Smith G. & Rowbotham, D.J. (eds) *Textbook of Anaesthesia*, 5th edn. Churchill Livingstone, Edinburgh.

National Institute of Clinical Excellence (NICE) (2007) *Inadvertent Perioperative Hypothermia: The Management of Inadvertent Perioperative Hypothermia in Adults*. NICE Guideline. Draft for Consultation. October 2007. NICE, London.

Oakley, M. & Van Limburgh, M. (2005) Care of the patient undergoing anaesthesia. In: Woodhead, K. & Wicker, P (eds) *A Textbook of Perioperative Care*. Elsevier, Edinburgh, pp 147–160.

O'Higgins, F. (2003) An introduction to mechanical ventilation in the intensive care unit. Update. *Anaesthesia* **16** (9). www.nda.ox.ac.uk/wfsa/html/u16/u1609_01.htm

Olympus Ltd (2009) *How to Get the Best Out of Your Camera System*. Olympus, Southend.

Phillips, N. (2004) *Berry and Kohn's Operating Room Technique*, 10th edn. Mosby, St Louis.

Sinclair, C.M., Thadsad, M.K. & Barker, I. (2006) Modern anaesthetic machines. *Continuing Education in Anaesthesia, Critical Care and Pain* **6** (2), 75–78.

Scott, E., Beswick, A. & Wakefield, K. (2004) Hazards of diathermy plume. *British Journal of Perioperative Nursing* **14** (9), 409–414 (part 1); **14** (10), 452–456 (part 2).

United Kingdom (UK) Anaesthesia (2003) Principles of ventilators. www.frca.co.uk/article.aspx?articleid=100419

Perioperative Pharmacology

3

Paul Wicker and Africa Bocos

LEARNING OUTCOMES
❑ Understand the *principles of pharmacokinetics* and *pharmacodynamics*.
❑ Discuss the *routes of drug administration*.
❑ Describe the *actions of* some of the *important perioperative drugs*.

PRINCIPLES OF PHARMACOLOGY
Drug errors account for much of the litigation against the NHS. The reasons for this are obvious – the factors involved in drug administration are complex and the margins for error are usually small. A minute quantity of a drug could also have a great effect on the body. Therefore, the slightest error in calculation of dosage, route of administration or wrong choice of preparation can have a fatal effect on the patient.

There are several common problems with drug administration. For example, an error in a prescription might result in the practitioner giving the wrong dose. Alteration of the distribution or elimination of the drug may cause complications in a patient with a particular condition. Failure to anticipate the side effects of drugs can lead to many unwanted results. It is possible to give the wrong drug, especially in emergency situations where mistakes can easily occur if the practitioner does not follow strict protocols. It is even possible to cause nerve damage because of wrongly sited injections. Casualties litter the fields of drug administration, so it is imperative to encourage good practice during early training into post-registration practice.

Most accidents happen because of human error. Legislation aims to reduce drug errors and increase patient safety. Current legislative framework involving drugs use within the perioperative field includes:

- the Medicines Act 1968, as amended, which regulates the manufacture, distribution, import, export, sale and supply of medical products. It also allows exemptions for the general restrictions on the sale, supply and administration of medicines; for instance, it allows midwives to supply and/or administer diamorphine, morphine or pethidine;
- the Misuse of Drugs Act 1971, which controls the availability of drugs liable to misuse. These are divided into three classes (A, B and C) for the purpose of establishing the maximum penalties which can be imposed;
- the Misuse of Drugs (Safe Custody) Regulations 1973, which controls the storage of controlled drugs (CDs);
- the Misuse of Drugs Regulations (MDR) 2001 (Home Office 2001), which enables named healthcare professionals to possess, supply, prescribe and administer CDs in the scope of their practice. The MDR 2001 divide CDs into five schedules, each of which indicates the degree to which a CD is regulated. Schedule 2 covers drugs more commonly used in perioperative practice (opioids). The MDR are amended and revised periodically. Currently (2009), the MDR in force are the Misuse of Drugs and Misuse of Drugs (Safe Custody) (amendment) Regulations 2007. These regulations are of special relevance to Operating Department Practice in that for the first time in their history, Operating Department Practitioners (ODPs) are allowed to order, posses and supply CDs (Home Office 2007), a legal recognition hitherto attributed to registered nurses only;
- the Health Act 2006, which provides for regulations to be set up in order to strengthen governance and to monitoring arrangements for CDs. For instance, it requires both public and private healthcare organisations to appoint an Accountable Officer (AO). The AO is responsible for the monitoring and safe and effective use of CDs, and has to nominate a person or group of persons to witness the destruction of CDs since

he or she is not authorised to witness it personally. It also places a duty of collaboration between healthcare organisations, responsible bodies and other local and national agencies to share information on CDs issues; and gives the police and other nominated people a power of entry and inspection of stocks and CD records (Home Office 2007).

The introduction of a whole raft of government guidelines has improved drug safety.

The National Prescribing Centre explored the issue of drug safety and published guidelines in response to the high cost of drugs-related litigation, and the human suffering caused by drug errors (National Prescribing Centre and National Primary Care Research and Development Centre 2002). The NHS Executive (2002) also published comprehensive guidelines for managing drugs under their *Controls Assurance Standards*. While these provided useful advice, on the whole users found the standards to be too prescriptive and complex. Therefore, from August 2004 the important elements of the standards have been incorporated into the *Standards for Better Health* (Department of Health 2004). This document encourages NHS organisations to bring together good risk-management practice linked to continuous quality improvement and improved patient care.

Trust drug policies, which are the mainstay of error prevention and patient safety, should incorporate and support these government guidelines, directives and legislation. Often these policies act at two levels – a trust-wide policy and a local implementation of this policy. A good evidence-based drugs policy should contain sections on topics such as ordering, receipt and storage of drugs; procedures for administration of drugs; emergency procedures (such as cardiac arrest); and management of controlled drugs.

Safe practice during drug administration

Practitioners must know which drug to give, the quantity, when to give it and the route of administration. A suitably qualified person, in a perioperative setting normally a surgeon or anaesthetist, achieves this with a prescription. It is also becoming more common practice for suitably qualified practitioners to order drugs as required. Prescriptions are most often used outside the hospital; within the perioperative setting, drugs are usually ordered either verbally or with the anaesthetic chart. The chart records the administration of the drugs. The use of the anaesthetic chart to order drugs during the postoperative period is also common practice. It is therefore essential for the practitioner to be familiar with its use as a tool for recording and administering drugs.

Accuracy in drug administration is always the mainstay of safety. The practitioner should read drug labels at least three times – before removing the drug from the shelf, before opening the container and before giving it to the patient. Most institutions have a protocol for administering drugs; however, different rules often apply to the operating department. For example, it is normal practice in wards for two qualified practitioners to check drugs; however, in the operating department often only the anaesthetist will give a drug, without checking the drug with a colleague. Similarly the anaesthetist may sometimes order a drug verbally, or prepare a drug for use, but be unable to administer it. For example, during induction of anaesthesia, the anaesthetist must maintain the patient's airway and may not be able to free a hand to administer the drug. It is also possible for a member of the circulating staff to prepare a drug for use by the operating team during surgery. It is therefore important to identify working policies that identify the normal scope of practice, minimum safe practice and allow the effective working of the perioperative team. This will involve developing safe working practices in areas such as:

- preparation of drugs before the operating list;
- preparation of drugs by one professional for administration by another professional;
- identification of routes of accountability for drug administration;
- defining the scope of roles for practitioners in drug administration;
- identifying the knowledge required, e.g. actions, uses, side effects or dosage.

PHARMACOKINETICS AND PHARMACODYNAMICS

Pharmacokinetics is the study of how the body manages the absorption, distribution, metabolism and excretion of drugs. Pharmacodynamics is the study of the actions and effects which the drugs have on the body.

Pharmacokinetics

Absorption

The route of administration of the drug can affect the rate of absorption – this is known as bioavailability. The intravenous route gives the highest possible bioavailability of 100%. For example, an intravenous dosage of a drug will be much more quickly available to the body than a subcutaneous or oral dosage. Hence the use of intravenous analgesia throughout all areas of the operating department, where it is often preferential to use rapid-acting analgesia.

Distribution

Following absorption, drugs distribute themselves throughout the tissue of the body in various quantities. For example, a lipid-soluble drug may quickly leave the circulation and be absorbed by fat cells where it would become inactive towards its intended target. All drugs eventually leave the bloodstream and therefore patients need repeated doses to maintain a therapeutic level. The term used to describe the dose of drug required to maintain this therapeutic level is the 'maintenance dose'.

Metabolism and excretion

To maintain homeostasis, the body immediately starts to eliminate the drug from the bloodstream. It does this by metabolising the drug in the liver or other organs such as the lungs, and then excreting it through organs such as the kidneys, lungs or skin. The half-life of the drug is the time taken to remove half the dose given. Various factors can affect elimination of drugs from the perioperative patient, including, for example, cardiac failure, hypovolaemia, drug interactions and hypothermia.

Pharmacodynamics

Drugs affect the body by acting on receptors either on cell membranes or within the cells themselves. Blocking or activating receptors leads to specific cellular responses which create particular effects on the system as a whole. The drug only becomes active when it reaches its therapeutic level – too little is ineffectual, too much is toxic.

The therapeutic ratio is the ratio of the therapeutic level to the toxic level – a drug with a wide therapeutic ratio is safest. Too little of a drug will not produce the desired effect. Overdose, producing drug levels outside the therapeutic level, may produce side effects or toxicity, leading to patient harm or even death. The range between these margins is called the therapeutic margin. Some drugs, for example digoxin, have a narrow therapeutic margin, while many modern drugs have a safer, wider therapeutic margin.

Paediatric considerations

Children are not small adults and this is a particular consideration when it comes to drug dosages. Calculations of drug dosages are based on body weight or surface area. Calculating paediatric drug dosages from weight is inaccurate at best, and may even be dangerous. For example, for an overweight child, calculation of the dosage by weight does not necessarily give the correct dosage. Age factors such as the maturity of the system, the relatively large surface area of children when compared with adults, and pre-existing conditions all have a relatively greater effect on drugs in children than in adults. These factors become increasingly important with lower age groups, such as neonates. Drug calculation is therefore often based on knowledge of drug reactions, therapeutic levels, and surface area and body weight of children. Most situations require specialist advice to manage drug treatment for paediatric patients.

Body-weight considerations

Calculation of drugs dosages in adults sometimes uses 'expected lean body weight'. This is an estimate of what the patient's body weight would be if he or she were not thin or fat. Lean body mass depends on height and build – ectomorphs (light), meso-morphs (medium) or endomorphs (large). An obese patient, for example, would fall into one of these categories, but with extra fatty tissue. So, for example, it is possible to have an obese endomorph or an obese ectomorph. Fat is usually irrelevant in relation to drug *action* since the target is not usually fat cells. Drug dosage based on expected lean body mass therefore more closely reflects the dosage of the drug required to produce the therapeutic level. Increased distribution of drugs that are lipid soluble may occur in obese patients, requiring alteration of the frequency with which the drug is given, even though the thera-peutic level remains the same.

Considerations in elderly patients

External controllers have an increased effect on the homeostasis of elderly patients. For example, the physiological responses of organs vary with advancing age for reasons such as anatomical and physiological changes, lifestyle, and concurrent diseases and conditions. Hypothermia and declining liver and renal function lessen the rate of elimination, prolonging the effect of the drugs. Elderly patients also have a relatively low water content, leading to increased drug concentrations when com-pared with younger people. This often means that a reduced dose of drug will produce the required therapeutic level, whereas a normal dosage will produce toxic effects. Potency of drugs is also often increased because elderly less well-nour-ished patients have lower levels of circulating plasma protein, which normally binds drugs and makes them ineffectual. Also, elderly patients are often on various drugs because of pre-exist-ing conditions and the chance of adverse drug interactions is thus raised.

MAJOR CHANNELS OF DRUG ADMINISTRATION

Administration of drugs is often oral. Until the 20th century, this route was the only route available for most drugs. However, it is now possible to use almost every available tissue, tract and orifice. Available routes fall into two main channels of admin-istration – local and systemic.

Local channels of administration

Skin

Drugs can be administered via the skin by a number of routes. Painted or sprayed drugs include iodine and other antiseptics. These produce a local effect and include several solutions and lotions. The skin is also a valuable route of administration for topical local anaesthetics such as lidocaine and tetracaine (see later in this chapter). Swabbing and painting of drugs result in direct action at the point of contact with the skin. Antibacterial skin preparation solutions, such as chlorhexidine and iodine solutions used preoperatively, are good examples of this route of administration. Rubbing ointments (oil based), creams (water based) and liniments (fluids) onto and into the skin results in local action, for example, on skin lesions.

Skin lesions can also be covered with plasters, poultices or moist dressings which contain substances that act locally – although systemic effects are possible following absorption of substances into the circulation.

Mucous membranes

Mucous membranes offer a versatile and rapid route for drug administration which can lead to either local or systemic effects. Inhalations include sprays or nebulae, which are fine particles of a drug in a suspension of water. An example is a local anaesthetic spray used before intubation. Inhalations are normally effective at the point of contact with mucous membranes, but may also act systemically; for example, the action of glyceryl trinitrate on the heart, or the action of inhalational anaesthetics on the central nervous system (CNS). It is also possible to use drugs in a suspension of steam (water vapour).

Aerosols are fine particles suspended in air which are drawn or forced into the respiratory tract; examples include drugs such as salbutamol or formoterol.

Cavities that communicate externally, such as the vagina, rectum, eyes or bladder can be irrigated with drugs suspended in fluids. Gargles contain drugs in fluid and are useful for conditions affecting the mouth and throat. Drugs can also be dropped directly onto mucous membranes such as the eyes (eye drops) or ears. Packs or tampons can be soaked in drugs and inserted into cavities such as the nose, ears or vagina.

Systemic channels of administration

Alimentary tract

Absorption of oral drugs occurs via the mucous membrane of either the stomach or the intestines. Specially coated drugs are absorbed selectively by the intestines and act directly on the digestive tract or are absorbed into the circulation and act systemically. Longer acting drugs tend to be absorbed via the intestines, whereas short-acting drugs tend to be absorbed via the stomach lining. Oral drugs come in various forms, including, for example, powders, tablets, capsules, pills, syrups, elixirs, spirits, emulsions or mixtures.

Sublingual drugs, such as digoxin, are usually tablets which, when placed under the tongue, are absorbed directly into the bloodstream, producing a rapid systemic effect.

Suppositories are drugs that are solid at room temperature but which melt at body temperature or dissolve in body fluids. They are used either rectally or vaginally and include, for example, diclofenac (Voltarol).

Parenteral routes

A parenteral route refers to all other routes of systemic administration other than the alimentary tract. Parenteral routes are usually more complex and therefore involve more training and equipment for administration. The drugs also work much more quickly and have a shorter onset of action; they could therefore need a greater degree of care during administration and are more dangerous to administer.

Subcutaneous (SC) injection

This route involves injecting drugs into the fatty layer just underneath the skin. It can allow delivery of drugs that are low volume, cannot be used by the oral route, and when a more rapid onset than is possible orally is required. Injection of the drug is through a small gauge needle, by angling the needle in a shallow angle, just penetrating the skin into the adipose layer. It is usually possible to see a small blister of the drug fluid.

Intramuscular (IM) injection
Rapid absorption and distribution of the drug occurs with IM injection because muscle has a good blood supply. Administration of large volumes of a drug is possible because of the large muscle mass when compared with adipose tissue used for SC injection. The practitioner can give IM injections in many areas of the body, the favourite sites being the upper arm (deltoid), lateral anterior side of the thigh (quadriceps) and the buttocks or gluteus muscles.

The practitioner should take special precautions when injecting into the gluteus muscles because of the proximity of the sciatic nerve. The correct site of injection into the gluteus maximus is identified by dividing the buttock into quarters and injecting into the inner angle of the upper outer quadrant. Access to the gluteus minimus is from below the outer portion of the iliac crest. The practitioner places the first two fingers of the non-dominant hand along the angle of the iliac, with the fingers following the crest, and then carefully inserts the needle.

There are two common techniques for carrying out IM injections. The Z technique involves sliding the skin to one side with the fingers of the non-dominant hand, inserting the needle, drawing back to make certain that it is not in a blood-vessel, injecting the drug and then releasing the skin. This procedure ensures that fluid cannot leak out of the injection line into the surrounding SC tissue. The pinch technique has the same effect of separating the skin from the underlying tissues. This technique involves pinching the tissue between the forefingers and injecting the bunched up tissue.

Whichever technique the practitioner uses, it is essential that the drug enters the muscle, not the SC tissues. Consideration should be given to aspects such as the length of needle required and the depth of injection. Changing the site of injection for subsequent injections helps to avoid excessive damage to tissue and may prevent potential drug interactions caused by mixing of drugs within the tissues.

Intraperitoneal administration

Drugs are administered directly into the peritoneal cavity. Delivery of antibiotics using this route is common during surgical procedures on the digestive tract. Absorption is quick because of the contact with large areas of mucous tissue.

Intravenous (IV) administration

This technique involves administering a drug directly into a vein. It is possible to use many veins, with the favourite sites being the crook of the elbow, the back of the hand or other veins of the forearm, such as the accessory cephalic and the median anterior brachial. In difficult cases, when it is not possible to find suitable veins, cut-down access may be required for deeper veins such as branches of the femoral, popliteal or brachial veins.

For multiple injections, venflons, butterflies or other IV cannulae provide semi-permanent access. Learning the technique of IV cannulation is relatively easy, although the outcomes of improper technique can be painful, dangerous and disturbing for the patient, especially in the perioperative setting.

An IV infusion is the administration of a large quantity of fluid which may or may not contain drugs. For this procedure, the practitioner attaches an IV giving set to the IV cannula; for example, to combat amoebic infections using a metronidazole infusion. Drugs can also be added to electrolyte infusions such as sodium chloride 0.9%. The drug is injected into a rubber bung close to the cannula, which then seals closed. If the cannula tip leaves the vein and enters the surrounding tissue, then fluid can build up in the area around the vein causing a painful localised oedema. This extravasation or 'tissuing' can be extensive and painful at times.

Other routes of parenteral drug administration include intracardial, intrapleural and drug implants (e.g. some long-acting contraceptives).

DRUGS USED DURING PERIOPERATIVE INTERVENTIONS

The discovery of ether in 1846 and chloroform in 1847 heralded the age of anaesthesia and with it the ability to perform ever more extensive surgical procedures on patients, without the fear of pain, sensation and awareness. Administering ever more complex and specific anaesthetic drugs achieves the triad of anaesthesia – narcosis, analgesia and relaxation.

The range of drugs used in today's perioperative interventions is huge. Each stage of the patient's perioperative experience requires the practitioner to administer drugs to produce a therapeutic effect or to support the body systems. Surgery and anaesthesia produce a huge degree of stress on the body resulting in physiological and emotional effects which, if left untreated, may result in harm to the patient (see Chapter 1). The rest of this chapter discusses some of the common drugs used in perioperative care.

Preoperative drugs

Giving drugs weeks or months before an elective procedure helps to ensure that the patient is in the best condition possible for the impending surgery.

Antianaemia drugs raise haemoglobin levels in blood. Preoperative anaemia is a risk because of the oxygen-carrying capacity of blood and the dangers of hypoxia and blood loss (see Chapter 1). Antianaemia drugs include, for example, iron, vitamin B_{12}, folic acid and liver or stomach extracts. For less extreme cases of anaemia or general malaise, vitamin complexes may improve general health.

Treatment of blood disorders, such as clotting problems, helps to reduce the risks associated with haemorrhage. Vitamin K, calcium gluconate or calcium lactate improve prothrombin times. Vitamin K is fat soluble and its absorption is dependent on the liver, especially the presence of bile. Dehydrocholic acid given with vitamin K improves absorption in patients with liver or gall bladder disease such as cholecystitis.

Patients may need prophylactic antibiotics if they are undergoing surgical procedures that carry a high risk of infection, such as abdominal or respiratory procedures. Broad-spectrum antibiotics protect the patient against a wide range of infections; however, if the procedure points to a particular infection risk, a specific antibiotic should be given.

Admission of the patient to hospital on the day before the procedure allows the administration of various drugs. These may include, for example, sedatives, antibiotics, analgesics or IV infusions such as electrolytes or blood or its derivatives. The purpose of these medicines is to increase the health of the patient's body systems in preparation for surgery. Specifically, preoperative drugs may:

- allay anxiety;
- provide a measure of amnesia;
- provide analgesia;
- reduce side effects caused by stimulation of the autonomic nervous system (mainly cardiovascular effects);
- reduce risk of nausea and vomiting;
- increase pH of gastric contents;
- reduce secretion in the airways.

The anaesthetist normally orders preoperative drugs related to the surgery since he or she is responsible for preserving the patient's condition during the procedure. Administration of a barbiturate, hypnotic or sedative (e.g. diazepam or temazepam) before induction of a general anaesthetic is common practice. Analgesia may take the form of an opiate such as morphine or fentanyl. Giving an antiemetic, such as cyclizine or ondansetron, helps to oppose the side effects of opioids or to reduce nausea and vomiting caused by the effects of surgery.

Parasympathetic depressants are naturally occurring alkaloids or synthetics, and include parasympatholytics and cholinergic blocking agents. The most common naturally occurring alkaloids are atropine, from the plant *Atropa belladonna*, and hyoscine, from *Hyoscyamus niger*. Both these drugs are readily soluble in water and body fluids since they are organic esters – a combination of an acid and organic base.

All parasympathetic depressants have a similar action, only varying in degree, onset or duration of action. They act by inhibiting acetylcholine action at nerve junctions and on smooth muscle which responds to acetylcholine. They dilate pupils, relax smooth muscle, decrease secretions and increase or stabilise heart rate.

In perioperative use, the decrease in oral and upper airway secretions is useful to reduce the incidence of partial obstruction of the airway and to reduce coughing on induction and reversal of the anaesthetic. Relaxing smooth muscle may aid in some surgical procedures and the extra sedative actions of hyoscine may help in producing a preoperative calming effect.

Administration of parasympathetic depressants is by most routes, although in the preoperative setting IM or SC injections are commonest. The preoperative dosage for atropine or hyoscine is normally between 0.3 and 0.6 mg. Combination of parasympathetic depressants in one syringe with an analgesic such as morphine can reduce the number of injections required. The most common side effects of this group of drugs are dilated pupils, blurred vision and dryness of the mouth, nose and throat. Exaggerated side effects may be early signs of toxicity and may progress to symptoms such as shallow respirations, disorientation, dizziness and tachycardia. In excessive doses, the toxic effects of these drugs can result in coma followed by respiratory and cardiac failure and death.

It is important to offer an explanation for giving the preoperative drugs – to calm the patient, reduce secretions, and ease induction and maintenance of anaesthesia. This may help the patient to tolerate the dryness of the mouth and the discomfort caused by slight tachycardia or hypotension. It is important to maintain the patient's safety, especially from injury because of falling, after giving these drugs. Similarly, because of the mild confusion or dizziness, gaining consent for surgery is good practice before their administration. With proper use, these drugs are invaluable in preparing the patient for impending surgery and anaesthesia.

ANAESTHESIA

Anaesthesia is the lack of awareness of sensation either locally or systemically resulting from drug administration. General anaesthetics affect the whole body and result in unconsciousness; local anaesthetics affect regions of the body while the patient remains conscious. Under many circumstances, anaesthesia uses a combination of the two approaches.

Anaesthesia therefore involves the use of drugs to induce the desired effects of the anaesthetic and to maintain or promote the health of the patient while protecting the body from the side effects of the anaesthetic or surgery. The most common drugs can be conveniently divided into three groups:

- drugs used during general anaesthesia;
- drugs used during local anaesthesia;
- drugs used to support body systems.

Drugs used during general anaesthesia

General anaesthetic agents target both the spinal cord and the brain to produce loss of consciousness, loss of explicit memory and lack of response to nociception (pain) (Peck *et al.* 2008). Recent studies show that there is still no general consensus regarding the mechanism of action of general anaesthetic agents. It appears, however, that patients go through four stages of anaesthesia following their administration – analgesia, excitement, surgical anaesthesia and overdose (see Chapter 8 for a description of these stages).

On completion of surgery, the anaesthetist reverses the anaesthetic by progressively reducing the administration of drugs and allowing the patient to regain consciousness. The stages of anaesthesia reverse until the patient returns to his or her normal state of consciousness, which can occur either within minutes for light anaesthesia or many hours later for deep anaesthesia. Administration of reversal agents can block the effects of some of the anaesthetic drugs and speed up the reversal. Reversal agents include: parasympathetic depressants which help to stabilise pulse and blood pressure; neostigmine which reverses the effects of non-depolarising muscle relaxants; and opiate antagonists which combat the side effects of opiates.

Oxygen and nitrous oxide

Giving oxygen for 5–10 minutes before starting surgery 'preoxygenates' the patient, which increases alveolar oxygen concentration and therefore raises pO_2. Nitrous oxide produces light anaesthesia and some analgesia which assists in the smooth transition of the fully awake patient into the first and second stages of anaesthesia. Nitrous oxide potentiates the use of general anaesthetic agents and so its use throughout surgery reduces the need for the more toxic volatile anaesthetic agents.

General anaesthetic agents
Delivery of general anaesthetics is either by inhalation or intravenously, or a combination of both. One of the skills of the anaesthetist is to manipulate drug dosages to produce specific effects. For example, it may be desirable to provide a light anaesthetic so that the patient awakes quickly, or a deep anaesthetic which produces the best degree of muscle relaxation.

Intravenous induction agents
Administration of IV agents is usually in one bolus which then travels around the circulatory system towards their target organ, the brain. Here they depress the CNS. The extent to which they limit neural function depends upon the drugs used.

These drugs also depress other body systems such as the cardiovascular and respiratory systems (Allman & Wilson 2006)

Because of the rapid onset, actions and potency of IV induction agents, it is essential to monitor the patient's vital signs during induction of anaesthesia. Monitoring allows for early interpretation of untoward signs and symptoms associated with cardiovascular and respiratory depression which can then be treated accordingly. As a minimum, it is normal to check electrocardiogram (ECG), SaO_2, blood pressure, CO_2 and respirations. The patient's condition and the anaesthetic may demand the use of other monitors (Simpson & Popat 2003).

Table 3.1 gives some examples of IV induction agents.

Volatile (inhalational) anaesthetic agents
Volatile anaesthetic agents perform the same role as IV agents, but are inhaled and absorbed by the respiratory system. Absorption thus depends in part on the health of the patient's respiratory system; they are also unpleasant and can be irritating to patients. Inhalational agents can be used for induction (e.g. in paediatric patients); however, they are more often used for maintaining and deepening anaesthesia following induction using IV agents. Inhalational agents have the capacity to

Table 3.1 Intravenous induction agents.

Name	Usual actions of this group of drugs, plus	Doses (in a 70 kg adult) and mode of administration	Uses	Usual side effects of this group, plus
Thiopental	Very short onset and action. 5–10 minutes duration, terminated by dilution and absorption by fat cells	3–6 mg/kg IV. Mixed with water to form a 2.5% solution for injection	Commonly used IV for induction of anaesthesia. Can also be given rectally or as an infusion	Severe hypotension, respiratory depression, laryngeal/bronchial spasm. Contraindicated in patients suffering from porphyria
Propofol	Non-barbiturate providing a smooth induction. Metabolised in the liver. Short acting	1–2.5 mg/kg IV	Used when rapid recovery is required. Effective in total IV anaesthesia (TIVA) because of short action, low incidence of side effects and lack of 'hangover effects'	Few side effects apart from respiratory depression when used as an infusion
Etomidate	Rapid onset, short-acting induction agent	0.2–0.5 mg/kg IV		Little effect on cardiovascular and respiratory systems
Ketamine	Short acting, rapid onset. Produces dissociative anaesthesia	1–2 mg/kg IV, 3–5 mg/kg IM	Induction of anaesthesia, short surgical procedures, burns dressings	Hallucinations and other emergence reactions. Hypertension and tachycardia. Post-anaesthesia nausea and vomiting

produce narcosis, relaxation and analgesia, although the concurrent administration of IV drugs potentiates the action of these drugs and reduces the effects on the cardiovascular system.

Cardiovascular effects include reduced heart rate, cardiac output and myocardial contractility, which results in lower blood pressure. This group of drugs causes increasing respiratory depression as dosage (and progression through the stages of anaesthesia) increases.

Removal of waste anaesthetic gases from the operating room is important because of the longer term dangers of these gases to staff working there. Effects of exposure to waste anaesthetic gases may include fatigue, nausea, headaches, increased risk of spontaneous abortion and other systemic effects on the organs of the body (Pressly 2000).

Table 3.2 gives some examples of volatile anaesthetic agents.

Muscle relaxants

Muscle relaxants commonly used in perioperative practice have mainly two indications: to facilitate controlled breathing and tracheal intubation and to improve tissue handling during surgery (Spry 2005).

Delivery of these drugs blocks the transmission of impulses at the neuromuscular junction (NMJ), meaning that impulses from motor nerves to skeletal muscle are suppressed. This explains why patients become paralysed.

The NMJ is the area of contact between the ends of a motor nerve fibre and a fibre of skeletal muscle. Normally, stimulation of a motor nerve causes the nerve endings to release the enzyme acetylcholine (AcH), which binds to receptors on the motor end-plate in the skeletal muscle fibre. Depolarisation (activation) of the muscle cells occurs and the muscle contracts. Acetylcholinesterase then metabolises the AcH to allow the muscle to repolarise and relax in preparation for the next contraction.

Muscle relaxants are either depolarising or non-depolarising. Depolarising muscle relaxants, such as suxamethonium, mimic AcH and bind to the receptors on the motor end-plate. Depolarisation occurs and the muscle contracts. However, ace-

Table 3.2 Volatile anaesthetic agents.

Name	Action: narcosis, relaxation and analgesia, plus	Uses: general anaesthesia, plus	Usual side effects of this group, plus
Sevoflurane	Widely used because it produces less irritation than other drugs of this group. Produces low levels of respiratory depression. Pleasant smell, fast induction and recovery	Induction of anaesthesia in paediatrics	Little or no nephrotoxicity
	Rapid onset and short duration of action. Irritant to inhale	Maintenance of anaesthesia in day-case surgery	Can cause a fall in blood pressure
Desflurane	Rapid onset, little analgesic action and around 0.3% metabolism in the liver	Used for repeated anaesthesia, especially when liver damage is a possibility. Also used to induce hypotension, when required, e.g. during some surgical procedures	Hypotension caused by peripheral vasodilation. Little effect on the heart

tylcholinesterase does not immediately metabolise the drug and so depolarisation persists, preventing the muscle from contracting a second time. The patient initially displays signs of muscle contractions (fasciculations), followed by paralysis. After between 2 and 5 minutes, plasma cholinesterase or pseudocholinesterase metabolises the drug, allowing the muscle to repolarise and normal function returns. Whereas its rapid onset explains why the drug is ideal for helping endotracheal intubation during emergency situations, its short duration explains why the drug does not require a reversal.

A decrease or absence of plasma cholinesterase activity can prevent or slow down the metabolism of suxamethonium, leading to a prolonged paralysis commonly called 'suxamethonium apnoea'. Normally, the metabolism of the drug will occur through natural degradation after several hours or even days. However, this block can be reversed by administering fresh frozen plasma since it contains a source plasma cholinesterase (Peck *et al.* 2008).

Non-depolarising muscle relaxants (such as atracurium and pancuronium) compete with AcH for the receptor site on the motor end-plate. Concentration of the drug increases and this results in displacement of AcH from the receptor site. However, in this case, the drug does not cause depolarisation of the fibre muscle cell and so the muscle cannot contract and paralysis of the muscle results. Metabolism of the muscle relaxants by cholinesterase does not occur; therefore, it remains bound to the receptors and paralysis persists. Eventually, however, AcH levels increase, displacing the muscle relaxant and leading to a return to normal muscle function. These drugs have a slower onset and longer duration of action when compared with the depolarising group and are therefore often used on induction for longer procedures and during longer periods of anaesthesia. Neostigmine reverses their action by inhibiting cholinesterase production, thereby allowing AcH to build up quicker than normal and speeding up the return to normal function. Table 3.3 gives some examples of muscle relaxants.

Analgesics

Analgesics are a complex group of drugs with poorly understood actions. They act by either reducing the capacity of the nerve fibres to sense pain or by reducing pain recognition by the higher centres of the brain. Anaesthesia often involves the use of other analgesics; however, this chapter will only discuss the use of opiates.

Opiates

Opiates are useful drugs for reducing pain, anaesthetic and surgical stress. Hence the reason they are used pre-, intra- and post-operatively to aid in relaxation, analgesia and postoperative pain management.

Table 3.3 Muscle relaxants.

Name	Action	Doses (in a 70 kg adult) and mode of administration	Uses: endotracheal intubation plus	Side effects
Suxamethonium	Depolarising agent with rapid onset (<1 minute) and short duration of action (3–5 minutes)	75–100 mg IV	To assist endotracheal intubation when short onset of action is required, e.g. rapid sequence induction	Increased intraocular pressure due to contraction of the intraocular muscles, increased serum potassium due to muscle fibre rupture, postoperative muscle pain, bradycardia
Pancuronium	Synthetic non-depolarising agent. Rapid onset (2–3 minutes) and medium duration of action (15–20 minutes)	8–10 mg with 4 mg incremental doses to maintain paralysis	Endotracheal intubation when a longer onset of action is required, e.g. elective procedures	Tachycardia, raised blood pressure
Vecuronium	Similar to pancuronium, but with a slightly longer action (20–30 minutes)	0.08–0.1 mg per kg body weight IV	Used for patients with unstable cardiovascular systems because normally has little effect on cardiovascular system	Can stimulate the vagal nerve leading to bradycardia
Rocuronium	Non-depolarising. Rapid onset and medium acting		Suitable for total IV anaesthesia (TIVA)	
Atracurium	Non-depolarising. Rapid onset and medium acting. Broken down in plasma by 'Hofmann elimination' independently of liver or renal function. Minimal effects on heart and blood pressure	40 mg IV	Especially useful for patients with hepatic or renal failure	May cause bradycardia

Opiates can be given via several routes, including, for example, IM, IV, topical and intrathecal (spinal and epidural).

Morphine, as one of the oldest and most effective analgesic agents, is a standard to measure opiates against. Development of new opiates aims to overcome or improve one or other of morphine's problems or actions. Morphine is a potent analgesic which also produces a characteristic euphoric effect favoured by drug addicts. Respiratory depression occurs at low dosages, and so spontaneously breathing patients usually receive only 10–15 mg IM. Morphine can also produce all the other side effects of the opiate group. Some of these include:

- analgesia – opiates are potent analgesics and many also produce a characteristic euphoric effect;
- respiratory depression – close monitoring of all patients is essential since all opiates result in a degree of respiratory depression;
- depression of the cough reflex – this may be important to consider during the patient's recovery;
- nausea and vomiting – giving antiemetics is common with opiates and may counteract this side effect;
- reduction of smooth muscle contraction – the bowel in particular is susceptible to this action, resulting in constipation, as is smooth muscle of the bronchus, resulting in bronchospasm and difficulty in breathing;
- cardiovascular depression – this may result in bradycardia and hypotension.

Morphine and pethidine have been the drugs of choice for many years. However, the wide therapeutic margin of modern drugs, fentanyl for instance, has resulted in the use of far greater doses of analgesics. These drugs help to produce anaesthesia in total IV anaesthesia (TIVA) or to support the body systems against the effects of perioperative stress. In the same way, opiates like remifentanil can also be used purposely to produce hypotensive anaesthesia (Allman & Wilson 2006) to lessen bleeding and therefore reduce the need for transfusion, to increase surgical visibility or to decrease operating times.

Table 3.4 gives some example of opiates.

Table 3.4 Opiates in common perioperative use.

Name	Action	Indicative dosage (in a 70 kg adult) and mode of administration	Uses	Side effects
Morphine	Opiate analgesic, sedative, actions on cardiovascular and respiratory systems	10–15 mg IM, incremental doses for IV or intrathecal administration	Perioperative analgesia, general anaesthesia, epidural and spinal anaesthesia	Respiratory and cardiovascular depression, addiction
Diamorphine	As for morphine plus potent respiratory depression	Twice as potent an analgesic as morphine, 5–7.5 mg IM, incremental doses IV	Perioperative analgesia, postoperative ventilation (because of its action of respiratory depression). Added to bupivacaine in continuous epidural infusion	As for morphine plus increased risk of inadvertent respiratory depression
Fentanyl	As for morphine, except little action on cardiovascular system. Wide therapeutic ratio	2–20 μg/kg to produce general intraoperative analgesia and with larger doses its effects can last 2–3 hours following IV administration	Drug of choice during many perioperative situations. Cardiac surgery (without concurrent cardiovascular effects). High doses given in total IV anaesthesia (TIVA)	
Alfentanil	Short-acting potent analgesic	Administered in doses of 6–8 μg/kg	Day surgery because of its short duration of action	
Remifentanil	Rapid onset, short-acting potent analgesic	Approx 50 μg/ml in a controlled infusion	TIVA and neurosurgery because it is very short acting and its effects wear off soon after administration is complete	Relatively low respiratory depression compared with fentanyl or morphine
Phenoperidine	Synthetic derivative of pethidine. Analgesic and respiratory depression. Duration of around 2 hours when given IM, 1 hour after IV administration	Dose varies. Can be given as a 1 mg bolus over 1 minute with 0.5 mg supplement every 30–60 minutes. A 2–5 mg bolus plus 1 mg every 30–60 minutes is used for ventilated patients	Prolonged ventilation and analgesia, e.g. for patients ventilated in intensive care	

Opiate antagonists

Opiate antagonists support the patient during reversal of anaesthesia and postoperative care by combating persistent respiratory or cardiovascular depression.

One of the most commonly used in perioperative practice is naloxone, a synthetic opiate antagonist derived from oxymorphone, with no opiate activity of its own. To treat opioid-induced respiratory depression, the drug is administered in small doses (0.1–0.2 mg) until respiratory depression is reversed. However, if opioid overdose is suspected, then 0.4–2.0 mg may be administered IV, IM or even SC. Something important to bear in mind is that naloxone reduces analgesia, as well as the fact that its duration of effect (approximately 20 minutes) may be shorter than the opioid whose effects are to be counteracted. This is why the practitioner may have to administer additional doses sometimes (Sasada & Smith 2003).

It is also possible to use respiratory stimulants such as doxapram to stimulate respiration while maintaining effective pain relief.

Drugs used during local anaesthesia

Local anaesthetics are drugs that reversibly block nerve conduction when applied locally to nerve tissue. One of the oldest drugs used for local anaesthesia is cocaine, which was first used for eye surgery in 1884. Cocaine has spawned several other drugs, including, for example, lidocaine and bupivacaine.

Most local anaesthetics have similar actions: rapid onset of action, short duration, low systemic toxicity, non-irritant, soluble in water and stable in solution (Simpson & Popat 2003). There are various routes for giving local anaesthetics:

- spinal block – useful for one-off injections during, e.g. gynaecological surgery;
- epidural block – injection into the epidural space which can produce blockade for surgery on the lower peripheries;
- nerve block – injection directly into a local nerve, e.g. femoral or ulnar nerve blocks;
- local infiltration – useful for minor surgery and IV cannulation;

- IV regional block – e.g. Bier's block, which is the injection of a drug into a limb and a tourniquet applied to limit its circulation;
- topical block – applied directly onto the skin or mucous membrane, e.g. the throat (lidocaine spray), or before cannulation (lidocaine cream), especially in children.

Local anaesthetics act by preventing the normal depolarisation and repolarisation of nerve cells. In its resting state, the inside of a nerve cell is positively charged compared with its outside. When a nerve cell is stimulated, the electrolyte balance changes, polarity reverses and the inside becomes positive relative to the outside. Local anaesthetics block conduction of the electrolytes (sodium channels, in particular) and therefore block the normal action of the nerve.

After absorption of the drugs into the systemic circulation, metabolism occurs either in the liver or in the plasma by pseudocholinesterase, and the drug then is excreted by the kidneys.

Toxicity occurs if there is a release of high levels of the drug into the systemic circulation. Factors such as age, body weight and poor liver function may worsen this effect. Systemic side effects can include numbness of the tongue, dizziness or muscular twitching progressing to convulsions. As the depressive effects on the CNS increase, the patient becomes unconscious followed by respiratory and cardiovascular arrest.

Treatment of toxic effects include preventing further local anaesthetic absorption, treating cardiovascular symptoms and controlling the convulsions by use of sedatives or tranquillisers.

The addition of vasoconstrictors to local anaesthetics can also cause toxicity; for example, 0.5 ml of 1:1000 adrenaline (epinephrine) is the maximum dose that should be administered subcutaneously to a man of 70 kg. More than this may result in increasingly dangerous side effects as the dose increases.

Local anaesthetic drugs such as lidocaine also have other uses, for example:

- antiarrhythmic – by preventing ventricular ectopic beats, ventricular tachycardia and ventricular fibrillation after myocardial infarction (Paw & Park 2006);

- reducing the pressure response of intubation – spraying the throat with lidocaine before intubation may block the reflex rise in pulse rate and blood pressure;
- an aid to minor surgery;
- extensively used in specific surgical procedures, e.g. eye surgery (Carroll 2002).

Table 3.5 gives some examples of local anaesthetic agents.

Drugs used to support the body systems

Antiemetics
Perioperative patients often suffer from nausea and vomiting, or acid reflux (Farman 2004), which are common side effects of many anaesthetic drugs. Vomiting in perioperative patients occurs because of stimulation of the vomiting centre in the brain or through direct irritation of the stomach lining. The phenothiazine group of drugs are the most common antiemetics. These drugs all produce different levels of sedation, hypotension, vasodilation, urinary retention, blurred vision, etc, as well as antiemesis. Long-term antiemetics also include anticholinergic agents (such as atropine or hyoscine), with side effects including CNS depression.

Table 3.6 gives some example of antiemetics.

Drugs affecting the autonomic nervous system
The autonomic nervous system controls smooth muscle, for example in the gut, bronchi and blood vessels, the endocrine glands such as the adrenal and pituitary glands, and the heart. The autonomic nervous system is divided into two systems – the sympathetic and parasympathetic nervous systems.

The role of the sympathetic nervous system is to prepare the body for 'fight or flight'. Effects include increased heart rate and blood pressure, vasoconstriction of skin, vasodilation of skeletal muscle and bronchi, and dilation of the pupil of the eye. The parasympathetic nervous system essentially stimulates the opposite reactions, for example, decreased heart rate, bronchoconstriction and increased gastrointestinal activity.

Table 3.5 Local anaesthetic agents.

Name	Action	Doses (in a 70 kg adult) and mode of administration	Uses	Side effects: usual systemic side effects including depression of central nervous system (CNS), depression of cardiac and respiratory systems, plus
Cocaine	Local anaesthetic, excitation of the CNS, vasoconstriction	Max: 150 mg in a 5% solution (50 mg/ml)	Topical anaesthesia in ENT surgery	Ventricular fibrillation, convulsions
Lidocaine (lignocaine)	Local anaesthetic, local vasodilatory effect	Max: 200 mg plain, 500 mg with adrenaline (epinephrine)	Versatile drug that can be administered via any route and is used for local analgesia and systemically as an antiarrhythmic	
Bupivacaine	Long-acting local anaesthetic. Effects of 'heavy' version can last 2–3 hours	Max: 150 mg	Epidural block, plexus blocks	
Prilocaine	Local anaesthetic	Max 300 mg plain, 600 mg with adrenaline (epinephrine)	Dentistry and Bier's block	Produces methaemoglobinaemia when given in high doses – possible effects on fetus in utero
Tetracaine (amethocaine) gel	Topical local anaesthetic	4% gel	Topical anaesthetic used before cannulation or venepuncture	Little risk of systemic side effects
Emla cream (lidocaine and prilocaine)	Topical local anaesthetic	5% cream	Topical anaesthetic used before cannulation or venepuncture	Little risk of systemic side effects

Table 3.6 Antiemetics.

Name	Action	Doses (in a 70 kg adult) and mode of administration	Uses	Side effects including: sedation, hypotension, vasodilation, urinary retention, plus:
Cyclizine (Valoid)	Powerful antiemetic	50 mg/ml IV. Often combined with an opiate such as morphine or as a ready-made preparation (Cyclimorph)	Perioperative antiemetic	
Prochlorperazine (Stemetil)	Antiemetic	12.5 mg IM, 25 mg rectally	Perioperative antiemetic	Fewer sedative properties than other drugs of this group. Antidote is atropine. Can cause constipation, dry mouth, hypotension if given IV
Metoclopramide (Maxolon)	Antiemetic which reduces the activity of the vomiting centre and reduces the peripheral stimulation to vomiting by increasing gastric emptying	10 mg orally or IM; 10–20 mg IV	Perioperative antiemetic	Fewer side effects than drugs in the phenothiazine group

The autonomic nervous system's three main transmitter substances are adrenaline (epinephrine), noradrenaline (norepinephrine)and AcH. Adrenoreceptors are the target for the actions of adrenaline (epinephrine) and noradrenaline (norepinephrine). Adrenaline (epinephrine) and noradrenaline (norepinephrine) attach to these specialised groups of cells, producing the effects of the sympathetic nervous system. Blocking of these agents reduces sympathetic activity. The actions of AcH are muscarinic (acting on parasympathetic nerves) and nicotinic (acting on neuromuscular and autonomic ganglia).

Drugs affecting the autonomic nervous system therefore have the following actions:

- cholinergic agents – enhance or mimic AcH and therefore stimulate the parasympathetic nervous system;
- anticholinergic agents – block AcH and therefore block the parasympathetic nervous system;
- adrenergic agonists – enhance the actions of noradrenaline (norepinephrine) and therefore stimulate the sympathetic nervous system. They are also called sympathomimetics or adrenoceptor agonists;
- adrenergic antagonists – block the actions of noradrenaline (norepinephrine) and therefore block the sympathetic nervous system. They are also called sympatholytics or adrenoceptor antagonists.

Cholinergic agents
This small group of drugs mimics the effects of AcH. A commonly used cholinergic agent in clinical practice is neostigmine. This drug is mainly used to reverse the blockade produced by muscle relaxants. It is also used in the treatment of paralytic ileus and urinary retention. It may cause bradycardia and also hypotension when administered in high doses (Sasada & Smith 2003).

Anticholinergic agents
Atropine blocks the effects of the parasympathetic nervous system, causing tachycardia, drying of secretions, relaxation of

the gut and dilation of pupils. Other drugs in this group include hyoscine and glycopyrronium bromide (glycopyrrolate). Atropine's main perioperative use in cardiovascular support is to reduce bradycardia caused by vagal stimulation, for example, during abdominal procedures or when caused by intubation. It also blocks the parasympathetic effects (bradycardia) of the muscle relaxant antidote neostigmine.

Adrenergic agents

This wide group of drugs has effects on the cardiovascular and respiratory systems and includes drugs such as adrenaline (epinephrine), noradrenaline (norepinephrine), dopamine, isoprenaline and salbutamol. Because of their effects on the cardiovascular and respiratory systems, these drugs are often used in severely ill patients or during emergencies such a haemorrhage and cardiac arrest. During surgery, they control blood pressure and pulse, and reduce the effects of anaesthetic drugs. This group of drugs represents possibly the largest group used in perioperative care. They have a multitude of uses, displaying both local and systemic effects. The effects of adrenergic agents on adrenoceptors are listed in Table 3.7.

Common adrenergic agonists are listed in Table 3.8 and adrenergic antagonists in Table 3.9.

Table 3.7 The effects of adrenergic agents on adrenoceptors.

Adrenoreceptor	Agonist activity	Antagonist activity
$\alpha 1$ – cardiac and respiratory	Coronary vasoconstriction, bronchial dilation	Coronary vasodilation
$\alpha 2$ – peripheral circulation	Peripheral vasoconstriction, intestinal sphincter contraction, sweat production	Peripheral vasodilation
$\beta 1$ – cardiac	Increases force and power of the heartbeat, increases blood pressure, coronary and peripheral vasodilation	Reduces heart rate and contractility
$\beta 2$ – bronchial	Bronchodilation	Bronchoconstriction

Table 3.8 Adrenergic agonists.

Name	Action	Doses (in a 70 kg adult) and mode of administration	Uses	Side effects as usual, plus
Adrenaline (epinephrine)	Stimulates α2, β1 and β2 receptors. Cardiac stimulant, peripheral vasoconstriction, bronchial dilation	For anaphylactic shock – 100–500 µg SC or IM, repeated as required every 20 minutes. 100–250 µg IV slowly. Bronchospasm – 100–500 µg SC or IM. Cardiac arrest – 0.1–1 mg IV or intracardiac (IC)	Treatment of cardiac arrest, reduces bronchospasm, local vasoconstrictor when used with local anaesthetic, reduces allergic and hypersensitivity reactions	Tachycardia, restlessness, weakness, pallor, hypertension, palpitation, sweating, nausea, cardiac arrhythmias
Noradrenaline (norepinephrine)	Stimulates α2 receptors. Peripheral vasoconstriction leading to increased blood pressure	4 µg/ml infusion delivered at 8–12 µg/min until patient is stable	Used in severely ill patients to increase blood pressure. Cardiac surgery	Poor renal and peripheral perfusion
Isoprenaline	Stimulates β1 receptors. Increases force and power of the heart beat, reduces bronchospasm, peripheral vasoconstrictor	0.1–0.2 mg by aerosol. 0.01–0.2 mg by slow IV	Treatment of low blood pressure, treatment of bronchospasm. Treatment of atrio-ventricular heart block	Atrial tachycardia, cardiac arrhythmias
Dopamine	β2 agonist, cardiac stimulant which increases pulse and blood pressure, renal vasodilator	200 mg added to 250 ml to give an IV infusion of 800 µg/ml. Administered at 2–5 µg/kg/min	Used to increase blood pressure and improve renal function	Peripheral vasoconstriction when used in large doses
Ephedrine	Stimulates α and β receptors to increase heart rate and myocardial contractility, and peripheral vasoconstriction. Also causes bronchodilation	15–50 mg SC, IM or slow IV	Used to reduce hypotension caused by general and local anaesthesia, especially following spinal or epidural anaesthesia	Interacts with monoamine-oxidase inhibitors
Salbutamol	β2 receptor stimulant which selectively targets bronchial muscle receptors to relieve bronchospasm	1–2 inhalations (100–200 µg) from metered dose aerosol. 500 µg SC or IM, 200–300 µg slow IV	Relief of bronchospasm in asthma, bronchitis and emphysema	Can cause cardiac stimulation and peripheral vasodilation

Table 3.9 Adrenergic antagonists.

Name	Action	Doses (in a 70 kg adult) and mode of administration	Uses	Side effects
Phentolamine	α2 receptor antagonist which produces vasodilation, resulting in falling blood pressure and lower central venous pressure (CVP). Short-acting drug lasting around 30 minutes	5–10 mg IM or IV	Vasodilator during cardiopulmonary bypass, to antagonise the effects of noradrenaline (norepinephrine) and as a vasodilator during cardiogenic shock	Hypovolaemia because of the larger extravascular fluid compartment results in tachycardia and hypotension. Can be treated with fluids
Propranolol	β1 receptor blocker which reduces heart rate and output. Reduces oxygen demands of myocardial muscle	20–40 mg orally. 1 mg by slow IV up to a maximum of 5–10 mg	To control ectopic beats and tachycardia, and to reduce incidence of angina	Bronchospasm because of effects on β2 receptors

CONCLUSION

Perioperative care involves the use of a wide range of drugs, many of which have not been touched on in this chapter due to space restraints and not because of lack of importance in their role of patient support.

The role of the practitioner in drug administration is to ensure that administering drugs is safe and effective, and to be able to recognise and react to the effects and side effects of the drugs. The result of good practice should be that the patient receives the correct drug, at the correct time and by the correct route. It is therefore essential that all practitioners are fully familiar with all drugs used in their area of practice to ensure safe and effective patient care.

REFERENCES

Allman, K.G. & Wilson, I.H. (eds) (2006) *Oxford Handbook of Anaesthesia*. Oxford University Press, New York.

Carroll, C. (2002) Local anaesthetic techniques in ophthalmic surgery. *British Journal of Perioperative Nursing* **12** (2), 68–74.

Department of Health (2004) *Standards for Better Health*. HMSO, London.

Farman, J. (2004) Acid aspiration syndrome. *British Journal of Perioperative Nursing* **14** (6), 266–74.

Home Office (2001) *The Misuse of Drugs Regulations 2001*. The Stationery Office, London.

Home Office (2007) *Explanatory Memorandum to the Misuse of Drugs and Misuse of Drugs (Safe Custody) (Amendment) Regulations 2007*. The Stationery Office Limited, London.

National Prescribing Centre and National Primary Care Research and Development Centre (2002) *Modernising Medicines Management: A Guide to Achieving Benefits for Patients, Professionals and the NHS (Book 1)*. The National Prescribing Centre and National Primary Care Research and Development Centre, London.

NHS Executive (2002) *Medicines Management (Safe and Secure Handling)*. Department of Health, London.

Paw, H. & Park, G. (2006) *Drugs in Intensive Care*. Cambridge University Press, Cambridge.

Peck, T.E., Hill S.A. & Williams, M. (2008) *Pharmacology for Anaesthesia and Intensive Care*. Cambridge University Press, Cambridge.

Pressly, V. (2000) Waste anaesthetic gases. *British Journal of Perioperative Nursing* **13** (5), 299–304.

Sasada, M. & Smith, S. (2003) *Drugs in Anaesthesia and Intensive Care*, 3rd edn. Oxford University Press, Oxford.

Simpson, P.J. & Popat, M. (2003) *Understanding Anaesthesia*. Butterworth Heinemann, London.

Spry, C. (2005) *Essentials of Perioperative Nursing*. Jones and Bartlett Publishers, London.

Perioperative Communication

Joy O'Neill

LEARNING OUTCOMES

❏ Understand the need for *effective communication* in relation to patient care within the operating room environment.

❏ Discuss the *different aspects of communication*.

❏ Have an understanding of the *legal issues* that affect the practice of the perioperative practitioner.

❏ Identify the different *members of the operating room team* and their roles and responsibilities.

❏ Understand the different *government agencies* that influence patient care within the operating room environment.

PATIENT COMMUNICATION

This chapter will discuss the different aspects of communication between members of the multidisciplinary team and patients, and between practitioners themselves. Communication is a key factor in:

- patient advocacy;
- patient consent;
- accountability;
- documentation;
- clinical supervision;
- information technology (IT) within the NHS;
- teamwork;
- the perioperative team;
- change management;
- clinical governance:
  — government agencies;
  — performance indicators.

Communication is the key to the quality and effectiveness of patient care within the NHS. Communication between patients and the operating room multidisciplinary team is important to allay the patients' fears (Mitchell 2005). Perioperative practitioners can reassure patients and provide a friendly face when they are at their most vulnerable.

Research has identified the value of communication in patient care. Various authors, including Bury (2005) and Berry (2007), discuss how practitioners use communication skills on a daily basis to: gather information, reassure, facilitate patient expression; harness attitudes, views and opinions; encourage critical thinking; reduce anxiety, facilitate liaison with other disciplines and promote continuity of patient care (Buresh & Gordon 2006). Buresh & Gordon (2006) also believe that nursing cannot be seen as a significant healthcare profession unless it is visible and vocal in connection with all the major healthcare issues of our time. This could also apply to all perioperative practitioners who need effective communication skills to provide optimum and safe patient care.

It is important for the perioperative practitioner to identify any concerns that the patient may have with their surgical procedure or care and if appropriate, inform the anaesthetist or surgeon to allay any worries. Having a better understanding of the procedure may help with their concerns and reduce anxieties. Fear of the unknown or experience from previous surgery can cause the patient to be nervous or have signs of stress.

The prospect of undergoing anaesthesia and surgery can be unsettling for patients. The combination of patient communication and ongoing physician education can help alleviate some of this anxiety (Guidry 2006).

The Royal Colleges of Surgeons and Psychiatrists (1997) carried out a survey to identify the concerns of patients undergoing surgical procedures. Patients expressed the following fears:

- fear of not waking up after surgery;
- fear of waking up during the surgery;
- anxiety because of the patient face mask;
- needle phobia.

Anxious patients require more knowledge about their illness and increased control of chronic illness not only before surgery but also, in the long run, in the advanced stages of disease and after extensive surgery. Thus, before surgery, information may decrease anxiety and increase patient satisfaction (Hawighorst-Knapstein *et al.* 2006).

Providing patients undergoing elective surgery with email access to their surgeon results in improved levels of communication without impairment of satisfaction, with outcomes. Although the impact of email remains unknown on the delivery of healthcare, potential advantages of its use include increased convenience of the communication tool, leading to higher probability of communication occurring, increased information sharing, higher satisfaction with services and improved quality of care. Potential disadvantages include absence of subtle emotive cues, inability to examine the patient at the time, threats to patient privacy and overwhelming of service providers by the bulk of emails received (Barclay & Nghlem 2008).

Communication is the basic element of human interactions that allows people to establish, maintain and improve contacts with others. It is a complex and multifaceted process that involves behaviours and relationships, and allows individuals to associate with others and the world around them (Potter & Berry 1989). In the operating room it is important to create an environment where there is effective communication between the patient and perioperative practitioner.

Communication is the basis of accurate hearing, defining, organising, interpreting and managing exchanges with patients, the operating room multidisciplinary team and other hospital practitioners. It can be either verbal (involving issues such as volume, quality of voice and tone rate) or non-verbal (involving eye contact, facial expression, posture, closeness and touch). The effective use of both verbal and non-verbal communication by the perioperative practitioners can establish a caring and empathetic impression with patients on their perioperative journey. Practitioners must not judge or discriminate against patients of different ages, genders and race. They should treat every patient with equal respect.

Communication is the channel by which the perioperative practitioner helps to deliver effective patient care throughout the operating room. It is a two-way process where both parties should understand each other for effective interactions to occur.

Many of the complaints brought against the NHS are still caused by poor communication by health service staff. If only all health service staff made sure that they listened to patients and their carers, communicated clearly with them and with each other, then made a note of what had been said, the scope for later misunderstanding and dispute would be reduced enormously (Abraham 2004).

Listening is an important facet of communication since practitioners who do not listen to patients will not understand their needs. Some patients are anxious and this will manifest itself in some by making them talkative, whereas others become more reserved. It is important that the practitioner can assess the patient's needs and be able to elicit the correct amount of information from them. Barriers can reduce the efficiency of this process and the practitioners need to analyse their own and the patients' interpretation of their conversation. They always need to listen to patients and answer any questions that arise.

Effective feedback to the communication is important to the patient and may relieve the patient's stress before anaesthesia and surgery. Breakdown in communications can intensify this stress.

It is desirable for the patient to form a trusting relationship with the practitioner at their first meeting. The initial meeting, in the reception area, is where the professional relationship between patients and practitioners begins. Patients may feel vulnerable while lying on the operating room trolley so it is important that practitioners introduce themselves to the patient in a non-intimidating way. Practitioners who can detect non-verbal signs from the patient are better able to understand the patient's needs and reduce anxiety. They need to have perception and be able to interpret the needs of the patient.

In the reception area practitioners should:

- introduce themselves to the patient respectfully;
- maintain effective eye contact, speak directly to the patient and listen to their responses;
- assess the personal needs of the patient – is the patient blind, deaf or physically disabled?
- display a reassuring and calm manner during communication with the patient.

During the preoperative check the practitioner should speak to the patient directly, using simple language to assess and confirm the patient's understanding of the questions on the checklist. It is important to arrange for the anaesthetist or surgeon to speak to the patient to allay any worries if the patient is upset and needs reassurance on specific issues. An interpreter may increase the effectiveness of the communication, although usually the ward practitioners will have arranged for the interpreter to escort the patient to the reception area.

Patients differ in the extent of information they need before their surgical procedure. Practitioners need to respect this difference and treat each patient as an individual.

Patients with a hearing impairment

Patients with impaired hearing may have communication problems throughout their perioperative care. Wearing a hearing aid may help the patient understand procedures better and may also help the recovery practitioner in the postoperative care of the patient.

If it is not possible for the patient to wear a hearing aid, the anaesthetic practitioner should speak slowly in order for the patient to be able to lip read the information. If the patient is awake in the operating room, practitioners need to remember that their face masks are an obstacle to communication.

Patients with poor eyesight or who are visually impaired

Practitioners should introduce themselves to patients, so that the patient knows who they are speaking to, and use the sense of touch to help in the communication process.

Non-English-speaking patients

Normally the ward practitioners will arrange for an interpreter to accompany the patient to the operating room environment. The practitioner needs to ensure that these patients understand, via the interpreter, all the details of their anaesthesia and surgical procedure. The interpreter may accompany the patient into the anaesthetic room to ensure that he or she understands and feels less stressed in preoperative care; and the interpreter may again be present in the recovery area for postoperative care.

Paediatric patients

For paediatric patients, one relative or carer may normally accompany the patient into the anaesthetic room if allowed by local policy.

Anxious adult patients

Local protocol may allow a relative to escort an anxious adult patient, but the anaesthetic practitioner needs to confirm this before taking the patient into the anaesthetic room.

Patients have the right to be treated with skill, consideration and dignity regardless of their age, gender, race, religion, disabilities, health and legal status (Shields & Werder 2002).

Effective communication is essential between all members of the perioperative team, ward practitioners and allied professions from other departments in order to deliver quality care to the patient throughout their perioperative journey. Perioperative practitioners maintain effective communication with their patients and the multidisciplinary team to ensure optimal patient care.

PATIENT ADVOCACY

An advocate is someone who pleads for or speaks up for another. Advocacy is at the heart of nursing's professional commitment and it plays an essential role when nurses are caring for patients and patients' family members. The American Nurses Association's Code of Ethics for Nurses with Interpretive Statements that as advocates, nurses must be alert to and take appropriate action regarding instances of incompetent, unethical, illegal or impaired practice by any member of the healthcare team or system on any act on the part of others that places the rights or best interests of a patient in jeopardy (American Nurses Association 2001).

Boyle (2005) states that patients depend on nurses to help them through the changing healthcare system. This is also true of practitioners working with patients in the perioperative area. Advocacy is a critical issue for surgical patients who are unconscious or sedated and unable to make decisions related to their care.

All perioperative practitioners are responsible for the patients' care and they need to be their ears and voice during their surgical procedures. They can help patients with communication barriers, clarification of their anaesthetic and surgical procedure, and provide support during their perioperative care. Effective professional relationships within the multidisciplinary operating room team can help all operating room practitioners to discuss pertinent issues with the appropriate personnel on behalf of the patient. The perioperative practitioner should act in the best interests of the patient when undertaking the advocate role.

There is little doubt that vulnerable patients need and deserve to be protected from harm and those advocating for them must contend with personal and professional challenges that may inhibit effective advocacy. Significant barriers exist for perioperative nurses taking the advocacy role. These include personal assertiveness, relationships among surgical teams and lack of support from managers. Identifying and addressing the personal, professional and organisational barriers may contribute to stronger practitioner advocacy (Bull & Fitzgerald 2004).

The registering bodies for both nurses and operating department practitioners (ODPs) states that they should (NMC 2008a, HPC 2008):

- treat people as individuals and respect their dignity;
- act as an advocate for those in their care, helping them to access relevant health and social care, information and support;
- listen to those in their care and respond to their concerns and preferences;

- make arrangement to meet people's language and communication needs.

PATIENT CONSENT

The Department of Health issued a range of guidance documents on consent in 2004 which set out the standards and procedures for all health professionals who undertake consent procedures. Valid consent to treatment is central to the patient's surgical procedure within the operating room. This document identifies the 12 key points of consent. The points cover the following areas:

- Points 1–4 When do health professionals need consent from patients?
- Point 5 Can children consent for themselves?
- Point 6 Who is the right person to seek consent?
- Point 7 What information should be provided?
- Point 8 Is the patient's consent voluntary?
- Point 9 Does it matter how the patient gives consent?
- Point 10 Refusal of consent.
- Points 11 and 12 Adults who are not competent to give consent.

There are four consent forms within the operating room:

- adult;
- paediatric – only people with parental responsibility are entitled to give consent on behalf of their children. The anaesthetic practitioner checks the confirmation of signature with the parent. Children over 16 can sign their own consent, while children under 16 can sign their own consent if deemed to be competent to do so (Gillick competence);
- consultant – they sign for patients who do not understand the implications of the surgical procedure;
- local anaesthetic.

Perioperative practitioners encounter consent issues constantly in their practice, both in terms of the main procedure listed and procedures they will undertake personally to enable the main procedure to be carried out safely. The law on consent has previously been governed by case (common) law but is now also partly governed by the Mental Capacity Act 2005 (MCA 2005).

In some circumstances where an adult patient is incapacitated to understand the consent process, they may require a surrogate or proxy decision maker. In 2007 the Mental Capacity Act 2005 came into force, allowing health or social care decisions to be taken by a proxy decision maker. Circumstances could involve patients with a brain injury, dementia or learning disabilities. There are also implications for cultural or religious preference in the consent process (Bernat & Peterson 2006).

The onus is on practitioners to ensure that their practice is legal. Valid consent not only serves to respect patient autonomy and improve compliance, but also protects the healthcare practitioner from a charge of battery (assault). For consent to be legally valid, it must be competent, voluntary and informed. All perioperative practitioners are confronted with consent issues on a regular basis. The onus is on the practitioner to have a sound knowledge of the law (ignorance is no defence). If a practitioner is in doubt about the lawfulness of a certain situation, they should recourse to senior and legal advice where appropriate (Corfield & Pomeroy 2008).

Consent should only be obtained from a patient following a full explanation of the procedure, its benefits, relevant risks, expected outcomes and alternatives. It should be obtained by the person performing the intervention or a designated deputy who is adequately familiar with the procedure. The patient must be assessed as having the mental capacity to comprehend and retain information with regard to the intended treatment and especially the consequences of having or not having the treatment (AfPP 2007).

It is the anaesthetic practitioner's responsibility to check the patient's consent form in the reception area and confirm with patients that they understand and are aware of their surgical procedure. They should ensure that the surgical procedure on the consent form correlates with the details on the operating list. If the surgeon adds any further details of the surgical procedure or other procedures, patients should sign again to ensure that they understand the additions.

Table 4.1 Problems with consent.

Problem with consent	Action to be taken
Consent form not signed by patient	Ask medical practitioners to undertake consent procedure with patient
Consent form signed in outpatients on a previous date	Consent confirmed and signed on day of operation by ward or perioperative practitioners
Wrong limb identified on consent form and operating list	Check patient notes to confirm correct limb. Contact surgeon to change consent form and mark the correct limb. In some operating rooms members of the perioperative team have a 'time out' to ensure all parties are happy to go ahead with the surgical procedure
Patient not aware of surgical procedure	Ask the ward nurse or surgeon to confirm patient was lucid and can understand nature of surgical procedure. If patient is confused or has symptoms of dementia, ask for consultant consent
Patient has dementia	Ask for consultant consent

Patients who have received a premedication cannot sign for any additions as the premedication drugs can affect their understanding of the implications of extension to the surgery and therefore the surgery reverts to what was originally agreed.

Scrub practitioners should check the consent and any allergies or medical condition before the commencement of the surgical procedure. Any discrepancies (e.g. correct site for the surgical procedure) should be sorted out with the perioperative team before the anaesthetist commences anaesthesia.

Problems with consent are identified in Table 4.1.

ACCOUNTABILITY

The term 'accountability' refers to the responsibility to undertake a particular role or task and the necessity to answer to an individual or body regarding its undertaking. Every individual in society is legally accountable to the laws of society. Employees are accountable to their employers. Professionals are accountable to their registering body, which has the power to maintain their registration or remove them from the register, thereby effectively preventing them from practising their profession. The purpose of professional accountability is, therefore, to maintain standards of practice, prevent inappropriate practice and ensure public safety. Each practitioner is responsible for their own practice. The Nursing and Midwifery Council (NMC 2008b) states that 'nurses and midwifery hold a position of responsibility and other people rely on them. They are professionally accountable to the NMC, as well as having a contractual accountability to their employer and are accountable to the law for their actions'.

All registered nurses are professionally accountable for their actions and must adhere to the NMC Code of Conduct. Registered nurses must assess the care to be given, who gives the care and the outcomes of that care. Registered nurses are professionally accountable but all employees, including healthcare support workers, are accountable to their employers and their patients (RCN 2008a).

The duty of care that health professionals owe to patients is a deep-seated core within their professional codes of conduct. The NMC Code of Professional Conduct: standards for conduct, performance and ethics (NMC 2004) states 'to practise competently, you must possess the knowledge, skills and abilities required for lawful, safe and effective practice without direct supervision, you must acknowledge the limits of your professional competence and only undertake practice and accept responsibilities for those activities in which you are competent'.

Similarly, the Health Professional Council (HPC) Standards of Conduct, Performance and Ethics (HPC 2008) states 'you must keep your professional knowledge and skills up to date. You must make sure that your knowledge, skills and performance are of a high quality, up to date and relevant to your field of practice'.'

The Accountability Code of the NMC (2008b) states that 'as a professional you are personally accountable for actions and omissions in your practice and must always be able to justify your decisions and you must always act lawfully whether those laws relate to your professional practice or personal life'.

Perioperative practitioners are responsible and accountable for the patients throughout their perioperative journey. They provide a safe environment for patients and check all relevant equipment for their anaesthetic and surgical procedures. They are also accountable to their employer, manager, the operating room multidisciplinary team, their work colleagues and to themselves.

Perioperative practitioners:

- have a duty of care to their patients;
- should respect, inform and protect the patient throughout the perioperative journey;
- should be aware of current legislation and implications of the law;
- keep accurate documentation;
- have loyalty to members of the multidisciplinary team;
- maintain confidentiality and dignity of the patient;
- only undertake roles and responsibilities in which they are competent;
- are accountable for their practice.

Doctors' views about the contribution of guidelines to safety and to clinical practice differ from those of healthcare practitioners. Doctors reject written rules, instead adhering to the unwritten rules of what constitutes acceptable behaviour for members of the medical profession. In contrast, healthcare practitioners view guideline adherence as synonymous with professionalism and criticise doctors for failing to comply with guidelines (McDonald *et al.* 2005).

Lack of experience, ability or competence is not acceptable as a form of defence, and neither is team liability. Qualified practitioners are accountable not only for their own interventions but also for those of support staff and students. Therefore, they should refer to their standards for practice, which clearly illustrate their roles and responsibilities (Dimond 2004).

All perioperative practitioners and members of the multidisciplinary team should be aware of the issues of accountability, vicarious liability and indemnity. The employing authority is liable for the negligence of their employees and the NHS indemnity covers their employees for negligence claims. Accountability, responsibility and legal issues should be taken very seriously as litigation costs are increasing each year. Accountability is entailed in responsibility and anyone who is responsible is thereby accountable (Hunt 2005).

Regulation of perioperative practitioners is undertaken by the NMC for nurses and by the HPC for ODPs, and these bodies have the power to strike a professional off their registers if the practitioner is found guilty of malpractice. In this event, it would be illegal for that practitioner to practise in healthcare in the future. Some of the main reasons for litigation include:

- ignorance;
- poor communication between health care practitioners;
- incompetence;
- lack of resources.

DOCUMENTATION

Nursing documentation has a high priority in all trusts because analysis of records of care and observations has revealed that use of multiple charts and repetitive recording causes practical and legal problems. It should be comprehensive and accurately reflect the patient's care during the practitioner's time with the patient.

All records during the perioperative period are potentially legal documents in that they could be used in complaint investigations, professional conduct enquiries, coroner's courts and civil law-suits. In particular, with ever-increasing litigation, it is even more important that perioperative records reflect the highest standards of care. Ensuring that accurate and comprehensive perioperative records are kept is a key aspect of accountability. Perioperative records should be factual and informative about the events/incidents and should detail the responses and patient's progress. They should serve to clarify the care that was given and not be difficult to understand (Hind 2005).

High quality, relevant and appropriate documentation is central to the art and science of nursing and is fundamental in recording changes that happen during a patient's health and social care journey (RCN 2003b).

Patient documentation within the operating room gives a written account of the patient's care through the perioperative journey from the reception area until the handover to the ward nurse in the recovery area. It also gives postoperative instructions for the immediate and postoperative care on the ward or on discharge.

The perioperative practitioner completes several legally important records during the delivery of perioperative care:

- computer records;
- operation register;
- patient's care plan;
- information of surgical procedure on the operative list;
- confirmation of specimen information;
- checking of equipment, stocking up, blood and blood products.

In the event of a complaint, legal case or attendance at the Coroner's Court practitioners have to defend any missing information of care that they did not record on the patient's care plan. The accuracy of the documentation will support the practitioner's defence of the patient's care.

Verbal communication between patients and healthcare providers does not provide strong legal evidence in a court of law – it is difficult to prove because there is no permanent record of what was said. The patient's medical records are the best evidence of care received or omitted and are often relied on heavily during legal cases. Entries by practitioners and physicians in the record provide a history of the patient's clinical course and responses to treatment.

Documentation of care is summarised in Box 4.1.

The reporting of injuries, diseases and dangerous occurrences regulations (RIDDOR) require the reporting of work-related accidents, diseases and dangerous occurrences. The Act (HMSO 1995) applies to all work activities but not to all incidents. Reporting incidents and all health at work is a legal requirement as described by RIDDOR. The information enables the enforcing authorities to identify where and how risks arise and to

---

Box 4.1 Documentation of care

The practitioner should record care following local policy:

- Information should be written in a legible fashion and in black ink.
- Do not cross out, use Tippex or use abbreviations.
- Record all care given to patients, before, during and after the surgical procedure in a logical order with times if relevant.
- Only record relevant information (record facts and not opinions).
- Identify any instructions from the anaesthetist or surgeon.
- Identify patient's requests, important medical facts about patients (e.g. allergies).
- Sign for delivery of care.

---

investigate serious accidents. The enforcing authorities can then help and advise on preventative action to reduce injury, ill health and accidental loss. Employers have duties under the RIDDOR to report accidents or major injuries resulting in 3 days off work, dangerous occurrences or disease or related deaths (AfPP 2007)

The member of staff, if necessary, should seek medical assessment if he or she sustains any injury. Local reporting protocols should be adhered to and all the documentation should go to an agreed central collecting point and photocopies kept within the department.

The operating room manager may launch an internal enquiry into incidents where he or she identifies a problem. Any member of the perioperative team completes an incident report when there is a problem or incident during patient care. The incident report is a valuable tool in reporting a problem. All members of the perioperative team should complete this form in black ink and include all evidence of their patient care on the care plan.

CLINICAL SUPERVISION

Incidents such as the Bristol heart surgery tragedy, the failures of cervical screening at Kent and Canterbury Hospital and the case of Beverley Allitt have all caused widespread public and political concern and heightened general awareness of the potential harm when health services go awry. These incidents have also engendered a period of deep reflection and critical analysis among the health professions and fostered growing support for major changes in the way quality health services are managed (Smith 1998).

The Department of Health (2003) in its white paper entitled *A Vision for the Future* described clinical supervision as 'a formal process of professional support and learning which enables individual practitioners to develop knowledge and competence, assume responsibility for their own practice and enhance consumer protection and safety of care in complex situations'.

Clinical supervision allows a registrant to receive professional supervision in the workplace by a skilled supervisor. It allows them to develop their skills and knowledge and helps them to improve patient/client care. It enables registrants to:

- identify solutions to problems;
- increase understanding of professional issues;
- improve standards of patient care;
- further develop their skills and knowledge;
- enhance their understanding of their own practice.

Clinical supervision should be available to registrants throughout their careers so they can constantly evaluate and improve their contribution to patient/client care. Along with the NMC's PREP (continuing professional development) standard, clinical supervision is an important part of clinical governance (NMC 2006).

The operating room can be a stressful environment and the introduction of clinical supervision can provide a support mechanism for the operating room practitioners, enable individual practitioners to highlight and meet specific training and development needs, and help in the delivery of clinical excellence for patients. Issues that might be discussed within clinical supervision include:

- professional issues;
- clinical issues;
- roles;
- personal issues;
- environmental issues;

- educational issues;
- support and nurture;
- critical incidents;
- reflection.

A confidential contract will be completed at the end of the clinical supervision meeting between the clinical supervisor and supervisee. If anything is disclosed in the meeting which is illegal, which breaks the relevant code of professional conduct, which relates to potential or actual harm to a patient or colleague, or which constitutes misconduct, it should be reported to the operating room manager or relevant personnel to take the appropriate action.

Wood (2004) believes that clinical supervision supports practice, enabling practitioners to maintain and improve standards of care. To facilitate clinical supervision, a culture of lifelong learning needs to be embraced as an integral part of daily working life within the NHS. Education, training and lifelong learning can support perioperative practitioners' improvement in competence and delivery of patient care. Clinical supervision can also enhance patient care by perioperative practitioners supporting each other, discussing practice issues and improving teamwork and quality within the NHS.

INFORMATION TECHNOLOGY WITHIN THE NHS

Information and communications technology is a new component within patient healthcare to modernise the storage of patient information. All practitioners require basic computing skills as information on the patient's healthcare is input on computers by all practitioners within the NHS. Practitioners need to feel comfortable using computers and have the ability to input the relevant information.

Individual managers can arrange training for their practitioners but there is an opportunity to undertake a recognised training programme of IT skills. The European Computer Driving Licence course is a national scheme to equip all practitioners with a comprehensive practical knowledge of basic computing skills. The NHS Information Authority tracks and monitors registrations of practitioners and has access to the learning and testing materials.

Electronic storage of information is becoming more prominent within all areas of patient care and can give valuable information to all NHS agencies. It is an innovation to provide electronic health records, evidence-based decision making and valuable resources for NHS practitioners.

In the operating room, computer information can provide names of individual practitioners who undertake the different roles in each theatre discipline and time of the patient entering and leaving all areas of the operating room environment. It can also be used to record information on:

- type of anaesthesia;
- identification of laryngeal mask airway (LMA) number and the number of times it has been used during anaesthesia;
- time of commencement and completion of anaesthesia and surgical procedure;
- planned surgical procedure and details of any changes to it;
- any extra equipment necessary for the surgical procedure (e.g. TV and laparoscope);
- any change of ward on discharge;
- cancellation of surgical procedure with the identification of the reason.

The NHS is trying to improve clinical performance within the operating room environment and reduce cancelled surgical procedures. Effective utilisation of the operating room sessions is critical to the provision of efficient surgical procedures and to achieve full capacity and use of the operative lists. Computer information can identify an individual patient's surgical procedure cancellation and allow managers to reschedule the procedure within the specified government time limits.

The implementation of the electronic patient record systems has modernised patient information within the NHS. It allows practitioners and medical practitioners to access patient information to aid delivery of patient care, audits or incident reports. It can improve multiagency information and minimise frustration for all.

Computer reports can provide:

151

- for the patient:
  - satisfaction – arrange suitable appointments, admissions and discharge;
  - reduction of delays in their surgical procedures;
  - reduction of cancelled surgical procedures.
- for the practitioners:
  - patient care information;
  - laboratory results, x-ray reports.

Access to computers for training purposes is becoming the norm for all operating room environments. All practitioners can access the intranet and internet services for information on patient care issues and also for their own professional development. They can prepare presentations for teaching and assessment of students and research information for university courses, and enhance their own and others' knowledge of patient care issues.

TEAMWORK

Perioperative practitioners have complementary skills within their theatre disciplines and have a commitment to the operating room performance goals, and the delivery of quality care to their perioperative patients.

Effective teamwork of the multidisciplinary team can help to improve quality patient care and can also enhance patient and staff safety. Clear aims and objectives assist effective communication, team coordination and active participation in patient care. Successful teams support each other and recognise the importance of personal and professional competence and development.

The new General Medical Services (GMS) contract challenges traditional attitudes and working practices, embracing a whole team approach in improving the quality of care. It will be important for practice teams to work together effectively to identify patient needs, plan work and involve all members in decision making and developments in order to fulfil the requirements of the contract. Effective teamwork is underpinned by effective two-way communication.

An effective team can be defined as one where:

- roles and relationships are accepted;
- there is mutual support, openness and trust among members;
- task expectations and accomplishments are high with members taking initiative and energy being channelled into effective work;
- there is respect for individual differences;
- Individual needs are met.

For teams to function effectively:

- the team needs to have a reason for working together;
- members need to be interdependent, i.e. they need each others' expertise;
- members need to be committed to the idea that working together as a team leads to more effective decisions than working in isolation;
- the team needs to be accountable as a functioning unit (NHS Scotland 2009).

Until relatively recently, surgical performance and surgical outcomes were mostly understood and modelled as a function of first, the surgical patient's risk factors and second, the technical expertise and ability of the surgeon. In the last few years, however, there has been a shift in the conceptualisation of surgical competence. The shift involves a system-oriented approach to surgery, in which multiple determinants of surgical outcomes are considered alongside the manual dexterity of the operating surgeon –including the perioperative environment and the ability of the surgical team to work effectively as a team (Calland et al. 2002, Vincent et al. 2004, Yule et al. 2006).

A number of recent reports from professional associations emphasise the importance of effective teamwork in surgery. A report by the National Confidential Enquiry into Perioperative Deaths (NCEPOD 2002) states that 'the continuity of quality patient care throughout the patient's journey depends largely on interdisciplinary teamwork'.

Successful teams have a strong and effective leader. Team members have clear views, are clear about their roles and responsibilities, share objectives, discuss and resolve problems, value and respect each other and encourage development and growth of the team.

The team consists of a mix of people with individual personalities and talents who blend to work together effectively. Managers and team leaders should recognise the strengths and weaknesses of their team members and ensure that they make the best use of their resources to develop them into a cohesive team. All these issues encourage team cohesiveness and therefore encourage the delivery of effective patient care.

THE PERIOPERATIVE TEAM

The roles and responsibilities of the operating room are diverse and at times overlap within the different areas of the operating room environment (reception, anaesthetic room, operating room and recovery). Members of the operating room team have different levels of qualifications and experience, but they pool these in the care of the perioperative patient.

Operating room support worker

There are different names for the unqualified practitioner who cares for the operating room equipment: assistant operating room practitioners, operating room technician or operating room orderlies.

Their roles and responsibilities include:

- check, prepare and monitor the relevant equipment and accessories for the surgical procedures on the operative list following manufacturer's recommendations and local policies;
- position patients safely on the operating room table;
- maintain the patient's dignity and ensure the patient's limbs are free from pressure and the patient is comfortable;
- prepare and clean the theatre at the relevant times and ensure the waste bags, linen and needle sharp boxes are available following local policies of infection control, waste management and health and safety.

Operating room orderlies

Orderlies are the first members of the operating room team to meet the patient. They can help allay the patients' fear and anxieties with effective communication.

Their roles and responsibilities include:

- collect patients from the ward and return them after their surgical procedure accompanied by the ward or theatre escort nurse;
- take the patients' specimens to the pathology department;
- collect blood or blood products from the pathology department following local policies;
- collect and return any relevant equipment to the hospital departments when necessary.

They have the opportunity for further development within the operating theatre. They have the potential to increase the flexibility of the theatre team and aid retention of critical staff.

The number of support staff employed within the NHS and independent sector has increased rapidly in recent years across all elements of healthcare. As the numbers of staff employed as support workers within perioperative teams has increased, the Perioperative Care Collaborative (PCC 2007) has observed diversity in their roles and in the standards and quality of underpinning education and training. The PCC recommends that to promote public confidence, patient safety and clinical excellence, employing organisations must ensure that:

- support workers are competent for the role they undertake, having been trained and assessed in accordance with the requirements of the National Qualification Frameworks and the relevant NHS Knowledge and Skills Framework outline for their job;
- they are provided with a detailed job description, specification/contract of employment outlining the parameters of their approved sphere of practice;
- they are supervised by a registered nurse or ODP in the delivery of patient care tasks commensurate with their approved sphere of practice;
- they are provided with instruction regarding the principles of vicarious liability, teamwork and delegation, and the accountability owed to the patient and employer through civil, criminal and employment law.

In March 2005, Skills for Health launched a range of new Health NVQs. The entry level NVQ Level 2: Health (Perioperative Care Support) award is an introduction to care in the perioperative environment. The NVQ Level 3: Health (Perioperative Care – Surgical Support) award should be the default qualification for experienced health care assistants (HCAs) who regularly undertake the circulating role for a wide range of procedures (Huddleston & Scoins 2006).

Pirie (2005) states that the PCC recommends a thorough risk assessment of each potential procedure that may be delegated to a support worker in the scrub role. It is advisable and essential that all practitioners are aware of their limitations with these new developments and that practitioners are not pressured to undertake more duties than those detailed in the policy.

This is a controversial issue as qualified practitioners are taking responsibility for the theatre support worker during their scrub role. All perioperative practitioners' roles (qualified and ancillary) are expanding, but guidelines and policies must be in place, and training and support must be given to all the support workers undertaking this new role.

Scrub practitioner

Nurses qualify and undertake an in-house scrub training programme on entry to the operating department before they work autonomously within this role. ODPs undertake the scrub discipline within their 3 years' training and can work autonomously immediately after qualification. Both types of practitioner are supported by their senior colleagues during the first few months of their scrub practice. Both are practitioners who prepare the equipment and surgical accessories for surgeons and are aware of their surgical preferences during the procedures.

Their roles and responsibilities are to:

- check all relevant equipment for the different operations for the individual patients on the operative list;
- maintain a safe operating room environment and sterile field for surgical patients;
- ensure the theatre team position the patient safely and comfortably on the operating room table;

- maintain the patient's dignity and ensure the rest of the operating room team observes this;
- provide the swabs, needles, instruments and accessories for surgeons. Anticipate their needs to facilitate an efficient and safe surgical procedure. Undertake counts at the beginning, commencement of closure and the end of the surgical procedure;
- communicate effectively with the theatre team throughout the patient's perioperative journey to provide holistic and efficient patient care;
- check the specimens from the operative list following local policy and ensure the specimens go to the correct department for examination;
- complete the relevant documentation following local policy.

Circulating practitioner

A qualified scrub practitioner or an operating room support worker can undertake this role. Circulating practitioners perform an important role as they are the eyes and ears of the scrub practitioners. They assist them to prepare the theatre, ensure the operating room environment is clean and tidy, and stock the operating room after the operative list.

Their roles and responsibilities are to:

- prepare the surgical gown and gloves, and tie up the surgical gowns of the surgical team when relevant;
- open the sterile instruments sets for the scrub practitioner, check the integrity and expiry dates of the sterile swabs, needles, instruments and accessories before delivering them to the scrub practitioner;
- provide the swabs, needles, instruments and accessories for surgeons. Anticipate their needs to facilitate an efficient and safe surgical procedure. Undertake counts at the beginning, commencement of closure and end of the surgical procedure;
- pour the skin preparation into the relevant galley pots, maintaining the sterile field and ensuring that all the surgical team also observes this;

- assist the theatre team to position the patients and maintain their dignity;
- collect the specimen or specimens from the scrub practitioner, label the specimen container, use the correct medium and complete the specimen card following the local specimen policy;
- communicate effectively with the operating room team, giving any messages to the surgeon or scrub practitioner in a respectful manner and at a convenient time;
- clean the operating room table, positioning equipment and other equipment after each patient following local infection control policies.

Advanced scrub practitioner

In 2003, the PCC reviewed the role of the non-medical periop-erative practitioner working as first assistant to the surgeon, and redefined the role and job description title of the first assistant to that of the advanced scrub practitioner (ASP). The ASP role can be defined as that undertaken by a healthcare practitioner providing competent and skilled assistance under the direct supervision of the operating surgeon, while not performing any form of surgical intervention. It is important that the ASP works within a local clinical governance framework, albeit primarily within the intraoperative phase. The PCC (2003) recommends that the ASP undertaking this role should have demonstrable comprehensive skills, competencies and underpinning knowl-edge beyond the standard level expected of a newly qualified theatre practitioner. Therefore, registered practitioners are expected to produce evidence of lifelong learning within the perioperative field before undertaking a validated programme of study for this role. It is a clearly defined role and must not be undertaken at the same time as the scrub role.

The scope of the ASP role (PCC 2003, 2007):

- enhancing communication between the patient, ward and theatre, including preoperative assessment and postoperative evaluation of care;
- assisting with positioning the patient, including assessment of tissue viability;

- skin preparation and draping prior to surgery;
- skin and tissue retraction;
- handling of instruments;
- male/female catheterisation;
- cutting of sutures and ties;
- assisting with haemostasis, including use of suction;
- indirect application of electrocautery;
- camera holding;
- use and maintenance of specialised equipment;
- assistance with wound closure and application of wound dressings;
- transfer of patient to post-anaesthetic care unit.

The role has moved forward and evolved, but it is important to acknowledge that the practitioner remains accountable for his or her own actions (NMC 2008, HPC 2008).

Surgical care practitioner

The surgical care practitioner (SCP) role is defined by the Royal College of Surgeons Curriculum Framework as a non-medical practitioner working in clinical practice as a member of the extended surgical team who performs surgical intervention pre-operative and postoperative care under the direction and supervision of a consultant surgeon. Sixty per cent of an SCP's role involves routine procedures, preoperative and postoperative care, assisting with surgery, diagnostic procedures and supervised operative care (Skills for Health 2009).

Reception practitioners

Qualified anaesthetic practitioners or ancillary practitioners can undertake this role.

Their roles and responsibilities include:

- ask the porters to collect patients from the relevant wards;
- greet patients on their arrival in the operating room reception area;
- allay the patients' fears and anxieties with effective communication;
- check their identification in line with the operative list;

- check the preoperative document and request any missing information for the anaesthetic practitioner;
- monitor the patient's physiological readings if relevant;
- communicate with the patients while they are waiting for their surgical procedures.

Anaesthetic practitioners

Nurses qualify and undertake a competency-based anaesthetic training programme or university anaesthetic course on entry to the operating department before they work autonomously within this role. ODPs undertake the anaesthetic discipline during their 3 years' training and can work autonomously immediately after qualification. Both types of practitioner are supported by their senior colleagues during their first few months of practice.

Their roles and responsibilities include:

- prepare, check and stock the anaesthetic equipment and accessories for the anaesthetist for the operative list;
- prepare equipment for the relevant technique of anaesthesia for each patient. Preparation is the key to effective anaesthetic practice;
- undertake the preoperative checklist and inform the anaesthetist of any patient allergies, loose teeth, etc;
- assist the anaesthetist to establish and maintain anaesthesia;
- complete the patient documentation to identify patient care throughout the anaesthetic phase;
- give an effective handover to the recovery practitioner.

The roles and responsibilities of the anaesthetic practitioner are further discussed in Chapter 8.

Recovery practitioners

Nurses qualify and undertake an in-house recovery training programme on entry to the operating department before they work autonomously within this role. ODPs undertake the recovery discipline within their 3 year's training and can work autonomously immediately after qualification. Both types of practitioner are supported by their senior colleagues during their first few months of practice.

Their roles and responsibilities include:

- prepare, check and stock all relevant recovery equipment before patients arrive in the recovery area;
- check the patient's airway and maintain it throughout his or her stay in the recovery area;
- monitor the patient's physiological readings, intravenous infusion, dressing, drain, catheter, stoma, oxygen therapy and any other surgical or anaesthetic intervention;
- communicate with the anaesthetic team, patient, carer and ward nurse;
- complete effective documentation of the recovery care of the patient;
- give an efficient handover, to the ward nurse, of the patient's care throughout the operating room environment and the anaesthetist's and surgeon's instructions for the patient's postoperative care.

The roles and responsibilities of the recovery practitioner are further discussed in Chapter 9.

Both anaesthetic and recovery practitioners who acquire experience and competence within their operating room disciplines may undertake further roles within their practice. They undertake all these roles following local policies.

These roles include:

- intravenous cannulation;
- administration of intravenous drugs;
- administration of boluses for patient's pain management machines (patient controlled analgesia [PCA] and epidural machines);
- programming of pain management machines: patient controlled administration machines (PCAs and epidural machines).

Non-medical anaesthetist

Several recent reports have focused on the need to improve the efficiency of operating departments (Audit Commission 2002). Due to the European Working Time Directive and its implications for the reduction in doctors' hours, non-medical practitioners have been considered for a role in anaesthesia, in line with the expanding roles being introduced within the operating room environment.

Within Europe nurse anaesthetists undertake the direct care of the patient, chiefly during the maintenance of anaesthesia. An anaesthetist supervises them when they establish and reverse anaesthesia.

In the USA there are two types of nurse anaesthetists: certified registered nurse anaesthetists (CRNAs) and anaesthetic assistants (AAs). The CRNA may undertake relatively independent anaesthetic practice under the supervision of a non-anaesthetist (surgeon or general practitioner) and the AA is supervised on a one to two (1:2) basis, as are the majority of CRNAs in large hospitals when they practise anaesthesia. An anaesthetist, again, is present when they establish and reverse anaesthesia.

Rod (2003) believes that a nurse anaesthetist is someone who 'provides or participates in the provision of specialist nursing and anaesthetic services to patients requiring anaesthesia, resuscitation or any other life sustaining interventions'.

The Royal College of Anaesthetists (2003), in collaboration with the Changing Workforce Programme, undertook visits to several countries (Sweden, Holland and the USA) and its views on non-medical anaesthetists were highlighted in their report.

A National Curriculum Framework has been developed which sets out a competency-based education programme for the role. The Framework was developed with the Royal College of Anaesthetists, NHS University and University of Birmingham together with other major stakeholder groups, including nurses, patients and trainee anaesthetists. Nurses and ODPs can be seconded from their current roles for this training. A case for the regulation of anaesthesia practitioners was fed in to the Foster Review of Non- Medical Regulation (2006) and the Anaesthesia Practitioner Stakeholder Board are awaiting the outcome of the review in order to proceed towards regulation of the role (Copley *et al.* 2006).

In Scotland, the physician assistant – anaesthesia (PA–A) is a new member of the anaesthesia team. To become a trainee PA–A, an individual must either have a biomedical science degree (2nd class honours or better) or be a registered healthcare professional with at least 3 years' experience and evidence of relevant academic achievement or a first degree in a health-related subject (Chambers 2009).

CHANGE MANAGEMENT

Changes can be political, economic, social, technological, legislative or environmental. It is important to acknowledge and respond to changes and identify ways of communicating changes to all NHS practitioners.

Efficient change management results in the successful implementation of change by practitioners in the organisation, systems, procedures or work practices. Managers need to have commitment to the changes, integrity, and effective negotiation and communication skills to ensure that practitioners adopt the changes without too many problems. Problems of poor communication, acceptance and resistance to change can be possible stressors to all parties.

To accept change all practitioners need to have an awareness of the reasons for the change and the benefits that it can bring them. Commitment and communication need to be effective to achieve success. Effective communication on the reasons and strategies for achieving the change can make practitioners more receptive to change. Any change in working practices or threats to job security may meet with opposition and reduce job satisfaction. Managers need support and commitment and a willingness to listen to the reasons for the change from the practitioners. Time should be allowed to secure a discussion for the timetable of potential changes; and practitioners need to own the changes and feel that they have had an input into the final implementation.

The NHS is currently undergoing a period of intensive change and there is a real need for all managers to facilitate this change within their organisations and the wider NHS environment. Delivering and managing change is an especially important part of the health informatics role, but staff need to be supported through change and to be helped to understand the implications on their roles and responsibilities. Change management entails thoughtful planning and sensitive implementation, and above all, consultation with, and involvement of, the people affected by the changes. If change is forced on people, problems normally occur. Change must be realistic, achievable and measurable, and these aspects are especially relevant to managing personal change (NHS Connecting for Health 2009).

Political power refers to the ability to shape and influence policy and processes, including people, for developing and implementing policy. Healthcare practitioners must have an opportunity to shape policies that determine the quality of care, and the quality of life to which patients, people and communities are entitled. Without this opportunity, healthcare practitioners are continually working at a disadvantage, waiting for others to make policy decisions that nurses are then expected to implement, regardless of the consequences. This not only undermines the patient–healthcare practitioner relationship, but also diminishes morale among nurses (Hakesley-Brown & Malone 2007).

The RCN mission statement states 'The RCN represents nurses and nursing promotes excellence in practice and shapes health policy' (RCN 2003a, p2). This proactive mission is reflective of the determination by UK nurses to be involved in decision making early in policy development through think tanks, government task forces and commissions, and any other power shaping groups.

Recent changes within the NHS are the empowerment of patients and the public, and the extension of traditional roles undertaken by all practitioners, both qualified and unqualified.

Agenda for Change

Agenda for Change (AFC) is the most radical shake up of the NHS pay system since the NHS began in 1948. It applies to over one million NHS staff across the UK. NHS employers are responsible for representing the views of employers in national negotiations on AFC, and provide support and assistance for trusts introducing the new systems through the AFC Implementation Team. The NHS Employer's Pay and Negotiations Team offers support and advice to employers in the NHS. Individual members of staff are advised to seek advice from their employer, professional representatives or trade union as written information.

The NHS Knowledge and Skills Framework (NHS KSF) is the career and pay progression strand of AFC, the NHS pay system. It is mandatory for all AFC staff and should be fully implemented by all NHS organisations.

The KSF:

- defines and describes the knowledge and skills that staff need to apply in their work to deliver quality services;
- provides a single consistent, comprehensive and explicit framework for staff reviews and development;
- allows the operation of the AFC pay progression system, without which the contractual commitment to an equitable pay system cannot be met;
- is a generic competency framework developed from existing good practice.

The KSF is applied by identifying the knowledge and skills requirements for each NHS post (the KSF outline) and ensuring that each post holder has an annual review against their KSF outline to identify any development needs. A personal development plan is then agreed and carried out. At two points on each of the AFC pay bands, incremental progression is dependent on fulfilling the appropriate KSF outline for the post (NHS Employers 2009).

CLINICAL GOVERNANCE

Clinical governance is how health services are held accountable for the safety, quality and effectiveness of clinical care delivered to patients. It is the statutory requirement of NHS boards and is achieved by coordinating three interlinking strands of work: robust national and local systems and structures that help identify, implement and report on quality improvement; quality improvement work involving healthcare staff, patients and the public; and establishing a supportive, inclusive learning culture for improvement (NHS Scotland 2009).

NHS providers are responsible for ensuring that patients receive adequate and appropriate care. The national clinical governance agenda identifies seven 'pillars' of activity (clinical evidence and research, audit, risk management, education and training, patient and public involvement, using information and IT, staffing and staff management) that are required to achieve this including the 'use of information' and key to monitoring the quality of service provided is accurate and timely data collection (The Information Centre for Knowledge and Care 2006).

Patients and public involvement is vital to improving the quality of health services and opportunities can be provided to make sure that patients are able to contribute to a range of activities, including planning new services, staff training and education, and the development of information (RCN 2003b). This guideline was published 6 years ago but was still valid in January 2009 (NHS Evidence [2009] – National Library of Guidelines 2009).

The government created the following to ensure commitment to patient healthcare and commitment to clinical governance:

- the National Institute for Clinical Excellence;
- the Commission for Healthcare Audit and Inspection;
- the Modernisation Agency;
- the National Patient Safety Agency;
- Patient Advice and Liaison Service and user involvement groups;
- the Clinical Negligence Scheme for Trusts;
- performance indicators.

Clinical Negligence Scheme for Trusts (CNST 2009)

The CNST handles all clinical claims against member NHS bodies where the incident in question took place on or after 1 April 2005 (or when the body joined the scheme, if that is later). Although membership of the scheme is voluntary, all NHS trusts (including foundation trusts) and primary care trusts (PCTs) in England currently belong to the scheme.

The CNST is a scheme of risk pooling. It provides indemnity cover for NHS bodies in England that are members of the scheme against clinical negligence claims made by or in relation to NHS patients treated by or on behalf of those NHS bodies. It exists to provide a fair and cost-effective means of handling clinical negligence claims against NHS trusts in England and also to provide risk management guidance, so that adverse incidents and hence claims are reduced in number. CNST contributions are significantly lower than the equivalent commercial insurance schemes. This scheme handles claims and indemnifies NHS bodies in respect of both clinical negligence and nonclinical risks. It also has risk management programmes in place against which NHS trusts are assessed. CNST agencies are accountable to central government and provide effective strategies for and regulate and audit patient care. When a claim is made against a CNST member, the NHS body remains the legal defendant. The NHS Litigation Authority (NHSLA) takes over full responsibility for handling the claim and meeting the associated costs (NHSLA 2009).

National clinical audit
Clinical audit is a quality improvement process that seeks to improve patient care and outcomes through systematic review of care against explicit criteria and the implementation of change. Clinical audit and outcomes measurements are quality improvement tools that can help close the gap between what is known to be the best care and the care that patients are receiving. They aim to ensure that all patients receive the most effective, up-to-date and appropriate treatments, delivered by clinicians with the right skills and experience. Clinical audit against good practice criteria or standards answers the question – are patients given the best care? Clinical outcomes measurement answers the questions – are they better, and do they feel better? (www.dh.gov.uk/en/Publichealth/patientsafety/Clincalgovernance/DH_114).

The Healthcare Commission (2005)
The Healthcare Commission, Commission for Social Care Inspection and the Mental Health Act Commission ceased to exist on 31 March 2009. The Care Quality Commission (CQC) is now the independent regulator of health and social care in England. Its aim is to make sure better care is provided for everyone, whether that is in hospital, in care homes in people's own homes or elsewhere (CQC 2009).

The Healthcare Commission is committed to making a real difference to the delivery of healthcare and to promote continuous improvement for the benefit of patients and the public. In England, it assesses and reports on the performance of healthcare organisations on an annual basis. For NHS trusts this involves issuing an annual performance rating. The overall performance rating of an NHS trust is made up of a number of performance indicators. Performance indicators show how trusts are doing in relation to some of the main targets set by the government for the NHS, as well as other broader measures of performance. They include information from surveys of staff and patients and other measures useful to patients and carers (Healthcare Commission 2005).

NHS Constitution

The NHS Constitution was published in 2009. It was one of a number of recommendations in Lord Darzi's report, *High Quality for All*, published on the 60th anniversary of the NHS. This set out a 10-year plan to provide the highest quality of care for patients in England. The NHS belongs to us all. The NHS Constitution brings together in one place, for the first time in the history of the NHS, what staff, patients and public can expect from the NHS.

The NHS Constitution was developed as part of the NHS Next Stage Review led by Lord Darzi. Lord Darzi was asked to conduct a wide ranging review of the NHS as a 'once in a generation opportunity to ensure a properly resourced NHS that is clinically-led, patient-centred and locally accountable.' The review aims to protect and renew the enduring principles of the NHS. It will empower staff, patients and the public by setting out existing legal rights and pledges for the first time in one place and in clear and simple language. It also sets out clear expectations of government agencies about the behaviours and values of all organisations providing NHS care (RCN 2008b).

The NHS Litigation Authority (NHSLA (2009)

The NHSLA is a Special Health Authority (part of the NHS) responsible for handling negligence claims made against NHS bodies in England. In addition to dealing with claims, when they arise, it has an active risk management programme to help raise standards of care in the NHS and hence reduce the number of incidents leading to claims (NHSLA 2009).

The National Institute for Clinical Excellence (NICE 2009)

NICE is the independent organisation responsible for providing national guidance on the promotion of good health and the prevention and treatment of ill health.

NICE produces guidance in three areas of health:

- public health – guidance on the promotion of good health and the prevention of ill health for those working in the NHS, local authorities and the wider public and voluntary sector;
- health technologies – guidance on the use of new and existing medicines, treatments and procedures within the NHS;
- clinical practice – guidance on the appropriate treatment and care of people with specific diseases and conditions within the NHS.

NICE guidance is developed using the expertise of the NHS and the wider healthcare community, including NHS staff, healthcare professionals, patients and carers, industry and the academic world (NICE 2009).

The NHS Modernisation Agency (2007)

The NHS Modernisation Agency has been a catalyst for change and service improvement. The Agency's work has focused on the four main elements which are key to developing and delivering a truly patient-centred service (Department of Health 2007):

- to help speed up access to services for patients, the Agency is assisting in every part of the NHS to deliver national waiting and booking targets, introduce patient choice and emergency care service;
- to increase support at a local level by supporting organisations and leaders in new roles, helping them to join modernisation activity up to a local level, building networks and

working towards the establishment of local modernisation support teams and networks in every community;

• to enable equality of healthcare, the Agency provides rapid support to under-performing parts of the NHS and promotes leading-edge practice for those wanting to accelerate improvements;

• to create a comprehensive library of good practice resources which support organisations by giving practical help, spreading good practice and helping everyone share their knowledge and learning.

The National Patient Safety Agency (NPSA 2005)

The NPSA and the Royal College of Surgeons (RCS) launched new advice to the NHS in 2005 to help make surgery safer. The recommendations promoting correct site surgery encourage a consistent approach to marking the patient for surgery and provide staff with a checklist to ensure important steps have been taken to protect the patient. Lilleyman (2005) stated mistakes during surgery can have devastating emotional and physical consequences for patients and their families. For the staff incidents can be distressing and members of the clinical teams and the wider organisation can become demoralised and disaffected. The RCS collaborates with other medical and academic organisations in the UK and worldwide and seeks to convey the importance of good, effective communication and interpersonal relationships between patients and surgeons through its patient liaison group.

The NPSA helps the NHS learn from things that go wrong and develop solutions to prevent harm in the future. It works with patients and staff locally and nationally to foster a culture where errors can be investigated and innovative solutions developed. It collects and analyses information from staff and patients via the national reporting and learning system and other sources.

Advances in technology and knowledge in recent decades have created an immensely complex healthcare system – this complexity brings risks and challenges for healthcare staff in continuing to keep patients safe (NPSA 2005).

The National Clinical Assessment Service (NCAS 2008)

The NCAS was established following recommendations made in a report by the Chief Medical Officer for England in 1999 and its follow up report in 2001. There was concern that tackling problems with medical performance needed specialist skills which were not always available in individual NHS trusts. The NCAS helps to resolve concerns about a practitioner's performance. NCAS offers advice, specialist interventions and shared learning. Its guiding principles are to be effective, authoritative, objective and fair. It does not take on the role of an employer, nor does it function as a regulator. It is established as an advisory body, and the referrer retains responsibility for handling the case throughout the process (NCAS 2008).

Patient Advice and Liaison Service (PALS 2007)

PALS is a central part of the new system of Patient and Public Involvement (PPI). PALS (2007) provides:

- confidential advice and support to patients, families and their carers;
- information on the NHS and health-related matters;
- confidential assistance in resolving problems and concerns quickly;
- information on and explanations of NHS complaints procedures and how to get in touch with someone who can help;
- information on how to get more involved in your own health-care and the NHS locally;
- a focal point for feedback from patients to inform service developments;
- an early warning system for NHS trusts, primary care trusts and PPI forums.

Performance indicators (2002)

The indicators are an important part of the government's commitment to improve the quality of clinical and other performance information that patients receive. Patients and public have the right to know how well different NHS organisations are performing. Different NHS organisations also need to know how well they are doing in comparison with others, so success can be shared and weaknesses can be identified and acted on (see www.performance.doh.gov.uk/nhsperfomanceindicators/index.htm).

The Department of Health performance indicators are part of an intensive process of publishing information on the performance of NHS organisations in order to provide comparisons and improve performance over all NHS trust hospitals and PCTs. These indicators were first introduced in 1997.

The publication of the *Kennedy Inquiry Report* on the Bristol Royal Infirmary has reinforced the need to make more information on NHS performance available in more easily accessible formats (Department of Health 2005). Performance indicators focus on the issues that matter most to patients and the public, and are there to encourage an open and honest debate about the state of the NHS.

Perioperative practitioners deliver quality care (clinical governance strategies) to the patient with the consideration of:

- risk assessment strategies;
- incident reporting;
- evidence-based practice;
- clinical effectiveness;
- education and training and professional development;
- clinical supervision;
- effective communication;
- collaboration between allied professions.

Government policy concerned with the modernisation of the NHS has urged nurses and others working in the health services to become more collaborative, adopt a flexible approach to role boundaries and establish clear lines of accountability for the quality of clinical care. However, the government's clinical governance agenda gives little recognition of the ways in which healthcare professions have been hierarchically ordered in the past and how these historical relationships may continue to shape multidisciplinary working in the modernised NHS (Savage & Moore 2004).

Figures 4.1 and 4.2 are examples of clinical governance and effective patient care.

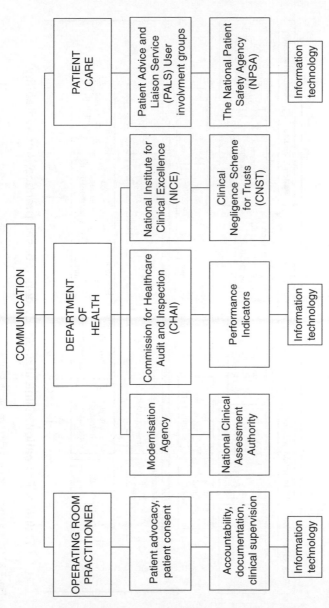

Fig. 4.1 Organisations and agencies involved in clinical governance.

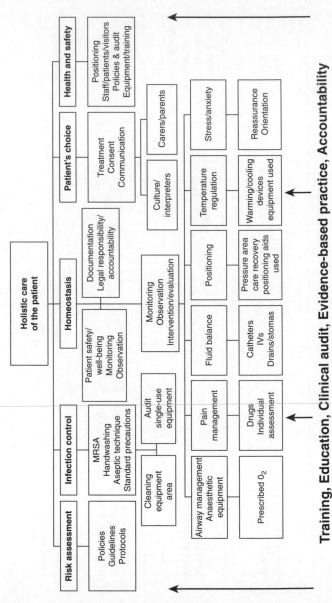

Fig. 4.2 Clinical governance and effective patient care.

CONCLUSION

Effective communication between the patient, perioperative practitioner, anaesthetist and surgeon, all allied professions and NHS agencies will enhance patients', their relatives' and carers' understanding of the care delivered to them within the operating room. Patient involvement, choice and opinions can help the NHS to develop and shape ongoing clinical practice.

REFERENCES

Abraham, A. cited in Pincock, S. (2004) Poor communication lies at the heart of NHS complaints, says Ombudsman. *British Medical Journal* **328** (742), 10.

American Nurses Association (ANA) (2001) *Code of Ethics for Nurses with Interpretive Statements*. American Nurses Association, Washington, DC.

Association for Perioperative Practice (AfPP) (2007) *Standards and Recommendations for Safe Perioperative Practice*. Harrogate, AfPP.

Audit Commission (2002) *District Audit – Operating Theatres. A Bulletin for Health Bodies*. Audit Commission, London.

Barclay, L. & Nghlem, H. T. (2008) Patient Email to surgeons may improve communication. Medscape. *Medical News*. CME released 2.19.2008.

Bernat, J. & Peterson, L. (2006) Patient-centered informed consent in surgical practice. *Archives of Surgery* **141** (1), 86–92.

Berry, D. (2007) *Healthcare Communication: Theory and Practice*. Open University Press, London.

Boyle, H. J. (2005) Patient advocacy in the perioperative setting. *AORN Journal* **8** (2), 250–262.

Bull, R. & Fitzgerald, M. (2004) Nurses' advocacy in an Australian operating department. *AORN Journal* **679** (6), 1265–1274.

Buresh, B. & Gordon, S. (2006) *From Silence to Voice: What Nurses Know and Must Communicate to the Public*. Cornwell University Press, New York.

Bury, M. (2005) *Health and Illness*. Blackwell Scientific Publications, UK.

Calland, J., Guerlain, S., Adams, R., Tribble, C., Foley, E. & Chekan, E. (2002) A systems approach to surgical safety. *Surgical Endoscopy* **16** (16), 1005–1014.

Care Quality Commission (CQC) (2009) www.cqc.org.uk

Chambers, A. (2009) Physician's Assistant – Anaesthesia – introduction www.nes.scot.nhs.uk/paa/introduction/

Clinical Negligence Scheme for Trusts (CNST) (2009) www.nhsla.com/Claims/Schemes/CNST

Copley, S., Ottley, E. & Rigby, J. (2006) Anaesthesia practitioner role development. *The Clinical Services Journal* May, www.clinicalservicesjournal.com/Story.aspx?Story=982

Corfield, L. & Pomeroy, A. (2008) Perioperative consent: How to make sure your practice is legal – Part one. *The Journal of Perioperative Practice* **8**, 326–328.

Department of Health (2003) *A Vision for the Future*. Department of Health, London.

Department of Health (2005) *NHS Performance Indicators Health Authorities*. Department of Health, London.

Department of Health (DH) (2007) www.dh.gov.uk/en/Publicationsandstatistics/…/DH_4907637

Dimond, B. (2004) *Legal Aspects of Occupational Therapy*. Blackwell Science Limited, Oxford.

Guidry, O. F. (2006) *Pre-Surgery Communication Comforts and Empowers Patients*, www.asahq.org/news/asanews040306.htm

Hakesley-Brown, R. & Malone, B. (2007) Patients and nurses; A powerful force. *OJIN: The Journal of Issues in Nursing* **1** (1). www.nursingworld.org.ojin/topic32/tpc32_4.htm

Hawighorst-Knapstein, S., Brueckner, D.O., Schoenefuss, G., Knapstein, P. G. & Koelbl, H. (2006) Breast cancer care: Patiernt information and communication as a preventive educational process. *Breast Care* **1**, 375–378.

Healthcare Commission (2005) ratings 2005. healthcarecommission.org.uk/

Health Professions Council (HPC) (2008) *Standards of Conduct, Performance and Ethics*. HPC, London.

Hind, M. cited in Woodhead, K. & Wicker, P. (2005) *A Textbook of Perioperative Care*. Elsevier Health Sciences, London.

HMSO (1995) *Reporting of Injuries, Diseases and Dangerous Occurrences Regulations (RIDDOR)*. HMSO, Norwich.

Huddleston, M. & Scoins, H. (2006) Assistant theatre practitioners: 'Must have' or needs must'? *The Journal of Perioperative Practice* **16** (10), 482–486.

Hunt, G. (2005) www.freedomtocare.org/page15.htm.

Information Centre for Knowledge and Care (2006) www.icservices.nhs.uk/clinicalgovernance/pages/default.asp

Lilleyman, J. cited in *The National Patient Safety and The Royal College of Surgeons of England Act to Protect Surgical Patients* (2005). www.reseng.ac.uk/media/medianews/National patientsafetyagency

McDonald, R., Waring, J., Harrison, S., Walshe, K. & Boaden, R. (2005) Rules and guidelines: a qualitative study in operating theatres of doctors' and nurses' views. *Quality and Safety in Health Care* **14**, 290–294.

Mental Capacity Act (MCA) (2005) www.opsigov.uk/ACTS/acts2005/ukpga_20050009_en_1

Mitchell, M. J. (2005) *Anxiety Management in Adult Day Surgery. A Nursing Perspective*. Whurr, London.

Modernisation Agency (2007) www.dh.gov.uk/Publicationsandstatistics/Publications/AnnualReports

National Confidential Enquiry Into Perioperative Deaths (NCEPOD) (2002). *Functioning as a Team: the 2002 Report of the National Confidential Enquiry into Perioperative Deaths*. NCEPOD, London.

National Clinical Assessment Service (NCAS) (2008) www.ncas.npsa.nhs.uk

National Institute for Health and Clinical Excellence (NICE) (2009) www.nice.org.uk

NHS Connecting for Health (2009). *Change Management*. www.connectingforhealth.nhs.uk/systemsandservices/capability/phi/personal

NHS Employers (2009) www.nhsemployers.org/PayAndContracts/AgendaForChange/KSF/Pages/Afc)

NHS (2009) Evidence – National Library of Guidelines. www.library.nhs.uk/GuidelinesFinder/View/Resiurce.aspx

NHS Litigation Authority (NHSLA) (2009) www.nhsla.com/Claims/Schemes/CNST

NHS Scotland (2009) Educational Resources Clinical Governance. www.clinicalgovernance.scot.nhs.uk/section1/introduction.asp

National Patient Safety Agency (NPSA) (2005) www.ncas.npsa.nhs.uk/news

Nursing Midwifery Council (NMC) (2004) *Code of Professional Conduct*. NMC, London.

Nursing Midwifery Council (2006) A–Z Advice Sheet; Clinical Supervision. London NMC. www.nmc.uk.org/aFrameDisplay.aspx?documentiD=1558

Nursing Midwifery Counci, (NMC) (2008a) *The Code: Standards of Conduct Performance and Ethics for Nurses and Midwives*. NMC, London.

Nursing Midwifery Council (NMC) (2008b) *Accountability*. NMC, London.

Patients Advice and Liaison Services (PALS) and User Involvement Groups (2007) www.dh.gov.uk/en/Managingyourorganisation/PatientAndPublicInvolvement

Perioperative Care Collaborative (PCC) (2003) Position statement. *British Journal of Nursing* **13** (9), 404–408.

Perioperative Care Collaborative (PCC) (2007) *Position Statement. Optimising the Contribution of the Perioperative Care Support Worker*. PCC, Harrogate.

Pirie, S. (2005) Support workers and the scrub role. *British Journal of Perioperative Nursing* **15** (1), 22–6.

Potter, P.A. & Berry, A.G. (1989) *Fundamentals of Nursing*. Mosby, St Louis.

Rod, P. (2003) Nurse Anaesthesia: Implications for the UK. Presentation given at the NATN. Managing Modernisation Conference, Olympia, London 16–17 May.

Royal College of Anaesthetists (2003) *The Role of Non-Medical Practitioners in the Delivery of Anaesthesia Services*. RCA, London.

Royal College of Nursing (RCN) (2003a) *Strategic Plan 2003–2008*. RCN, London.

Royal College of Nursing (RCN) (2003b). *Clinical Governance: An RCN Resource Guide*. RCN, London.

Royal College of Nursing (RCN) Direct (2008a) *A RCN Toolkit for School Nurses*. RCN, London.

Royal College of Nursing (RCN) (2008b) *Health Select Committee Inquiry Review*. RCN, London.

Royal College of Surgeons of England and Royal College of Psychiatrists (1997) *Report on the Working Party of Psychological Care of Surgical Patients (CR55)*. RCS and RCP, London.

Savage, J. & Moore, L. (2004) *Interpreting Accountability: An Ethnographic Study of Practice Nurses, Accountability and Multidisciplinary Team Decisionmaking in the Context of Clinical Governance*. RCN, London.

Shields, L. & Werder, H. (2002) *Perioperative Nursing*. Greenwich Medical Media, London.

Skills for Health (2009) Showcasing general surgery. www.healthcareworkforce.nhs.uk

Smith, R. (1998) All changed, changed utterly. British medicine will be transformed by the Bristol case. *British Medical Journal* **316** (7149), 1917–1918 (editorial).

Vincent, C., Moorthy, K., Sarker, S., Chang, S. & Darzi, A. (2004) Systems approaches to surgical quality and safety: From concept to measurement. *Annals of Surgery* **239** (4), 475–482.

Wood, J. (2004) Clinical supervision. *British Journal of Perioperative Nursing* **14** (4), 151–156.

Yule, S., Flin, R., Paterson-Brown, S. & Maran, N. (2006) Non-technical skills for surgeons in the operating room: A review of the literature. *Surgery* **139** (2), 140–149.

Managing Perioperative Risks

5

Joy O'Neill

LEARNING OUTCOMES
❏ Understand the principles of *risk assessment strategies* within the operating room.
❏ Understand the different *types of hazard* involved in risk assessment.
❏ Identify the *strategies for effective patient care* and the implications of poor practice in the following areas:
  ❏ *maintenance and use of equipment and manual handling;*
  ❏ *temperature management;*
  ❏ *pressure area care;*
  ❏ anaesthetic agents;
  ❏ latex allergy;
  ❏ *smoke inhalation;*
  ❏ deep vein thrombosis;
  ❏ infection control including *surgical site infections, methicillin-resistant* Staphylococcus aureus, Clostridium difficile.
❏ Be aware of the principles of *infection control* and the implications for the NHS if these are not observed.

RISK ASSESSMENT
The Healthcare Commission's Core Standard, C2 (2006) states that personnel working in the perioperative setting are aware of their legal and professional obligations for health and safety. There are systems in place to ensure a safe environment for patients, staff and visitors. Healthcare services are provided in environments which promote effective care and optimise health outcomes by being well designed and well maintained, with cleanliness levels in clinical and non-clinical areas that meet the national specification for clean NHS premises.

Perioperative personnel, like any other healthcare professionals, are personally accountable and, therefore, have a duty to carry out a risk assessment of all situations that may potentially cause harm to patients, or indeed, practitioners. In order to minimise any risk to patients, it is essential that there is a control mechanism for authorisation of people visiting the operating department.

The Management of Health and Safety at Work Regulations (MHSWR) imposed a responsibility on the employer to undertake risk assessments in its workplace to ensure risks are identified and reduced as much as possible. It places an obligation on the employer to actively carry out a risk assessment of the workplace and act accordingly (Beesley 2005).

In the modern, highly technical operating room environment, there is a need for perioperative practitioners to undertake risk management strategies to assess, monitor, control and prevent risks within their workplace. This will help retain quality practitioners, ensure patient safety and limit litigation costs in this complex and technical area. Risk assessment has an increasingly greater importance in the NHS as it grows more technical in nature. Strategies can identify danger or problems to healthcare practitioners, patients and visitors, and reduce financial loss to hospitals by reducing accidents.

The Association for Perioperative Practitioners (AfPP 2007) defines the following terms:

- hazard – represents the existence of an unsafe system of work, which encompasses a risk to health and safety of an employee, patient or visitor. A hazard may also involve equipment or fabric of a building which has become unsafe;
- risk – defined as the potential for harm to arise from a hazard. The extent of the risk will depend on the likelihood of that harm arising. Employers are expected to use all available information about the risks, such as relevant legislations, controls assurance, medical products, device manuals and safety instructions. The risk must be recorded either in writing or electronically and be available for risk managers and visiting inspectorates and auditors;

- patient safety incident – any unintended or unexpected event that could or has lead to harm for one or more patients receiving NHS-funded care (NPSA 2004);
- risk management – all department managers are responsible for ensuring that risk assessments are undertaken and that all staff are aware of the principles of risk management and their individual roles and accountability in reporting incidents, accidents and near misses. Organisational culture is at the heart of the learning process in risk management.

The key to effective risk management strategies for all perioperative practitioners is to be able to identify, evaluate, lessen, manage and treat any potential risks within the operating room. There is a Risk Management or Health and Safety Department within each hospital to guide all employees on safe patient and healthcare practice. Each trust devises policies that aim to prevent risks or to keep them to a minimum. Education and training are necessary to inform all practitioners of their roles and responsibilities. Perioperative practitioners should keep themselves up to date with safe practices within the operating room environment.

A risk assessment evaluates whether harm can occur because of hazards in the workplace. Health and Safety Departments in the hospitals can assess hazards and potential risks following these five steps:

1 identify the hazard and assess the harm that may occur (to practitioners, patients, carers and visitors to the operating room);
2 evaluate the risks;
3 assess existing precautions and the need for new ones;
4 identify risks as high, medium and low, and record the results;
5 review and revise the assessment, if necessary, annually or whenever relevant.

Figure 5.1 provides a flowchart of this assessment process.

In addition, managers and all members of the perioperative team have a responsibility to identify risks. Managers should:

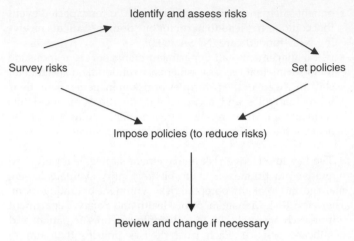

Fig. 5.1 Procedure for risk assessment.

- encourage the perioperative team to identify and analyse potential risks in their department;
- clarify risks and achieve better risk management strategies and results;
- write and revise, if necessary, protocols and policies for the perioperative team to follow;
- identify training that is necessary to ensure safe patient practices.

The effective management of risks can prevent problems from occurring and, in turn, produce efficient and cost-effective care. Risk assessment strategies recommend procedures for technical and professional perioperative practices. The health and safety of the perioperative multidisciplinary team and patients is a responsibility of employers.

Managers should:

- develop recommendations and guidelines, local policies and procedures, to prevent occupational hazards which might occur;
- recommend and produce policies and guidelines for all practitioners on equipment, medical devices and holistic patient

---

Box 5.1   Classification of hazards within the operating room environment

Accidental hazards
- Needle-stick injuries from sharps: blades and needles.
- Falls and slips on wet floors.
- Electrical shock from equipment.
- Injuries to staff and patients resulting from manual handling of patients.

Physical hazards
- Exposure to radiation (x-ray machine).
- Temperature control.

Chemical hazards
- Anaesthetic agents.
- Cleansing agents.
- Chronic poisoning due to anaesthetic gases and chemicals in cleansing agents.
- Latex allergy – exposure to latex gloves and latex-containing devices.

Biological hazards
- Exposure to blood-borne products – blood, body tissue, leading to possible hepatitis B and C, and HIV infection.
- Needle-stick injury from syringe and needle – infectious hepatitis, syphilis, malaria.
- Possibility of contacting palm and finger herpes (herpes whitlow).
- Increased hazard of spontaneous miscarriage.

Organisational factors
- Stress.

---

practices to deliver optimal care. These recommend and impose achievable practices and guidelines for the safety of patients and help to identify potential hazards in perioperative practice settings.

Hazards are classified under different headings as illustrated in Box 5.1.

Preventive measures

It is important for every member of the perioperative team to be aware of the potential hazards within the perioperative environment. They should have knowledge of the risks, preventive measures to avoid them and the procedures to follow if an incident occurs.

Safe work practices are developed within the framework of risk identification, risk assessment and risk control. Storage and ventilation of hazardous substances is a priority and all practitioners should be aware of these issues. All members of the perioperative team should adhere to protective measures that minimise risks to and from patients and equipment. Perioperative practitioners face a wide range of occupational hazards that can create risk to themselves and to their patients.

ACCIDENTAL HAZARDS

Protective clothing and safety equipment should be available for all members of the perioperative team. The aim of the principles of standard precautions is to limit the exposure of the perioperative team to blood-borne infections and spillages of blood and bodily fluids. The transmission of viruses (hepatitis B and C, and human immunodeficiency virus [HIV]) can occur in several ways: penetration of the skin by contaminated needles, splashing into the eye or through cuts and grazes.

These precautions recommend safe practices to protect the perioperative team and patients. Practitioners adopt these practices for each individual patient regardless of diagnosis. If practitioners observe these precautions within their practice, they can reduce the risk of transmission of blood-borne diseases such as hepatitis B and C, and HIV between patients and members of the perioperative team.

Hepatitis B (HepB) is a viral hepatitis caused by the virus HBV. It is transmitted by: blood or blood products, by sexual contact with an infected person or by the use of contaminated needles and instruments. Severe infection can cause prolonged illness, destruction of liver cells, cirrhosis and increased risk of liver cancer or death. A HepB immunoglobulin, a passive immunising agent, can be prescribed for exposure to the HepB virus.

Hepatitis C (HepC) is a type of hepatitis transmitted most commonly by blood transfusion or percutaneous inoculation (sharing of needles by drug users or when they share straws for nasal inhalation of cocaine). It is transmitted less commonly by sexual intercourse. The disease progresses to chronic hepatitis in up to 80% of patients who are acutely infected.

HIV is a retrovirus that causes acquired immunodeficiency syndrome (AIDS). HIV is transmitted through contact with an infected individual's blood, semen, breast milk, cervical secretions, cerebrospinal fluid or synovial fluid (Mosby's Medical, Nursing and Allied Health Dictionary 2002).

Perioperative practitioners should regard all patients as potentially infectious and should adopt standard precautions in their care. The surgeon and anaesthetist will schedule patients who are known to have an infectious disease at the end of the operating list to ensure effective management of their care.

Guidelines include:

- use of protective clothing, including gowns, gloves, eye protection (goggles, glasses with side shields, face masks with visors), aprons and shoes. These all protect the perioperative team from hazardous substances and exposure to blood-borne products;
- wash hands before and after contact with individual patients, and before putting on and removing gloves;
- the surgeon should adopt double gloving if applicable;
- cover all cuts and grazes;
- wear gloves and other protective clothing when handling swabs, instruments and specimens;
- clean up any spillages of blood or bodily fluids. Dispose of wipes into the clinical waste bag;
- take care when filling the specimen containers with formalin as this can be hazardous. Practitioners should report any accidents or spillages and take the appropriate action to ensure their health (normal saline should be available as an eyewash);
- observe safe practices with sharps, blades and needles. It is the responsibility of the individual members of the perioperative team to dispose of their own sharps;
- use a 'hands-free' technique when handing scalpel blades or syringes and needles to the surgeon. Place them in a receiver from which the surgeon can take them and replace them after use. When two surgeons are operating, each must have their own receiver;

- rinse off excessive blood from the surgical instruments before sending the instrument sets to the Hospital Sterilisation and Decontamination Unit (HSDU);
- dispose of all protective wear in the clinical waste bin and linen bag. Each patient has an individual bag or bags and the perioperative practitioner can identify the clinical waste bag by an individual number which matches the patient's linen bag.

To prevent exposure to blood and bodily fluids and needle-stick injuries from sharps (blades and needles), all perioperative practitioners should follow their 'local sharps policy.' Members of the perioperative team should handle, remove or dispose of any sharps safely in a sharps container. They should:

- avoid sharps use where possible;
- place the sharps bin near the point of use if possible (anaesthetists undertaking venous and arterial cannulation);
- take responsibility when using sharps and during their disposal into the sharps bin. If other practitioners dispose of the sharps or needles they should inform the user of their disposal;
- not resheathe, bend or break needles before disposal;
- change the sharps bin when it is three-quarters full and replace it. No member of the perioperative team should ever put their hands in the sharps bin to recover any item.

If perioperative practitioners suffer a needle-stick injury, they must follow their local policy. They have to gain the patient's consent to take a sample of his or her blood for testing. If the patient undergoes a general anaesthetic, it is important to wait several hours until the patient is fully awake and *compos mentis* before a member of the perioperative team informs the patient of the incident. The patient has the right to refuse. The practitioner also informs the Occupational Health Department and completes an incident report to the operating room manager.

It is essential that there is effective communication between all relevant departments. If there is a positive exposure to an infectious virus of a member of the perioperative team, professional counselling and follow-up services should be available.

Standard precautions are summarised in Box 5.2.

WASH HANDS
Hands should be washed:

- before and after individual patient care;
- before setting up a trolley using an aseptic technique;
- after contact with blood or bodily fluids;
- before handling food;
- after personal contact (blowing your nose or toileting).

MAINTENANCE OF EQUIPMENT
Perioperative practitioners use, clean and store all medical equipment following the manufacturer's instructions and receive training on how to operate it and care for it. Any faults are reported to the appropriate practitioner and they ensure that the Medical Electronic Department checks it before reuse. Appropriate documentation is completed to ensure effective tracking of faulty equipment following local policies. The management provides service agreements for all equipment.

Perioperative practitioners should report any faults in electrical equipment to avoid the hazard of electrical shock.

All practitioners must be aware of the location and use of emergency equipment. They must attend annual mandatory lectures on resuscitation, fire and manual handling.

See Chapter 2 for further discussion on managing perioperative equipment.

MANUAL HANDLING
It is the employer's responsibility to ensure that all employees are not exposed to a foreseeable risk of injury from manual handling as set out in the Health and Safety at Work Etc Act 1974 and the Manual Handling Operations Regulations 1992 (HSE 1992).

Employer's measures to minimise risks for practitioners are to:

Box 5.2   Standard precautions

Gown, apron, shoes
- Wear these when necessary to protect against blood and bodily fluids.
- Dispose of them in the clinical waste bag after use.

Gloves
- Wear gloves before handling blood or bodily fluids.
- Do not go from one care intervention to another on the same patient wearing the same gloves.
- Dispose of the gloves in the clinical waste bag after use.

Eye protection
- Wear a face mask with visor, goggles and glasses with side shields to protect you from any splashes of blood or bodily fluids.
- Dispose of them in the clinical waste bag after use.

Cuts and grazes
- Cover all cuts and grazes.
- Protect your skin from any infection.
- Wear gloves if relevant.
- After use wash your hands.

Sharps: blades or needles
- Dispose of sharps in a sharps bin according to local policy.
- Wear gloves if relevant.
- After use wash your hands.

Waste and linen
- Dispose of clinical waste following local policy.
- Dispose of linen in a red alginate bag (water soluble) and a laundry bag.
- Wear gloves if appropriate.
- After use wash your hands.

Equipment
- Wear gloves and appropriate clothing when cleaning equipment.

Cleaning the theatre
- Clean the operating table and any relevant equipment between operations.
- Use mops for floors. Clean them following local policies.
- Use warning signs to advise the perioperative team of wet floors.

Specimens
- Wear appropriate clothing when handling specimens and specimen containers.

- implement a local policy;
- induct all new practitioners;
- provide annual mandatory manual handling tutorials and training on new equipment;
- identify personnel's health problems and injuries from manual handling.

Employee's responsibilities are to:

- take reasonable care with his or her own and patient safety during manual handling;
- use equipment in accordance with local policy;
- have sufficient personnel present when transferring patients;
- report any incidents involving patients or perioperative personnel;
- attend an annual mandatory lecture on manual handling.

Factors that predispose practitioners to injury during patient handling are:

- lifting patients;
- working in an awkward, unstable or crouched position, including bending toward, sideways or twisting the body;
- lifting with a starting (or finishing) position near the floor, or overhead or at arm's length;
- handling an uncooperative patient or falling patient (RCN 2003).

The manual handling of patients is a potentially hazardous procedure to both patients and staff. The incidence of manual handling accidents is higher in the health service than in the rest of the working population. Safe positioning requires competent skills and an underpinning knowledge of the physiological implications of the patient's position. Therefore, no member of the perioperative team, regardless of his or her designation, should be allowed to take part unsupervised in the positioning of patients until they have received instruction, and have been assessed as proficient in the techniques involved. A record of proficiency in manual handling techniques is kept on the individual employee training file and updated annually (AfPP 2007).

The Association of Perioperative Registered Nurses' (AORN) recommended practices for positioning the patient in the perioperative practice setting (AORN 2005) state that the patient's position should provide optimum exposure for the procedure and access to intravenous (IV) lines and monitoring devices. Attention must be given to patient comfort and safety, as well as circulatory, respiratory, musculoskeletal and neurological structure. The procedure, surgeon preference and patient condition determine the equipment used for positioning. Working as a member of the team, the perioperative practitioner can minimise the risk of perioperative complications related to positioning. Positioning devices should be readily available, clean and in proper working order before placing the patient on the procedure bed. Policies and procedures related to positioning should be developed and reviewed annually, revised as necessary and be available in the practice setting.

The perioperative team coordinates the transfer of the patient from the operating trolley to the operating room table and *vice versa* following local policy. The aim of patient positioning is to provide optimal exposure of the surgical operative site and also to prevent any complications to the patient caused by nerve or tissue damage.

There should always be a sufficient number of the team available to transfer the patient to ensure his or her safety and that of the perioperative team. Practitioners should not move the patient until this is achievable. They should consult their operating room coordinator or person-in-charge. All members of the operating room team have individual and collective responsibility for patient well-being (Wilson 1995).

Patient assessment and continuous monitoring throughout the procedure for the risk of pressure injury to tissue and pressure or stretching injury to nerves are key concepts that should be included when designing education for perioperative practitioners on preventing operating room acquired injuries. In addition to the surgeon's history and physical assessment, it is important for the perioperative practitioner to perform and record a preoperative assessment to determine the patient's tolerance for the planned operative position and to identify pre-existing conditions. Additional precautions should be taken when positioning the patient for the surgery or invasive procedure if he or she is (Denholm 2009):

- 70 years of age or older;
- morbidly obese;
- thin, small in stature or has a poor preoperative nutritional status;
- diabetic or has a history of vascular disease;
- at a noted risk for pressure sores;
- undergoing a procedure planned to last more than 4 hours.

For a bariatric patient, the perioperative practitioner should communicate with the perioperative team to ensure the operating table can take the weight of the patient safely and all the appropriate devices are available for the operative procedure.

Safe and successful treatment of the morbidly obese patient requires a level of organisational commitment, protocols, expertise and staff training. These are commonly available in those hospitals that have a bariatric surgery programme, but may not necessarily be in place in hospitals that occasionally treat morbidly obese patients for non-bariatric surgical procedures, whether elective or emergency. Local protocols or policies should be in place. The risk of injury to patients and staff or damage to equipment is decreased by appropriate staff training. Special equipment may be required, as standard equipment (operating tables and transfer trolleys) is often rated to a maximum safe weight well below that of the morbidly obese patient. Wherever possible, equipment should be electronically operated, although a manual option is an essential safety feature in case of electronic failure (AAGBI 2007).

The transfer
- There should be effective communication with patients:
  — if they are awake, sedated or under regional anaesthesia to inform them of the transfer procedure;
  — between the perioperative team for general anaesthetic patients.
- The patient trolley should be as near to the operating room table as possible and in the correct position for the identified patient position.

- Anaesthetists should coordinate the transfer as they are in charge of the patient's airway and have an overall view of the patient in the transfer.
- The team should be aware of any intravenous infusions, catheters, arterial and/or central venous pressure lines, etc, medical problems or injuries (unstable limb fractures, arthritis, etc) of the patient before surgery and it should take these into consideration during the transfer.
- Practitioners should use appropriate aids to relieve pressure on the patient's nerves and tissues.

Whichever transfer equipment the perioperative team uses during transfer, it must ensure it supports the patient's head and feet and does not drag the patient across from the operating room patient trolley to the operating room table. Effective moving and handling of patients has a role to play in the prevention of pressure areas for perioperative patients. Uncoordinated or ineffective transfer can result in patient discomfort, tissue damage or formation of pressure sores.

Patient positioning is an important aspect of the care plan for patients who are undergoing surgical or other invasive procedures, and it requires a collaborative effort between the surgeon, the anaesthesia care provider and the perioperative practitioner. Aligning the patient, redistributing pressure, protecting the patient from tissue and nerve injuries, preserving IV access and physiological monitoring, and providing appropriate exposure for the procedure are all important considerations for safe and effective positioning (Denholm 2009).

PRESSURE AREAS/ULCERS

As the population ages, the incidence of pressure ulcers will increase. By 2020 those over 65 are forecast to increase from 9.2 million to 11.3 million, an increase of 23%, and they will comprise one in five of the total population (United Nations 2004).

The development of pressure ulcers is of enormous concern in all healthcare settings. A pressure ulcer is any lesion (i.e. localised area of tissue necrosis) caused by unrelieved pressure or pressure in combination with friction or shearing that results in damage to the skin or underlying tissue (Padula *et al.* 2008).

Pressure ulcers can occur any time body tissue is compromised, causing skin breakdown. Monitoring and maintaining skin integrity is an essential component of defining a patient's health status and evaluating the quality of perioperative care (Montalvo 2007).

Treating pressure ulcers represents a very significant resource cost to the health and social care system in the UK. The actual costs of preventing and treating pressure ulcers in hospitals are not readily identifiable because costs are distributed across many aspects of clinical care.

The cost of treating a pressure ulcer varies from £1064 (Grade 1, Table 5.1) to £10,551 (Grade 4, Table 5.1). Costs increase with grade because the time to heal is longer and because the incidence of complications is higher in more severe cases. The total cost in the UK is £1.4–2.1 billion annually (4% of the total NHS expenditure). Most of this cost is practitioner time and it is clear that reducing the incidence of pressure damage will

Table 5.1   Grades of pressure ulcer (European Pressure Ulcer Advisory Panel 1999).

Grade	Short Description	Definition
Grade 1	Non-blanchable erythema of intact skin	Non-blanchable erythema of intact skin. Discolouration of the skin, warmth, oedema, induration or hardness may also be used as indicators, particularly in individuals with darker skin
Grade 2	Blister	Partial thickness skin loss involving epidermis, dermis or both. The ulcer is superficial and presents clinically as an abrasion or blister
Grade 3	Superficial ulcer	Full thickness skin loss involving damage to or necrosis of subcutaneous tissue that may extend down to, but not through, underlying fascia
Grade 4	Deep ulcer	Extensive destruction, tissue necrosis or damage to muscle, bone or supporting structures with or without full thickness skin loss

not release substantial cash resources. However, practitioner time is a valuable resource with significant (and increasing) alternative uses.

Pressure ulcers represent a very significant cost burden in the UK. Without concerted effort this cost is likely to increase in the future as the population ages. To the extent that pressure ulcers are avoidable, pressure damage may be indicative of clinical negligence and there is evidence that litigation from this could soon be a significant threat to healthcare providers in the UK, as it is in the USA (Bennett *et al.* 2004).

Pressure sores may be a complication of inpatient care. All surgical patients are at risk during their perioperative journey. There is the possibility of reduced mobility as a result of circulatory and metabolic changes from anaesthesia and surgery. Pressure sores may result from compromised circulation over bony prominences, nerves or other pressure points when the practitioner and operating room team position the patient. Pressure sores can possibly go down into the muscle or even to the bone. These may become infected. It is essential that perioperative staff assess their patient and his or her risk so steps can be taken to prevent a pressure sore forming or reduce its severity.

Positioning is recognised as a crucial component of surgical care. Positioning for surgery depends on the surgeon's preference, the anaesthesia care provider's needs, the procedure being performed, the need for exposure of the surgical site and the patient's predisposing conditions (Phillips 2004 cited in Walton-Geer 2009, Montalvo 2007, AORN 2008a).

Guidelines for healthcare staff have been produced by government agencies and other professional bodies to direct them in effective patient care. The providers of these guidelines include The European Pressure Ulcer Advisory Panel (EPUAP, 1998), National Institute for Health and Clinical Excellence (NICE 2005) and the Royal College of Nursing (RCN 2005a). They have issued guidelines to assist healthcare staff with their patient care regarding pressure sores. Information on pressure sore formation and the use of pressure risk assessments are important, in conjunction with clinical judgments to understand the underlying causative factors of pressure sore for perioperative patients. These guidelines will aid healthcare staff to assess causes and identify practices to minimise the development of pressure sores in the perioperative environment.

There are multiple factors that may increase a person's risk of developing a pressure ulcer. These can be broadly separated into two categories: extrinsic, which are external to the body and can be influenced by the practitioner, and intrinsic, which are within the body and often cannot be influenced by the practitioner (Guy 2007).

Extrinsic factors
Three factors that can influence the development of pressure sores are pressure, shearing and friction.

Pressure
Pressure can be defined by its intensity and its duration. Pressure ulcers are caused by compression of soft tissue between a bony prominence and an external surface. Muscle is more sensitive than skin, underlying pressure may become necrotic by the time a lesion presents on the skin surface (Lee & Ostrander 2005 and Pieper 2007 cited in Walton-Geer 2009).

Pritchett & Mallett (1993) state the blood pressure at the arterial end of the capillaries is approximately 30 mmHg, while at the venous end this drops to 10 mmHg (the average mean capillary pressure is about 17 mmHg [Guyton 1984]). Any external pressure exceeding this will cause capillary obstruction so that tissues depending on these capillaries are deprived of their blood supply. Eventually the ischaemic tissues will die (Waterlow 1985, David 1986, Department of Infection Control, Memorial Hospital 1989, Johnson 1989). However, research has demonstrated that with constant pressure a critical period of 1–2 hours exists before pathological changes occur (Kosiak 1958, 1976).

Shearing
Shear is defined as the applied force that can cause an opposite, parallel, sliding motion in the planes of an object. Shear is affected by the amount of pressure that is exerted (Pieper 2007 cited in Walton-Geer 2009, Nix 2007).

Shearing can occur when the operating room team has to adjust the patient's position on the operating table; for example, if they drag the patient up the table instead of lifting shearing can occur. Pritchard & Mallett (1993) believe as the skeleton moves over the underlying tissue the microcirculation is destroyed and the tissues die of anoxia. In more serious cases, lymphatic vessels and muscle fibres may also become torn, resulting in a deep pressure ulcer (Waterlow 1985, Department of Infection Control, Memorial Hospital 1989, Johnson 1989).

Friction
Friction, which is the resistance created when one surface is rubbed against another, is generally acknowledged as one of the main mechanical causes of pressure ulcers (Sharp & McLaws 2005). Pritchard & Mallett (1993) believe that friction is a component of shearing which causes stripping of the stratum corneum, leading to superficial ulceration (Waterlow 1985, Johnson 1989).

Intrinsic factors
Intrinsic factors that affect the development of pressure sores in the perioperative patient include: age, level of consciousness, immobility, medical conditions (e.g. vascular disease and diabetes), malnutrition, previous pressure damage, chronic or terminal illness, smoking, alcohol abuse, neurological disease, impaired circulation and moisture. Regional anaesthesia and anaesthetic drugs may also be contributing factors (Walton-Geer 2009).

Peritoneal washout may cause the patient's canvas to be damp postoperatively and the perioperative team should either change the canvas or remove it (and dry the patient's skin) before the transfer of the patient into the recovery area.

Positioning is an important role of the perioperative practitioner in the prevention of pressure sores. When a patient has inadequate arterial blood flow, improper positioning can cause complications with blood pressure, decrease tissue perfusion and venous return, and cause thrombus formation. The patient's skin is at increased risk of tissue damage when his or her body weight is not distributed evenly on the operating table or bed or if poor perfusion is present (Phillips 2004 and O'Connell 2006 cited in Walton-Geer 2009).

Despite surgical patients' vulnerability, they do not all develop pressure sores during their perioperative journey. Waterlow (1985) states the operating room is, however, sometimes seen as the cause of any pressure sores that a surgical patient might develop. Underweight and overweight patients undergoing lengthy surgical procedures may be more at risk. It is the practitioner's responsibility to minimise this risk.

The Nursing Midwifery Council (NMC 2008) Code of Professional Conduct states that nurses should be open and honest, act with integrity and uphold the reputation of the profession; work with others to protect and promote the health and well-being of those in your care, and provide a high standard of practice and care at all times. The Health Professions Council (HPC 2008) states operating department practitioners must make sure that their knowledge, skills and performance are of a good quality, up to date and relevant to their scope of practice.

The preoperative checklist should identify the patient's vulnerability to pressure sores. An assessment of the patient's skin is essential on arrival in the operating room. Anaesthetic practitioners should assess the patient's skin integrity (heels, sacrum, elbows, shoulders, toes and any other area of the body where protection is necessary to prevent pressure occurring). They should document any problems on the patient's care plan before the surgical procedure begins. They should maintain the patient's dignity and privacy during transfer to the operating room table and inspect the patient's skin for any redness, discoloration, oedema, local indurations or pressure ulcer formation already present. If they use any pressure relieving equipment, they must record its use in conjunction with the recognised pressure-sore scale. If patients are wearing antiembolism stockings, practitioners will check that they fit properly and no pressure is placed on their skin. Stockings should be removed if necessary.

The perioperative team will position patients to avoid pressure, shearing or friction and any damage to their limbs or nerves. The operating room table should have a pressure-relieving mattress. All operating room table accessories should be made of suitable padding material to alleviate any pressure on the patient's body: heels, arms or head or relevant area. Practitioners should follow local policies and manufacturer's recommendations in the use, cleaning and storage of these accessories.

Prevention of pressure sores involves moving the patient frequently to relieve pressure on the limbs and circulation. Practitioners cannot alter the patient's position once the surgical procedure commences unless for access for the surgeon. Therefore, it is essential to position the patient correctly before surgery.

The perioperative team will inspect and assess the patient's skin for any deterioration during the surgical procedure. Practitioners will then record the results on the patient's care plan and hand over this information to the recovery practitioner.

Flanagan (1995) states that the identification of risk factors has helped the healthcare professional understand in more detail the complex aetiology of pressure sore formation. Pressure sore risk assessment scales represent an attempt to determine an individual's risk status by quantifying a range of the most commonly recognised risk factors affecting the patient at a given time. There are many risk assessment scales for practitioners to use (Norton *et al.* 1962, Gosnell 1973, Pressure Sore Prediction Scale 1975, Waterlow 1985, Braden & Bergstrom 1989).

The Waterlow Score remains the most widely used risk assessment tool in the UK as it has raised awareness of pressure sore prevention and offers practical guidelines for the management of patients. It was developed as a result of a pressure sore audit and its design offers guidelines on the selection and use of preventative equipment and dressings. It includes a pressure sore classification model which can help to improve consistency when grading and auditing tissue breakdown. The Gosnell and Braden Scales are used in the assessment and prevention of pressure sores (Flanagan 1995).

Perioperative practitioners should attend mandatory annual manual handling lectures and be able to position patients correctly following hospital local policies and guidelines. There should be relevant training in pressure sore or ulcer assessment and prevention, which identifies the risk factors, skin assessment and care, the use of pressure-relieving equipment and documentation of care. The prevention and management of pressure sores remains a high priority for all healthcare workers. In the operating room all members of the perioperative team aim to reduce patients' vulnerability to pressure area formation. Pressure relieving equipment plays an important role in the prevention and treatment of pressure sores.

RADIATION HAZARDS

To protect ovaries, testes or thyroid all members of the perioperative team use protective x-ray shields for themselves or the patient when radiological procedures are in progress. They handle, clean and replace the shields following local policy to ensure their maximum efficiency. The x-ray technician should never take an x-ray if any member of the perioperative team is not wearing a shield. Pregnant practitioners should not be present in the operating room when the patient undergoes x-rays.

If it is necessary to use x-ray equipment in the recovery room, it is essential that protective shields are worn by all recovery practitioners and patients, if appropriate. No other patient should be in the recovery room during this procedure.

AfPP (2007) states that all staff have a responsibility to protect themselves and others. They should not knowingly expose themselves or others to radiation more than is necessary. Staff must not stand in the direct primary beam and must maintain a desired distance from the beam, consistent with relevant duties. Only authorised personnel who are trained and assessed may use x-ray equipment. It is their responsibility to ensure a safe environment for all patients and staff. Protective garments, lead aprons, should be uniquely identified with a code in order that faulty equipment may be withdrawn from use, safeguarded from damage and cleaned after use – it is the responsibility of the user to return the garment in a clean condition and store appropriately. The lead apron should be examined visually at frequent intervals to ensure that it remains undamaged.

TEMPERATURE CONTROL

Patients need to maintain their normal temperature at around 37° C to ensure their organs function efficiently. The induction of anaesthesia can alter this temperature, either by raising it (malignant hyperthermia) or by lowering it (hypothermia).

Malignant hyperthermia

Malignant hyperthermia (MH), also known as malignant hyperpyrexia, is a rare inherited autosomal dominant myopathy. It is characterised by a hypermetabolic state which is triggered by exposure to some anaesthetic agents. The syndrome is thought to be due to a reduction in the reuptake of calcium by the sarcoplasmic reticulum. The reuptake of calcium is necessary for the termination of muscle contraction. Consequently, muscle contraction is sustained, resulting in signs of hypermetabolism, including acidosis, tachycardia, hypercarbia, glycosis, hypoxaemia and hyperthermia.

Some patients may develop MH despite multiple prior uneventful exposures to triggering drugs. Typically, MH is triggered by suxamethonium chloride or volatile anaesthetic agents. Some other drugs have been found to be safe in patients susceptible to MH (AfPP 2007).

It is difficult to identify patients susceptible to MH; 75% of those who develop the condition have had uneventful previous anaesthesia (Halsall & Ellis 2005).

The symptoms can cause muscle rigidity, tachycardia, unstable blood pressure and a rapidly increasing temperature. In order to combat this, anaesthetists discontinue the use of the anaesthetic agents and muscle relaxant and oxygenate (100% oxygen) the patient. They intubate the patient if necessary; administer dantrolene sodium to reduce the rapidly increasing temperature; use ice packs to help to reduce the temperature; and monitor temperature during treatment.

Hypothermia

In the perioperative environment between 60% and 90% of patients inadvertently become hypothermic (Kiekkas *et al.* 2005).

Hypothermia not only has significant negative consequences for the health of the patient, but also incurs economic expense for society in terms of increased hospital stay and additional procedures and diagnostic tests. Thus, it is paramount that all perioperative practitioners possess an in-depth understanding of inadvertent hypothermia, including risk factors, complications, and methods of prevention and treatment. It is only through use of this knowledge that practitioners can effectively fulfill their roles in the assessment, treatment and prevention of hypothermia.

The prevention and management of hypothermia centres on the correct assessment of each individual's risk for hypothermia, use of preventative strategies, monitoring of patients' temperatures routinely during the perioperative period and the employment of appropriate re-warming strategies. Clinical guidelines for the prevention and management of inadvertent hypothermia need to be readily available for practitioners and adopted for use in the perioperative environment (Hegarty 2009).

Hypothermia can be a result of impaired thermoregulation. The patient's temperature can decrease because anaesthesia inhibits the protective reflexes that generate heat (shivering). It also depresses the thermoregulating centre in the hypothalamus, decreases the basal metabolic rate and increases vasodilatation for heat loss by radiation and conduction. The exposure to the operating room environment (temperature and humidity) when the perioperative team opens and closes the operating room doors, movement of personnel, the surgical excision and skin preparation products can all help to decrease the patient's core temperature.

There are many causes cited for hypothermia. A primary cause is the cold temperature maintained in most operation rooms (i.e. below 21° C [68.8° F]). Other causes include open body cavities in abdominal and chest surgery, infusion of cold IV fluids and blood products, use of cooling irrigating solutions and skin preparations, and length of surgery. Hypothermia increases the risk of surgical site infections; increases hospital length of stay and subsequent costs and increases morbidity and mortality.

Hypothermia is one of the most preventable surgical complications and practitioners can proactively take charge to prevent it by implementing a variety of perioperative interventions. Maintaining normothermia in the surgical patient improves patient outcomes. Adverse outcomes of hypothermia include (Paulikas 2008):

- redistribution hypothermia;
- myocardial ischaemia;
- postoperative shivering;
- surgical site infection;
- blood loss and need for transfusion;
- altered medication metabolism.

Anaesthetists and anaesthetic practitioners usually measure the patient's temperature with a probe which they position in the patient's nasopharynx or oesophagus. Recovery practitioners may also use tympanic temperature monitors. To minimise and help to prevent hypothermia, the practitioner can begin care in the reception area and continue it throughout the anaesthetic room, theatre and recovery area.

Patients who are hypothermic on admission to the recovery area may have a prolonged recovery. Elderly patients can be at high risk of this anaesthetic and surgical complication. One of most important roles of anaesthetic practitioners is to maintain the patient's temperature regulation throughout his or her perioperative journey. They have a responsibility to be aware of all the complications that can occur and the correct treatment of hypothermia.

The RCN (2008) clinical guideline 'The Management of Inadvertent Hypothermia in Adults' was issued by the National Collaborating Centre for Nursing and Supportive Care (NCC-NSC) on behalf of the National Institute for Health and Clinical Excellence (NICE). Inadvertent hypothermia is a preventable complication of perioperative procedures. AORN also has issued 'Recommended Practices for Protecting Patients from Unplanned Perioperative Hypothermia' in 2007. The main aims of these guidelines are to inform perioperative practitioners of effective and cost-effective clinical management of inadvertent hypothermia issues in patient care. This is illustrated in Box 5.3.

Box 5.3   Temperature management by the perioperative practitioner

Reception
- Correct temperature of room.
- The use of blankets to ensure the patient is warm.

Anaesthetic room
- Blankets.
- Warmed intravenous fluids.

Theatre
- Correct temperature and humidity.
- Remove patient covers only before surgical procedure.
- Limit exposure to surgical site only.
- Warm irrigating fluids.
- Warmed intravenous fluids.
- Forced air skin surface warmer, e.g. Bair Hugger.
- Full monitoring body temperature.

Recovery
- Warmed intravenous fluids.
- Forced air skin surface warmer, e.g. Bair Hugger.
- Full monitoring body temperature.

CHEMICAL HAZARDS

The Health and Safety Executive (HSE 2002) states that the law requires employers to control exposure to hazardous substances in order to prevent ill health. They have to protect both employees and others who may be exposed by complying with The Control of Substances Hazardous to Health (COSHH) Regulations (2002). All members of the perioperative team should adhere to COSHH Regulations, which were introduced in 1988 and revised in 2002 by the HSE.

The employer must ensure that adequate control has been secured by:

- ensuring that all substances are COSHH-assessed in line with local guidelines;
- minimising the potential for exposure to hazardous substances by their removal or by using suitable alternatives;
- introducing measures other than personal protective equipment;

- using local exhaust ventilation during the preparation of bone cement.

Staff should be aware of procedures to be carried out in the event of injury related to such substances and suitable equipment should be available at all times (AfPP 2007).

The HSE (1999) issued guidance on the implementation of the regulations and recommended a seven-stage assessment guide for hazardous substances:

1. Identify hazardous substances in the work area and assess the risks to the employees' health.
2. Decide the precautions to take with their use.
3. Prevent exposure if possible or control the exposure.
4. Follow safe practices with their use.
5. Monitor their use and exposure to employees.
6. Carry out health surveillance where necessary.
7. Ensure all employees are aware of the hazards and safe use of the identified substances.

In the operating room environment practitioners will identify all hazardous substances and make an assessment to identify potential risks and preventive measures to limit these. Regular monitoring and documentation are necessary and named members of the perioperative team are responsible for this. They identify the hazardous substances in the operating room, which include anaesthetic vaporising agents and gases, cleansing agents, disinfectants and sterilants, and tissue preservatives.

To ensure safe practice all perioperative practitioners should store and use these products in the correct manner following local policies, wear protective attire if appropriate (standard precautions) and take care in their use. They will follow local policies if any spillages of anaesthetic agents occur. They will take care when they change any gas cylinders, following local policies and manufacturer's instructions.

Anaesthetic gases and agents
There has been considerable controversy regarding the risk to practitioners from atmospheric pollution by anaesthetic gases

and vapours. Earlier investigations suggested that perioperative practitioners are more likely than other hospital personnel to suffer from hepatic and neurological symptoms and for their children to have an increased risk of congenital abnormality. However, none of these problems has been substantiated. There was more convincing evidence from earlier studies that female practitioners who worked in the operating department during the early months of pregnancy suffered an increased incidence of spontaneous abortion. However, the most recent comprehensive and randomised prospective investigation of practitioners failed to demonstrate any increased health risk. Trace concentrations of anaesthetic gases have been implicated in impairment of professional performance. However, subsequent studies failed to confirm these findings. Nevertheless, it is sensible to minimise atmospheric pollution in the operating theatre and hospital regulations in Europe and North America require the installation of anaesthetic gas-scavenging systems in all areas where anaesthesia is administered (Aitkenhead 2007).

Perioperative practitioners must ensure that the scavenging system is working effectively. Female practitioners may have the choice to work in another area in the hospital in their first trimester if they have any concerns with their pregnancy.

The Occupational Safety and Health Administration (2002) states that potential adverse health effects of exposure to waste gases include loss of consciousness, nausea, dizziness, headaches, fatigue, irritability, drowsiness, problems with coordination and judgment, as well as sterility, miscarriages, birth defects, cancer and liver and kidney disease. Exposure to waste gases occurs from:

- poor work practices during anaesthetisation of patients;
- leaking or poor gas–line connections;
- improper or inadequate maintenance of the machine;
- patient exhalation in the recovery room or post anaesthesia care unit (PACU) during off-gassing of surgery patients.

Its recommendations to minimise this exposure are to:

- use appropriate gas scavenging systems in the operating rooms;

- provide enough ventilation in the surgical suite to keep the room concentration of waste anaesthetic gases below the applicable occupational exposure level;
- use a properly designed ventilation system;
- conduct periodic exposure monitoring;
- implement a routine ventilation system maintenance programme.

HMSO (2004) assesses and manages the potential risks of waste and anaesthetic gases in the perioperative setting by the statutory recommendations and guidance as provided by the COSHH Regulations (2004). The employer has a legal duty to inform, instruct and train individuals who are likely to be exposed to respiratory sensitisers, so they know and understand the risks to health, the symptoms of sensitisation, the importance of reporting even seemingly minor symptoms at an early stage, the proper use of control measures and the need to report promptly any failures in control measures (AfPP 2007).

LATEX ALLERGY
Latex is a natural substance which occurs in the sap of the rubber tree (*Hevea brasiliensis*). A water-soluble protein in natural latex contains an antigen that can cause a potentially fatal allergic response. Latex allergy is an allergic reaction to one or more of the components of natural rubber latex products. There are three reactions: irritation, delayed hypersensitivity (type IV) and immediate hypersensitivity (type I).

Irritation
Irritation is a non-allergic reaction which is usually reversible. A dry and itchy rash may occur after wearing gloves that contain natural rubber latex. Symptoms disappear or fade after discontinuation of use.

Delayed hypersensitivity
The accelerating agents used in the glove manufacturing process can cause contact dermatitis on the hands after glove use. This can appear after several hours and last for 24–48 hours. Further exposure can cause a rash that extends beyond the glove area.

Immediate hypersensitivity
This is a response to the protein in the natural rubber latex. It can produce a reaction after 5–30 minutes of latex exposure. The reaction will decrease after discontinuation of the latex contact. Local oedema can occur and, if the natural rubber latex comes in contact with mucous membranes, respiratory difficulties and anaphylactic shock can occur. Repetitive contact with latex can cause sensitisation. The signs and symptoms of the anaphylactic shock are hypotension, tachycardia, bronchospasm and generalised erythema.

The introduction of Universal Precautions in the late 1980s mandated that healthcare workers protect themselves against the risk of cross-infection from blood-borne pathogens such as HIV and hepatitis B. This led to an unprecedented demand for natural rubber latex (NRL) gloves, which was met by changes in some manufacturers' practice (i.e. high protein [allergen] examination gloves coming into the market place) and is believed to be the primary cause of the increased number of healthcare workers with NRL allergy. Most at risk are:

- healthcare workers;
- individuals undergoing multiple surgical procedures;
- individuals with a history of certain food allergies, such as banana, avocado, kiwi and chestnut.

Patients and staff alike are affected by latex allergy and the National Patient Safety Agency (NPSA) is working on a programme of initiatives to help to ensure that the dangers to latex-allergic patients in the NHS are minimised (HSE 2009).

Although latex gloves offer good defence against infection from blood or bodily fluids, allergy to latex is a serious health risk. It can lead to chronic ill health, early retirement or in extreme cases to death. As a result of an RCN campaign, hospitals in the NHS and independent sectors now place more emphasis on using non-powdered gloves and latex-free gloves (RCN 2002).

Because the number of individuals with latex allergy is growing around the world, it is important for medical personnel who work in areas in which NRL products are used know what NRL allergy is, which factors are associated with the allergy and what preventative measures healthcare workers can practise (Bundsen 2008).

Most of the surgical sterile gloves that the surgical scrub team wear are of natural rubber latex. All members of the multidisciplinary perioperative team may show signs of sensitivity to latex with frequent glove use. There is a risk of airborne exposure to latex allergens during the donning of pre-powdered gloves. Practitioners should be aware of this possibility through inhalation and direct contact with the glove powder.

Latex allergy protocols, for both patients and employees, are very important. Due to the potential risks associated with latex allergy and to help avoid further sensitisation, healthcare facilities should take steps to create a safe place for both patients and employees (Badger 2004).

Under Health and Safety Law (Health and Safety at Work Etc Act 1974), employers have a responsibility to reduce or remove risk as far as is reasonably practicable by establishing and maintaining a natural rubber latex safe environment. For this reason the NHS providers and trust hospitals have taken this health risk seriously and local policies are in place to minimise the risk to both patients and practitioners. Measures introduced into local policy to minimise this risk are:

Practitioners:

- to have a protocol and policy for latex allergy;
- to increase the awareness of the health risks of latex;
- to educate all practitioners of these risks;
- to reduce the use of powdered latex gloves and have non-latex gloves for latex-allergic patients. The awareness of healthcare practitioners of the potential risks of glove use and the introduction of local policies will assist in the control and decrease the prevalence of latex sensitisation and allergy;
- to purchase non-latex equipment. To identify within the operating room items of equipment (surgical and anaesthetic) that are latex-free;
- to support and test practitioners in liaison with occupational health departments;
- to advise management and practitioners of any adjustments to their perioperative practice;

- to arrange mandatory resuscitation lectures and guidelines for anaphylactic reactions.

  Patients:

- preoperative patient assessment by anaesthetists. This will identify patients who have a latex allergy;
- preparation of the theatre for the latex-allergic patient following local policy;
- effective communication of the multidisciplinary perioperative team;
- resuscitation equipment available.

Preparation for a latex-allergic patient
Measures are:

- all equipment containing latex is removed from the operating room;
- instrument sets are assessed by the Hospital Sterilisation and Disinfection Unit (HSDU) and identified as latex-free;
- non-latex gloves provided for the perioperative scrub team;
- resuscitation drugs are available;
- effective communication between the perioperative team – all are aware of the status of the patient;
- The patient is recovered within the operating room.

It is essential that a database detailing information obtained from manufacturers about the NRL content of specific products is maintained and reviewed annually. All records should be updated as new information is made available (AfPP 2007).

BIOLOGICAL HAZARDS
The risks to healthcare workers of occupational exposure to blood-borne pathogens from sharps injury have been documented since 1984, following the first reported occupational exposure to HIV. Consequently universal or standard precautions were implemented (Trim *et al.* 2003).

Herpes whitlow
The herpes simplex virus type 1 (HSV-1) causes infections of the lips, mouth and face. It is the most common herpes simplex

virus. Contact with saliva or the herpes sore can cause the perioperative practitioner to develop a herpes whitlow.

Professions at risk include health personnel and dentists exposed to oral or respiratory tract secretions. Preventative measures include avoiding treatment of patients with active infection and wearing of gloves during exposure prone procedures (Harries & Lear 2004). The wearing of gloves during intubation and extubation of the patient will help the practitioner to avoid this infection.

Smoke inhalation: surgical plume

The perioperative team and medical electrical departments take care with the use of electrosurgical equipment and the generation of smoke or plume. The thermal destruction of tissue creates a smoke by-product. This smoke may cause ocular or upper respiratory tract irritation in healthcare personnel.

Surgical smoke is the smoke produced when tissues are cut or coagulated during electrosurgery. There are three concerns that make plume and inhalation a problem:

- odour;
- particulate matter size;
- potential viability of the actual smoke.

Surgical smoke exposure can lead to hazardous chemical and biological effects on healthcare providers and patients (Barrett & Garber 2003), as well as a potentially debilitating allergic sensitisation for surgical staff members (Burge & Hoyer 1997). Perioperative practitioners and the other members of the surgical team are becoming painfully aware of the many hazards of inhaling surgical smoke. The offensive and pungent odour (caused from toxic gases that may be carcinogenic), the small size of the particulate matter and the potential for the transmission of pathogens that can cause disease are finally at the forefront of conversations in the operating room (Ball 2008).

AORN (2008b) believes that exposure to surgical smoke and bio-aerosols can and should be controlled. Healthcare professionals are responsible for learning about surgical smoke and bio-aerosols and taking steps to minimise the risks associated with these hazards.

When tissue is vaporised biological contaminants are released into the atmosphere. This can include carbonised tissue, blood or potentially infectious diseases and bacteria (Biggins 2002). Kokosa & Eugene (1989) and Ott (1994) suggest that over 80 chemicals have been identified in surgical smoke and many are known carcinogens.

Dedicated smoke evacuation machines must be used to remove the smoke, and the smoke evacuation filters should be checked and changed as per manufacturer's recommendations. The collection device should be placed as near as possible to the point where the plume is produced (AfPP 2007).

Surgeons and scrub practitioners wear face masks to protect the patient and themselves. Masks were originally designed to protect patients from the droplets expired by healthcare professionals, but today the focus of protection has shifted to how surgical masks can be used as a safeguard for the perioperative practitioners (Crook *et al.* 1996). In the future these practitioners may wear a special design of face mask to protect them, if necessary, after more research into this issue. The use of suction machines for the evacuation of the surgical smoke produced during invasive and laparoscopic surgery will also be a high priority for the safety of the perioperative practitioners.

Surgical smoke produced by an electrosurgical unit is not routinely evacuated because of factors that go beyond current guidelines and standards, and available equipment for the purpose (Dyke 1999). Local policies in the future will define practice for the disposal of surgical smoke and plume. Specialised filters may be incorporated into electrosurgery and suction machines to ensure safety for all operating room personnel.

Perioperative nurses routinely advocate for the welfare and safety of their patients. The time has come for them to be advocates for their own health and safety as well. Perioperative nurses working at healthcare organisations that have smoke evacuators should insist on using them (Bigony 2007).

ORGANISATIONAL HAZARDS

Stress

There are many reasons for stress within the operating room environment, including:

- lack of control over workload;
- time pressures;
- poor understanding of roles and competencies;
- management support;
- ineffective teams.

Recognising the signs and symptoms, and strategies to relieve stress can help the practitioner and his or her colleagues to lessen or overcome stress levels. Stress can impact on employees and patient care in the operating room environment. Support from the operating room manager and a culture of trust among work colleagues are necessary to achieve optimal patient care.

Stressors that perioperative practitioners may encounter include patient death or deterioration in the operating room, pressure to work more quickly, equipment that malfunctions, receiving contradictory instructions and working with others who are perceived to be incompetent (Kingdon & Halvorsen 2006). Practitioners' absenteeism, hostility and aggression, all of which may be signs of negative stress in the operating room, may eventually result in decreased productivity and efficiency, significantly diminishing patient safety efforts and the effective functioning of the organisation (Engel 2004).

Staff need to be valued, particularly in today's ever-changing healthcare environment (AfPP 2007). Occupational health departments have the facility for counselling services if staff become stressed. Confidential sessions can be arranged for staff if appropriate.

INFECTION CONTROL

The estimated cost of hospital-acquired infection (HACI) in 1986 was £111 million; moreover Dimond (2003) further compounds that the National Audit Office documented approximately 100,000 causes of HACI, costing the NHS £1 billion in the year 2000. Between 2004 and 2005 two outbreaks of

Clostridium difficile killed 30 people. The cost of human life forced new legislation with the publication of the Health Act 2006, which introduced the new Code of Practice for the Prevention and Control of Health Care Infections (Department of Health 2006a, Gilmour 2005).

Surgical site infections (SSIs) are a subset of a larger group of HACIs. SSIs affect many thousands of patients each year and contribute greatly to the morbidity and mortality associated with surgery (Barnett 2007). Many recent improvements in the delivery of perioperative care have focused on reducing SSIs, including using as many disposable products as possible in the operating room (Bush 2005).

The role of the perioperative practitioner is critical in the fight against SSIs. They can affect SSIs in a multitude of ways, beginning at the patient assessment and continuing through a patient's discharge from the operating room suite. Proper hand-washing is the most essential action perioperative practitioners can take to prevent SSIs. In addition, antibiotic prophylaxis, correct performance of surgical site skin prep to maintain the patient's skin integrity, maintenance of room temperature, the reduction of traffic through the operating room, the correct sterilisation of instruments and maintenance of the sterile field all contribute to prevention strategies and a comprehensive infection control plan (Plonczynski 2005).

SSI is one of the most common complications after surgery, and approximately 2.1–7% of surgical patients develop an SSI. SSI is known to increase morbidity, length of hospital stay, healthcare cost and mortality (Allen 2009).

The primary objective of infection control is to prevent the spread of infection by practitioners and patients. Practitioners have the responsibility to uphold high personal standards of infection control and to ensure that their colleagues also adhere to these. Practitioners should follow local policies and guidelines and may develop further knowledge by attending lectures to ensure optimal patient care within the perioperative environment.

The body deters infecting organisms by its defence mechanisms. The first defence is by the skin, eyes, reflexes, mucous membranes, cilia, secretions and muscular closures. The second defence incorporates inflammatory response, antibody production and temperature elevation. The third defence is by passive and active immunity. Infections can pass from patient to patient or from patient to practitioner or *vice versa* by direct (touch) or indirect contact (from equipment, linen or waste) or by droplet infection (sneezing, talking, dust).

The management strategies for infection control are to control, minimise, prevent and isolate any infection or infectious substances for all patients. Practitioners undertake interventions to prevent the infection; these include a high standard of personal hygiene, correct cleaning of the operating room, application of standard precautions and the use of anaesthetic filters with patients' breathing systems. Practitioners also maintain a clean operating room environment, set at the correct temperature and humidity.

SSIs are defined as infections related to surgical procedures that affect the surgical wound or deeper tissues handled during any given procedure. SSIs cannot be reliably identified from laboratory data alone as the diagnosis depends on the presence of signs and symptoms of infection in the wound. Therefore, surveillance to detect SSIs requires active monitoring of patients from the time of the operation until they are discharged (HPA 2007).

A major concern is that inpatient surveillance underestimates infection rates by failing to identify infections after hospital discharge (Scottish Centre for Infection & Environmental Health 2003).

Most infections in postoperative surgical wounds are acquired during surgery. They may be endogenous from the patient's own flora (i.e. from the skin, mucous membranes or gastrointestinal tract) or exogenous from the operating theatre personnel or, infrequently, from the environment. A policy for environmental cleaning in the operating theatres should be developed in collaboration with the local infection control team and housekeeping services. The policy should adhere to current microbiological recommendations and NPSA guidelines (NPSA 2007). Personnel should wear personal protective equipment, including gloves, eye protection, face mask or visor and disposable apron when cleaning (AfPP 2007).

All perioperative practitioners maintain effective principles of aseptic technique, sterile field and patient care. They should wear relevant operating room clothing and shoes and look after their own health. The length of the surgical procedure, skin preparation, the use of drains and catheters during the surgical procedure, and care interventions, such as the preoperative shave, can all increase the risk of postoperative infection.

Aseptic technique is a method employed to maintain asepsis and protect the patient HACIs. It protects the healthcare professional from being contaminated with the patient's blood, body fluids and toxic substances (Hart 2007). Aseptic technique is traditionally divided into two different processes: surgical aseptic technique and aseptic non-touch technique (ANTT) (Pratt *et al.* 2007). The perioperative practitioner should adhere to local policies for these practices.

Perioperative practitioners can be at risk from infections and it is important that they ensure their own skin integrity and cover any cuts and grazes. Exposure to infection from blood, blood-borne products and bodily fluids within the operating room environment is always a possibility. Therefore, all members of the perioperative team need to follow local infection control policies and recognise that they hope to minimise the sources of infection, interrupt their transmission and increase patient resistance. It is important that perioperative practitioners apply standard precautions to prevent contamination by any blood or blood products within their patient care.

Methicillin-resistant Staphylococcus aureus (MRSA)

In the last few years MRSA has become one of the major threats to inpatient care. *Staphylococcus aureus* is found naturally on the skin and in the nose. Sometimes these bacteria can cause an infection and in the past methicillin was given to treat these infections. Over the years resistance to this antibiotic has grown and hence it is more difficult to treat these infections now. These infections can cause skin, bone and severe blood infections and, if the postoperative patients are susceptible, the problem can be severe.

The control of MRSA in hospitals currently presents one of the most challenging aspects of infection control principles for all healthcare practitioners. It is an expensive problem for the NHS and, for the patient, the cause of skin and bloodstream infections. There is no risk to healthy people but young, old and immunocompromised patients undergoing invasive and surgical procedures are susceptible. The spread of infection is by close contact and it is transmitted between practitioners and patients by hands and also through contact with equipment, medical devices, bed linen and work surfaces.

A significant increase of MRSA during the 1990s led to infection control teams developing local policies and procedures for the management and control of the organism (RCN 2005b). Mortality rates for death involving MRSA increased over 15 fold during the period 1993–2002 (Office for National Statistics 2005).

Practitioners undertake optimal principles of infection control, including hand washing, ANTT and the surgical scrub procedure, to prevent or limit the infection by:

- placing the MRSA patient's surgical procedure last on the operating room list. The practitioner recovers the patient in the operating room and not in recovery, following local policy;
- taking simple precautions, universal or standard, which are the key to prevent the spread of MRSA;
- establishing effective communication between the perioperative team and ward practitioners;
- providing a clean operating room environment;
- being aware of local policies and guidelines

Data collection on MRSA cases in NHS acute trusts is undertaken by the Department of Health's MRSA Surveillance Scheme and results are available for the public, patients and healthcare practitioners to read.

The Department of Health's *Essential Steps to Safe and Clean Care* document represents a strategy that will assist local health economies to be mutually supportive in the commitment to reduce HACI (including those due to MRSA). Since the changes include mandatory data on *C. difficile*, it should be noted the framework contained within this document can also be used for investigation of contributing factors in the instance of *C. difficile* related-deaths (Department of Health 2006b).

The World Health Organization (WHO 2009) Surgical Safety Checklist is designed to reduce the number of errors and complications resulting from surgical procedures by improving team communication and by verifying and checking essential care interventions. It identifies a set of ten core standards to assist operating teams to reduce the number of patient safety events in the surgical environment. They can be applied universally within any healthcare setting to address issues including correct site surgery, haemorrhage risk, antibiotic prophylaxis, airway management and the risk of allergies.

DEEP VEIN THROMBOSIS (DVT)

A major risk to patients undergoing a surgical procedure is DVT – thrombo-occlusive disease of the peripheral veins. It occurs in the lower extremities and results from the reduction of venous flow due to the patient's positioning during surgical procedure. If these clots travel to the heart, lungs or brain, they can become life-threatening. A pulmonary embolism (PE) occurs when a clot travels through the heart and blocks the pulmonary arteries, and a cerebral embolism is when the brain arteries become blocked.

The '1000 Lives Campaign', launched in 2008, is aiming to improve patient safety by preventing a 1000 avoidable deaths and up to 50,000 episodes of harm across Welsh healthcare by April 2010. 'Reducing the Surgical Complications' has identified patients at risk of DVT and the provision of DVT prophylaxis interventions in order to reduce this surgical problem. DVT occurs in over 20% of surgical patients and over 40% of patients undergoing major orthopaedic surgery (NHS Wales 2008). The prevention of these complications could significantly contribute to the number of lives saved and the reduction in harm to patients.

In the WHO Surgical Safety Checklist perioperative practitioners ascertain if venous thromboembolism (VTE) prophylaxis has been undertaken. VTE is associated with inactivity during surgical procedures. The level of risk increases with the duration of the operation and period of immobility. NICE guidance advocates the documented risk assessment for every patient and provides recommendations on the most clinically and cost-effective measure for risk of VTE (NICE 2007).

AORN (2007) and NICE (2007) guidelines emphasise that an objective risk assessment for the prevention of DVT linked to appropriate thromboprophylactic interventions should be carried out for all patients. Risk assessment is an essential component in implementing care for patients perioperatively and this should be initiated on admission.

Perioperative practitioners play a key role in the prevention of DVT. They must first understand the significance of the problem, and communicate and discuss interventions with other members of the healthcare team to ensure that each patient receives the appropriate preventative interventions. When using the compression devices, practitioners need to ensure that they are able to use them competently. Policies and protocols should be in place for all staff to follow (Dipaola 2008).

Successful thromboprophylaxis is based on rigorous risk assessment and the compliance with local guidelines. The AORN (2007) and NICE (2007) guidelines are aimed at improving patient outcomes and minimising the risk associated with surgery. The use of risk assessment tools has been recognised as key to improving practice and effective thromboprophylaxis (AORN 2007, Autar 2007, NICE 2007). Early mobilisation, leg exercises, use of graduated compression stockings (GCS) and intermittent pneumatic compression devices (IPC) are examples of mechanical prophylaxis (Geerts *et al.* 2004, NICE 2007).

Antiembolism stockings

Patients wear support stockings (knee or thigh high) through their perioperative journey and postoperatively. It is important for the patient to wear the correct size and have no pressure from ruffled stockings at the top of the knee or thigh. Static compression on the legs helps to promote venous flow and reduce venous stasis.

GCS antiembolism stockings are designed to prevent blood from pooling in the veins of the leg, which may contribute to blood clot formation. These stockings are intended for use during the patient's hospital stay only. They can increase blood velocity, and reduce the incidence of venous stasis, DVT and

PEs. They should fit the patient and not cause any restriction to blood flow. GCS, once fitted, exert circumferential pressure, mechanically preventing venous distension, and reduce pooling of blood in the deep veins.

Their use, however, is contraindicated in some cases, but specifically in patients with peripheral vascular disease or diabetic neuropathy (MacLellan & Fletcher 2007, NICE 2007).

AORN (2007) and NICE (2007) guidelines advise perioperative practitioners in the safe use of mechanical devices and clinical risk assessment. Correct application and use is essential to the effectiveness of DVT mechanical prophylaxis. Practitioners need to develop their skills and keep their practice up to date. Patients wear inflatable woven leg wraps or boots during their surgical procedure. The tubing from these devices attaches to a pump which delivers compression and relaxation to the legs or feet at pressures that vary between devices. The garment inflates and deflates intermittently and has adjustable cycle times and pressures. The anaesthetic practitioner should ensure that the patient is not lying on the device tubing, as this could cause a pressure sore.

Intermittent pneumatic compression devices (IPC)
IPC devices are inflatable garments wrapped around the legs. The pneumatic pump provides an intermittent cycle of compressed air which alternately inflates and deflates the chamber garments, enhancing venous return and fibrinolytic activity (Comerota *et al.* 1997). The main contraindication to the use of these devices is peripheral vascular disease.

The DVT prophylaxis system, IPC apparatus, consists of inflatable leggings which are wrapped around the patient's calves preoperatively and fastened with velcro. Once the patient is on the operating table and has been positioned accordingly, he or she is then connected up to the pump, which can be placed under the table by tubing with snap-lock connectors, which help to prevent accidental disconnection. Should disconnection occur an alarm sounds. The pneumatic compression system inflates the stockings with air for 10–15 seconds followed by deflation of 45–50 seconds. The pump operates on a 60-second automatically timed cycle. This compresses the veins and aids return of blood to the heart, thus reducing stasis of the blood in the venous system. The recommended pressure required for DVT prophylaxis is 40 mmHg (Davis 1999).

To facilitate appropriate prophylaxis for patients a local thromboprophylactic team should be established to standardise care plans and develop a local risk assessment tool, protocols and guidelines. Local thromboprophylactic teams will have a key role auditing practice outcomes against national guidelines (Ryan & Johnson 2009).

DVT is common in hospital inpatients, both medical and surgical; for example, prior to specific prevention measures being introduced, around 30% of surgical patients developed a DVT. Furthermore, the patient often had no signs or symptoms of this serious complication. Around 100,000 people in England and Wales are estimated to suffer from venous leg ulcers often arising from a DVT. Various methods are used to promote healing but some ulcers are resistant, resulting in severe distress and often prolonged periods of hospitalisation. The NHS cost of treating venous leg ulcers is as high as £400 million per year (House of Commons 2009).

Preventive strategies

Ward assessment
Patients should be assessed to identify individual risk factors that, in addition to the proposed surgery, are known to increase the risk of developing venous thromboembolism (NICE 2007).

Positioning
The patient should be positioned using padded operating table accessories and ensuring the patient is comfortable (limbs and nerves) in the identified position.

Huntleigh Healthcare (2005) offers a comprehensive range of IPC systems for the prevention of DVT. The products are safe and help to reduce the incidence of DVT (Ginzburg *et al.* 2003). The lightweight garments (calf- or thigh-length garments, foot system or air-walk system) are made of soft, breathable fabric and have been shown to reduce oedema and postoperative pain, enhance circulation, provide a drier postoperative field and reduce wound haematoma.

Training
The perioperative practitioner should undertake training in the use of compression devices to ensure effective care of the patient. Then they will be aware of the indications, recommendations and contraindications of their single use and report any faults to the relevant personnel. They should also attend regular updates on DVT and the appliances available to reduce this disease.

CONCLUSION
All healthcare practitioners have a duty to deliver the optimum care to their patients. They must provide a safety culture within their theatre department and ensure professional development is promoted and undertaken. The safety of the patient and staff is paramount within the perioperative environment and all healthcare staff should be aware of their roles and responsibilities and be accountable for their practice. They should not be complacent and remain vigilant and focused during their clinical practice and patient care.

All members of the perioperative multidisciplinary team should adhere to policies and guidelines to promote patient and their own and colleagues' safety.

REFERENCES
Aitkenhead, A.R. (2007) Intravenous anaesthetic agents. In: Aitkenhead, A.R. & Smith, G. & Rowbotham, D.J. (eds) *Textbook of Anaesthesia*, 5th edn. Elsevier, Edinburgh, pp 34–51.

Allen, G. (2009) Evidence for practice: predictive factors for surgical site infection. *AORN Journal* **89** (2), 417–418.

Association for Perioperative Practice (AfPP) (2007) *Standards and Recommendations for Safe Perioperative Practice*. AfPP, Harrogate.

Association of Anaesthetists of Great Britain and Ireland (AAGBI) (2007) *Perioperative Management of the Morbidly Obese Patient*. AAGBI, London.

Association of Operating Room Nurses (AORN) (2005) *Recommended Practices for Positioning the Patient in the Perioperative Setting.* AORN, Denver.

Association of Operating Room Nurses (AORN) (2007) Recommended practices for prevention of unplanned perioperative hypothermia. *AORN Journal* **89** (5), 972–988.

Association of Operating Room Nurses (AORN) (2008a) *Recommended Practices for the Prevention of Unplanned Perioperative Hypothermia in Perioperative Standards and Recommended Practices.* AORN, Denver, 407–420, 497–520.

Association of Operating Room Nurses (AORN) (2008b) *AORN Position Statement on Surgical Smoke and Bio Aerosols.* AORN, Denver.

Autar, R. (2007) NICE Guidelines on reducing the risk of venous thromboembolism (deep vein thrombosis and pulmonary embolism) in patients undergoing surgery. *Journal of Orthopaedics Nursing* **11**, 169–176.

Badger, B. (2004) Latex allergy: still a challenge. *Canadian Operating Room Nursing Journal* **22** (3), 17–24

Ball, K. (2008) *Expert Advice.* www.becomenasti.com/main-content/ask-the-expert.htm

Barnett, T.E. (2007) The not-so-hidden costs of surgical site infections. *AORN Journal* **86** (2), 249–258.

Barrett, W.L. & Garber, S.M. (2003) Surgical smoke: A review of the literature. Is this just a lot of hot air? *Surgical Endoscopist* **17** (6), 979–987.

Beesley, J. (2005) Minimising the risk to patients. *Nurse 2 Nurse Magazine* **4** (1). www.n2nmagazine.co.uk/print.asp?ArticleID=297

Bennett, G., Dealey, C. & Posnett, J. (2004) The cost of pressure ulcers in the UK. *Age and Aging* **33** (3), 230–235.

Biggins, J. (2002) The hazards of surgical smoke – not to be sniffed at. *British Journal of Perioperative Nursing* **12**, 136–138, 141–143.

Bigony, L. (2007) Risks associated with exposure to surgical smoke plume: a review of the literature. *AORN Journal* **86** (6), 1013–1024.

Braden, B.J. & Bergstrom, N. (1989) Clinical utility of Braden scale for predicting pressure sore risk. *Decubitus* **2** (3), 44–46, 50–51.

Bundsen, I.-M. (2008) Natural rubber latex: a matter of concern for nurses. *AORN Journal* **88** (2), 197–209.

Burge, H.A. & Hoyer, M.E. (1997) In: DiNardi, S.R. (1997) *The Occupational Environment: Its Evaluation and Control.* 3rd Ed. AIHA Press, Fairfax, VA, p. 400.

Bush L.M. (2005) Disposable items help prevent healthcare-acquired infections. *Infection Control Today.* March 2005. http://www.infectioncontroltoday.com/articles/531feat2.html. Accessed January 26, 2010.

Comerota, A.J., Chouhan,V. & Harada, R.N. 1997 The fibrinolytic effects of intermittent pneumatic compression: mechanism of enhanced fibrinolysis. *Annals of Surgery* **228** (3), 306–313.

Control of Substances Hazardous to Health (COSHH) (2004) Amendment Regulations 2004. Her Majesty's Stationery Office (HMSO), Norwich.

Crook, B., Brown, R.C., Wake, D. and Redmayne, A.C. (1996) *Final Report to HSE. Efficiency of Respiratory Protective Equipment against Microbiological Aerosols*. HSL Report, Sheffield.

Davis, B. (1999) Towards 2000: A new age in DVT prophylaxis. *British Journal of Theatre Nursing* **9**, 116.

Denholm, B. (2009) Clinical issues: tucking patient's arms and general positioning. *AORN Journal* **89** (4), 755–757.

Department of Health (2006a) *The Health Act: Code of Practice for the Prevention and Control of Healthcare Associated Infections*. Department of Health, London.

Department of Health (DOH) (2006b) *Essential Steps to Safe, Clean Care*. www.dh.gov.uk/en/Publicationsandstatistics/Publications/PublicationsPolicyAndGuidance/DH_4136212

Dimond, B. (2003) Health and safety law: Infection control and maintaining hygiene and cleanliness. *British Journal of Nursing* **12** (1), 22–25.

Dipaola, C.A. (2008) Preventing deep vein thrombosis. *AORN* **88** (2), 283–285.

Dyke, C.N. (1999) Is it safe to allow smoke in the operating room? *Today's Surgical Nurse* March/April, 15–21.

Engel, B. (2004) Are we out of our minds with nursing stress? *Creative Nursing* **10** (4), 4–6.

European Pressure Ulcer Advisory Panel (EPUAP) (1998) *Pressure Ulcer Prevention Guidelines*. Available from: http://www.epuap.org/glprevention.html

European Pressure Ulcer Advisory Panel (EPUAP) (1999) *Statement on Pressure Ulcer Classification: Differentiation Between Pressure Ulcers and Moisture Lesions*. www.eupap.org/review6_3/page6/html

Flanagan, M. (1995) Pressure sore risk assessment. *Educational Leaflet* **3** (4), Smith and Nephew Healthcare.

Geerts, W.H., Pineo, G.F., Heit, J.A., Bergqvist, D., Lassen, M.R., Colwelt, C.W. & Ray, J.C. (2004) Prevention of venous thromboembolism. The Seventh American College of Chest Physicians conference on antithrombotic and thrombolytic therapy. *Chest* **126** (338S–400S), 1–114.

Gilmour, D. (2007) HCAIs: A statutory code of practice in England and Wales. *The Journal of Perioperative Practice* **17** (6), 266.

Ginzburg, E., Cohn, S., Lopez, J., Jackowski, J., Brown, M. & Hameed, S.M. Miami DVT Study Group (2003) Randomised clinical trial of intermittent pneumatic compression and low molecular weight heparin in trauma. *British Journal of Surgery* **90**, 1338–1344.

Gosnell, D.J. (1973) An assessment tool to identify pressure sores. *Nursing Research* **22** (1), 55–59.

Guy, H. (2007) Pressure ulcer risk assessment and grading. *Nursing Times* **103** (15), 38–41.

Guyton, A.C. (1984) *Physiology of the Human Body*, 6th edn. CBS College Publishing.

Halsall, P. & Ellis, F. (2005) Malignant hyperthermia. *Anaesthesia and Intensive Care Medicine* **6** (6), 192–194.

Hart, S. (2007) Using an aseptic technique to reduce the risk of infection. *Nursing Standard* **21** (47), 43–48.

Harries, M.J. & Lear, J.T. (2004) Occupational infections. *Occupational Medicine* **54**, 441–449.

Health and Safety at Work Etc. Act (1974) HMSO, London.

Health and Safety Executive (1992) *Manual Handling Operations Regulations*. HMSO, London.

Health and Safety Executive (1999) *Control of Hazardous Substances Hazardous to Health*. HMSO, London.

Health and Safety Executive (2002) *Control of Substances Hazardous to Health Regulations*. HSE, Suffolk.

Health and Safety Executive (HSE) (2009) *Patient Safety: Latex Allergy and Patient Safety*. www.hse.gov.uk/latex/patient.htm

Healthcare Commission (2006) *Criteria for Assessing Core Standards in 2006–2007 for Healthcare Audit and Inspection*. www.healthcarecommission.or.uk/_db/_documents/Criteria_assessing_core_standards_2006-2007.pdf

Health Professions Council (HPC) (2008) *Standards, Conduct, Performance and Ethics*. HPC, London.

Health Protection Agency (HPA) (2007) *Surveillance of Surgical Site Infection. Orthopaedic Surgery. April 2004 to March 2005*. London.

Hegarty, J. (2009) Nurses' knowledge of inadvertent hypothermia. *AORN Journal* **89** (4), 701–713.

House of Commons (2009) *Memorandum by Lifeblood: The Thrombosis Charity* (VT6).www.publications.parliament.uk/pa/cm200405/cmselect/cmhealth99/4120905.htm

Huntleigh Healthcare Ltd (2005) *Flowtron DVT Prophylactic Systems*. Huntleigh Healthcare, Luton.

Johnson, A. (1989) Granuflex wafers as a prophylactic pressure sore dressing. *Care – Science and Practice* **7** (2), 86–88.

Kiekkas, P., Poulopoulou, M., Papahatzi, M., Panagiotis, S. (2005) Effects of hypothermia and shivering on standard PACU monitoring of patients. *American Association of Nurse Anesthetists Journal* **73** (1), 47–53.

Kingdon, B. & Halvorsen, F. (2006) Perioperative nurses' perceptions of stress in the workplace *AORN Journal* **84** (4), 607–614.

Kokosa, J. & Eugene, J. (1989) Chemical composition of laser–tissue interaction of smoke plume. *Journal of Laser Applications* **July**, 59–63.

Kosiak, M. (1958) Evaluation of pressure as a factor in the production of ischial ulcers. *Archives of Physical Medicine and Rehabilitation* **40**, 62–69.

Kosiak, M. (1976) A mechanical resting surface: Its effects on pressure distribution. *Archives of Physical Medicine and Rehabilitation* **57**, 481–3.

MacLellan, D.G. & Fletcher, J.P. (2007) Mechanical compression in the prophylaxis of venous thromboembolism. *ANZ Journal of Surgery* **9** (6), 418–423.

Montalvo, I. (2007) The National Database of Nursing Quality Indicators (NDNQI) The Online Journal of Issues in Nursing 2007;**12** (3).

Mosby's Medical, Nursing and Allied Health Dictionary (2002). Elsevier Science, St Louis.

National Health Service (NHS) Wales (2008) *The 'How to Guide' for Reducing Surgical Complications*. nww.1000livescampaign.wales.nhs.uk

National Institute for Health and Clinical Excellence (2005) *Pressure Ulcers – Prevention and Treatment*. Available from: http://www.nice.org.uk/nicemedia/pdf/CG029publicinfo.pdf

National Institute for Health and Clinical Excellence (NICE) (2007) *Venous Thrombo Embolism: Reducing the Risk of Venous Thrombo Embolism (Deep Vein Thrombosis and Pulmonary Embolism) in Patients Undergoing Surgery*. www.nice.org.uk 2007

National Patient Safety Agency (NPSA) (2004) Seven Steps to Patient Safety. www.npsa.nh.uk/health/resources/7steps

National Patient Safety Agency (NPSA) (2007) *Colour Coding Hospital Cleaning Materials and Equipment*. Safer Practice Notice 15. London. NPSA. www.npsa.nhs.uk/site/media/documents/2140_0429colourcodingsp1D2F4.pdf

Nix, D.P. (2007) Patient assessment and evaluation of healing. In: Bryant, R.A. & Nix, D.P. (eds) *Acute and Chronic Wounds: Current Management Concepts*, 3rd edn. Mosby, St Louis, pp 566–578.

Norton, D., McLaren, R. & Exton-Smith, A.N. (1962) *An Investigation of Geriatric Nursing Problems in Hospitals*. National Corporation for the Care of Old People, London.

Nursing Midwifery Council (2008) *Code of Standards of Conduct, Performance and Ethics for Nurses and Midwives*. NMC, London.

Occupational Safety and Health Administration (OSHA) (2002) *Guidelines for Workplace Exposures in Surgical Suite Module*. www.osha.gov.SLTC.etools/hospital/surgical/surgical.html

Office for National Statistics (ONS) (2005) Deaths involving MRSA: England & Wales 1993–2003. *Health Statistics Quarterly*, No 25. ONS, London.

Ott, D. (1994) Smoke production & smoke reduction in laparo-scopic surgery procedures. *Surgical Services Management* **3** (3), 11–13.

Padula, C.A., Osborne, E. & Williams, J. (2008) Prevention and early detection of pressure ulcers in hospitalized patients. *Journal of Wound Ostomy Continence Nursing* **35** (1), 65–75.

Paulikas, C.A. (2008) Prevention of unplanned hypothermia. *AORN Journal* **88** (3), 358–364.

Plonczynski, D.J. (2005) In Barnett, T.E. (2007) The not-so-hidden costs of surgical site infections. *AORN Journal* **86** (2), 249–258.

Pratt, R.J., Pellowe, C.M. & Wilson, J.A. *et al.* (2007) Epic 2: National evidence-based guidelines for preventing healthcare associated infections in NHS hospitals in England. *Journal of Hospital Infection* **65S**, S1–S64.

Pressure Sore Prediction Scale (1975) Cited in Flanagan, M. (1995) Pressure sore risk assessment. *Education Leaflet* **3** (4), Smith and Nephew Healthcare.

Pritchett, A.P. & Mallett, J.M. (1993) *The Royal Marsden Hospital Manual of Clinical Nursing Procedures*, 3rd edn. Blackwell Science, Oxford.

Royal College of Nursing (RCN) (2002) *Working Well: A Call to Employers*. RCN, London.

Royal College of Nursing (2003) *Manual Handling Assessments in Hospitals and the Community. An RCN Guide*. RCN, London.

Royal College of Nursing (RCN) (2005a) *The Management of Pressure Ulcers in Primary and Secondary Care: A Clinical Practice Guideline*. RCN, London.

Royal College of Nursing (RCN) (2005b) *Methicillin-Resistant Staphylococcus Aureus (MRSA) Guidance for Nursing Staff*. RCN, London.

Royal College of Nursing (RCN) (2008) *The Management of Inadvertent Perioperative Hypothermia in Adults*. www.rcn.or.uk/development/practice/clinicalguidelines/perioperative_hypothermia_inadvertent

Ryan, K. & Johnson, S. (2009) Preventing DVT: a perioperative per-spective. *Journal of Perioperative Practice* **19** (2) 55–59.

Scottish Centre for Infection and Environmental Health (2003) *Surveillance of Surgical Site Infection*. SSHAIP, Glasgow.

Sharp, C.A. & McLaws, M.-L. (2005) *A Discourse on Pressure Ulcer Physiology: The Implications Of Repositioning and Staging. World Wide Wounds*. www.worldwidewounds.com/2005/october/Sharp/Discourse/On/Pressure-Ulcer-Physiology.html

Trim, J.C., Adams, D. & Elliott, T.S. (2003) Healthcare workers' knowledge of inoculation injuries and glove use. *British Journal of Nursing* **12** (4), 215–221.

United Nations (2004) *World Population Prospects*. United Nations (Annual), London.

Walton-Geer, P.S. (2009) Prevention of pressure ulcers in the surgical patient. *AORN Journal* **89** (3), 538–548.

Waterlow, J. (1985) A risk assessment card. *Nursing Times* **81** (49), 49–55.

Wilson, J. (1995) Clinical risk management in theatres. Professional practice. Are you a team player? *British Journal of Theatre Nursing* **4** (11), 5–7.

World Health Organisation (WHO) (2009) *Surgical Safety Checklist* www.who.int/patientsafety/safesurgery/...checklist/...index. html

Section 2

Perioperative Practice

6 | A Route to Enhanced Competence in Perioperative Care

Paul Wicker and Jill Ferbrache

LEARNING OUTCOMES

❏ Discuss the *developing role of the perioperative practitioner*.
❏ *Identify the competencies* displayed by experienced perioperative practitioners and anaesthetic assistants.

INTRODUCTION

Perhaps the greatest change in the perioperative environment has been in the roles of perioperative practitioners, who have now developed into integrated and autonomous members of the multidisciplinary team. The aim of this chapter is to discuss the competencies displayed by qualified perioperative practitioners and anaesthetic assistants.

This chapter is based on two important pieces of work to develop perioperative competencies which were carried out by NHS Education Scotland (NES) working parties (A Route to Enhanced Competence 2001–2002 [NES 2002] and Portfolio of Core Competencies for Anaesthetic Assistants 2006–2008 [NES 2008]). The working parties developed portfolios which guide professional development both in the early years of practice and when developing into the role of the anaesthetic assistant. Both portfolios can be downloaded in full from the NHS Education website (http://www.grafix2art.co.uk/qacpd/qacpdportfolios.html and http://www.nes.scot.nhs.uk/documents/publications/classa/260208_13358NESAA.pdf).

The perioperative care competencies have been used for many years in perioperative programmes throughout the UK, and there is now a need to update them in line with the developing role of perioperative practitioners. The anaesthetic assistant competencies were released in 2008 and are being used extensively in anaesthetic and recovery programmes in colleges and universities throughout the UK.

ROLE OF THE PERIOPERATIVE PRACTITIONER

The role of the perioperative practitioner begins even before the patient enters the operating department. Chapter 7 discusses the advantages of preoperative visiting by a practitioner. The main aims of this visit are to gain information which will help to plan the patient's care in the operating department. The visit can also help to educate the patient, which may help relieve anxiety. Chapters 4, 8, 9 and 10 explore aspects of the role of the perioperative practitioner in depth.

The role of the perioperative practitioner, when used to its full extent, can involve a huge range of influence extending well beyond the traditional boundaries of the 'theatre doors'. Figure 6.1 shows the wide range of areas where perioperative practitioners work.

Developing role of the perioperative practitioner

In common with many other clinical specialties during the 1970s and 1980s, the role of the perioperative practitioner came under increasing scrutiny. It appeared for a while as though the nurse

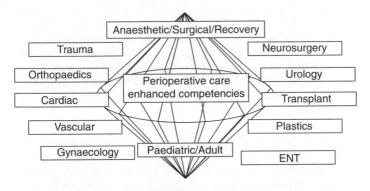

Fig. 6.1 Scope of the perioperative practitioner's experience.

as a member of the perioperative team might disappear altogether. This occurred because there was a general devaluing of what many saw as caring for an unconscious patient. Questions were being asked: 'Why is there a nurse in theatre?' and 'What is the nursing role?' The nurse's professional body, the National Association of Theatre Nurses (NATN), responded to this challenge and led the way in justifying the role of the nurse in theatre.

These questions were answered in full and even the authors of reports such as the Bevan report, which looked at the staffing and utilisation of theatres, eventually admitted there was a place for nurses in the perioperative team (Bevan 1989, 1994).

Concurrently, operating department assistants found themselves at a disadvantage because they were viewed as technical staff rather than professional practitioners. However, the increasing focus on the patient as the centre of approaches to care encouraged the move from theatre technicians, to assistants in the operating department, and finally to registered practitioners in their own right. The modern training for operating department practitioners (ODPs) provides a patient-centred approach to patient care which encourages harmony between these two professions. The Association of Operating Department Practitioners (AODP), now the College of Operating Department Practitioners (CODP), was vital in leading ODPs towards full professional registration.

The overlap in the roles and education of the two professional bodies, NATN and CODP, has continued to increase in recent years. The NATN has been proactive in this change in the perioperative team and increasingly looked at the role of the practitioner in perioperative care, rather than limiting itself to the role of nurses. This led to a change in name to the Association for Perioperative Practice (AfPP) and a redefinition of its membership to include nurses and ODPs.

The two groups of registered professionals who now perform the role of perioperative practitioner are ODPs and nurses. The ODP Diploma programme lasts either 2 or 3 years and provides the individual with a qualification tailored specifically to the perioperative environment. The courses are patient centred, evidence based, reflective and encourage autonomous practice.

They focus specifically on the care of the patient undergoing surgery or anaesthesia.

Nurses normally enter perioperative care with a preregistration Diploma or Degree in Nursing and with a broad range of experience which can include perioperative experience. Preregistration training equips nurses with transferable skills adaptable to various areas, including perioperative care; for example, airway maintenance, drug administration and pressure area care. However, nurses need to develop specific skills (e.g. anaesthetics, recovery, scrubbing and cirulating following registration and while working in the area.

The similarity between ODP diplomas and nursing diplomas, especially in the early modules, leads to greater opportunities for shared learning between the professions than was possible with the previous NVQ-based ODP courses.

Various post-registration courses are available for nurses and ODPs, none of which is essential for entry into the area, although most are required for career progression. Post-registration courses available in the UK include, for example, diplomas, degrees, postgraduate diplomas and masters in perioperative care. ODPs have had limited access to these courses in the past, mostly because their vocational background did not provide the necessary entry qualifications for higher education. However, with increasing access to preregistration education in universities and a greater familiarity with the higher education principles of teaching and learning, such access increased (Wicker & Strachan 2001) and is continuing to do so.

One of the most significant effects of this harmonisation of training has been a greater understanding of each profession's ethics of practice. Many barriers between the professions have dissolved because of the greater understanding of the approaches to patient care and the increased career opportunities that have resulted.

Practitioners now accept that the unconscious patient deserves at least as much care as the conscious patient. Perioperative practitioners, with their knowledge of the patient's preoperative and postoperative episodes of treatment and their holistic approach to patient care, are ideally placed to provide that care. Now the question that needs to be answered is 'What can registered perioperative practitioners do?' The answer can be found in the increasing number of roles that practitioners are now adopting. These include, for example, the role of advanced scrub practitioner, surgical care practitioner, the surgeon's assistant, non-medical anaesthetist and a myriad of role improvements such as cannulation, intubation, extubation and 12-lead electrocardiograph (ECG) recording.

Practitioners have adopted the role of advanced scrub practitioners in ever increasing numbers and in fact many now view this as an integral part of a scrub practitioner's role. For example, practitioners have for many years routinely prepared patients' skin with skin disinfectants, draped limbs and parts of bodies with surgical drapes, cut sutures, retracted tissues and applied dressings and bandages. These roles are now firmly embedded in practice and supported by appropriate education and a job description. This is essential both for the safety of the patient and the well-being of the practitioner.

The non-medical advanced scrub practitioner only helps the surgeon, and does not operate on the patient. However, surgical care practitioners perform surgery on the patient. There is normally a consultant surgeon available to help if necessary, possibly in another part of the hospital, but essentially the practitioner takes responsibility for undertaking the surgery alone. Well-established surgical care practitioner posts include cardiac surgeon's assistant, urology specialists who undertake cystoscopy lists and surgical practitioners who run minor plastic surgery lists using local anaesthesia.

Non-medical anaesthetists are not a new idea and have been in place in the USA and several European countries for many years. There is now a move to introduce anaesthetic assistant roles through direct entry to degree and master level programmes, without the need to go through nurse or ODP training.

The future of the perioperative team is complex. The two main groups of professionals now have the opportunity to develop closer links by harmonising their training. Into this arena also comes the generic healthcare worker, currently at NVQ Level 3, but now with increasing access to diploma and degree-level courses. The push towards patient-centred care is also obvious in this group, and developments in their training seem certain as the government strives to maintain the perioperative workforce across the country.

In response to these challenges, the main perioperative professional bodies – the AfPP, the CODP, the National Association of Assistants in Surgical Practice and the British Association of Anaesthetic and Recovery Nurses, among others, have combined in a group called the 'Perioperative Care Collaborative'. The purpose of this group is to provide a voice to represent the perioperative workforce and greater harmonisation of the workforce in the way that they work. Professional boundaries are fading fast – the emphasis must be on the roles that are provided and the care the patient needs.

ENHANCED PERIOPERATIVE COMPETENCIES

Developing the diverse and complex competencies required of an experienced perioperative practitioner starts with entry-level competence through nursing and operating department practice programmes of learning. However, it is only through experience and continuing professional development that the practitioner can develop and enhance such competencies. The experienced perioperative practitioner therefore has the potential to develop specialist knowledge and a complex portfolio of skills.

The five key areas of perioperative practice the NES Working Party (2002) identified and subdivided into their individual competencies are:

- communication;
- professional development;
- clinical leadership;
- clinical governance;
- perioperative care.

The work on the Enhanced Perioperative Competencies was developed in the form of a portfolio. It provides the framework to support a route to enhanced competence in perioperative care. The features of the portfolio are that it:

- meets the needs of perioperative practitioners from novice to experienced practitioner level;
- will have application for preparing in-house clinical courses as well as a place in informing curricula developed by higher education providers either in partnership with NHS trusts or independently;
- can be achieved as a work-based programme through rotational placements in identified, educationally audited, practice placements;
- supports programmes of preparation for qualifications in specialist practice;
- provides a bank of evidence of enhanced competence which could be presented for Accreditation of Prior Learning (AP(E)L) for specialist qualifications in perioperative care.

Completing the portfolio encourages reflection on past experience and learning to record enhanced clinical competence in perioperative care. It will help the individual practitioner to identify sources of learning and evidence of good practice for providing high-quality care. An electronic version of the NES Portfolio Route to Enhanced Competence can be downloaded from the NES Education website (www.grafix2art.co.uk/qacpd/qacpdportfolios.html).

PORTFOLIO OF CORE COMPETENCIES FOR ANAESTHETIC ASSISTANTS

In the UK a medical practitioner administers anaesthesia. As suggested by the Association of Anaesthetists of Great Britain and Ireland (AAGBI 2005b), the profession has a good safety record, with morbidity and mortality figures that compare favourably with other first-world countries. The anaesthetist is either a fully qualified specialist or an experienced anaesthetist working under supervision (AAGBI 2005a).

Anaesthetic assistants are members of the anaesthetic team. They are essential for the safe delivery of anaesthesia, which requires two practitioners with complementary skills and knowledge (AAGBI 2005a). Anaesthetic assistants are involved in many routine aspects of perioperative care and play an important role in the safe management of unforeseen clinical adverse events.

It is intended that the achievement of these competencies should form an overall level equivalent to level 9 of the Scottish Credit and Qualifications Framework (SCQF). The layout of this portfolio is intended to make it easy to use by the anaesthetic assistant in the clinical area. The anaesthetic assistant can also add evidence of learning, reflective commentary, etc into the loose-leaf format. Throughout the portfolio there are Internet links to relevant documents to aid the anaesthetic assistant in achieving the stated competency.

Utilising the reflective/competency-based elements of the portfolio, the anaesthetic assistant can accumulate evidence that may be useful for the KSF process and to satisfy the Nursing & Midwifery Council (NMC)/Health Professions Council (HPC) requirements for evidence of ongoing education for registration purposes.

Individuals already working as anaesthetic assistants can use the competencies to check their existing levels of knowledge and skill, and use the portfolio as evidence of continuing professional development.

The competencies meet the needs of the AAGBI referred to in the publication *The Anaesthesia Team* (AAGBI 2005a) and qualified in the statement issued in December 2006 and also the current NHS Quality Improvement Scotland (QIS) anaesthesia care standards (NHS QIS 2003). This document is also intended to build on such aspects of induction and orientation, rather than to replace them. It presents the competencies in two parts. Part A (Box 6.1) presents ten sections of competencies, which form the essential core required for anaesthetic assistant education and training. All competent anaesthetic assistants will be expected to have achieved all ten of these competencies or their equivalent as achieved in programmes such as the Diploma of Higher Education in Operating Department Practice.

Part B (Box 6.2) comprises a further ten sections of competencies which are specific to surgical and anaesthetic specialties.

Anaesthetic assistants working in these specialties must achieve and maintain the corresponding competencies. Not all anaesthetic assistants will be expected to have completed every

---

Box 6.1   Part A General core competencies

Section 1.1–1.8 Preparation of patients for theatre
Section 2.1–2.10 Aspects of patient care
Section 3.1–3.9 Involvement in common anaesthetic procedures
Section 4.1–4.17 Involvement in airway management
Section 5.1–5.13 Care of anaesthetic machine, monitoring and related
   equipment
Section 6.1–6.16 Care of equipment relevant to anaesthesia
Section 7.1–7.8 Participation in intra-operative patient care
Section 8.1–8.15 Involvement with routine drugs / fluid therapy
Section 9.1–9.8 Participation in post-operative patient care
Section 10.1–10.11 Involvement in emergency

Box 6.2   Part B Specialty-specific core competencies

Section 11.1–11.7 Obstetric anaesthesia and analgesia
Section 12.1–12.6 ENT
Section 13.1–13.6 Cardiac anaesthesia
Section 14.1–14.4 Thoracic anaesthesia
Section 15.1–15.3 Neurosurgery
Section 16.1–16.6 Paediatrics
Section 17.1–17.10 Anaesthesia in Remote Locations (Interventional radiol-
   ogy and ECT)
Section 18.1 Maxillofacial surgery
Section 19.1–19.3 Burns
Section 20.1– 20.5 Inter-hospital adult patient transfer

---

specific competency in this section as they may or may not have
had experience in that particular specialty.

The 20 sections of the portfolio are broken down further into
competencies. The number of competencies varies from section
to section, depending on the complexity of the competency. The
skills and knowledge required to achieve each of the competencies is provided beneath each competency.

The final aspect of the framework layout is the indicators
column. The indicators provide guidance as to what the trainee
would reasonably be expected to know or demonstrate in the
clinical setting. It also provides guidance to the clinical
assessor(s) in what they should be looking for when assessing
the trainee. The indicators provided are not exhaustive and
serve as examples. The trainee can demonstrate competency in

Box 6.3 Common themes

Theme 1 Patient care
Theme 2 Communication
Theme 3 Infection control
Theme 4 Consent to treatment
Theme 5 Manual handling
Theme 6 Professional issues
Theme 7 Clinical skills
Theme 8 Decontamination
Theme 9 Health and safety

---

other ways, provided that this fits into the overall framework and assessment process. The indicators should not be viewed as a tick list, but are used to ensure standardisation across the assessment. Some sections also contain an overview relevant to that area of practice.

Throughout the initial drafts of this document, many comments were made regarding repetition of a number of 'themes'. It was felt that to group these together would make the document more user friendly for practitioners and assessors.

Box 6.3 describes the common themes that are all applicable to achieving the competencies. Once these have been demonstrated to a competent level, they need not be reassessed. This is intended to make it easier for the practitioner to concentrate on the indicators specific to each competency in Part A and B (Boxes 6.1 and 6.2).

An example of Theme 1 can be found in Box 6.4 and an example of Competency 1 Preparation of patients for theatre in Box 6.5.

CONCLUSION

This chapter has introduced the full range of competencies – knowledge, skills and attitudes – that the experienced perioperative practitioner requires. The role of the practitioner is multifaceted – a diverse and challenging one which requires years of experience to develop fully. The following four chapters further develop some of the specific aspects of knowledge, skills and attitudes associated with the roles of anaesthetic, surgical and recovery practitioners.

Box 6.4 Theme 1 Patient care (*ensures patient care is satisfactory and individualised to each patient*)

Knowledge and skills	Indicators	Date	Performance criterion achieved	Trainee assessor
Interacts appropriately with patients Utilises appropriate aids to ensure patient comfort and safety Prepares anaesthetic room/ equipment appropriately Patient positioning	Assess, plan, deliver and evaluate individualised patient care in collaboration with all members of the multidisciplinary team Treat patient in a non-judgmental and accepting manner Demonstrate concern and respect for the individual patient and carers Maintain patient dignity at all times Demonstrate ability to use equipment/aids appropriately and effectively to reduce risk of harm to the conscious, sedated or unconscious patient Demonstrate and discuss appropriate listening and responding skills in developing relationships with patients Recognise patients' feeling of vulnerability Provide reassurance and comfort Provide appropriate physical/ psychological support and patient care to the anaesthetised, awake or sedated patient Prepare anaesthetic room to receive patient, ensuring all equipment and drugs are available for proposed anaesthetic Utilise knowledge to anticipate individual patient requirements Discuss the importance of correct positioning Discuss the term compartment syndrome and the appropriate prevention strategies			

Box 6.5   Section 1 Preparation of patients for theatre

Fitness for anaesthesia and surgery

Many clinical factors identified preoperatively have a bearing on perioperative anaesthetic care. The anaesthetic assistant (AA) must be aware of the factors, which affect patient care, and should be able to outline how these factors might influence choice of anaesthetic technique. Preoperative investigations are part of the perioperative safety net: clinically significant abnormal values should be identified by the AA and their risks understood. The AA should be able to identify many preoperative risks (e.g. a missed ranitidine pre-med) and bring these to the attention of the anaesthetist. The concept of the American Society of Anaesthesiologists (ASA) (www.asahq.org/clinical/physicalstatus.htm) scoring system is international, and a foundation for assessing fitness for anaesthesia and surgery. Airway assessment is an important part of anaesthetic assessment, and because the AA assists in securing the airway it is important that he or she understands how the anaesthetist anticipates difficulty with airway manipulations. Fasting protocols are designed to help protect patients from aspiration of gastric contents. These are part of routine preoperative assessment, and the AA should be aware of those situations where the benefits of fasting are unpredictable, or where fasting is inappropriate. Transferring, positioning and protecting the obese patient represents a shared challenge for the AA and the anaesthetist, as all aspects of local and general anaesthesia are made more difficult and more prone to complications.

1.1 Competency Understands the assessment, significance, and limitations of the ASA score

Knowledge and skills	Indicators	Date performance criterion achieved	Trainee	Assessor
The ASA score, including its correlation with operative mortality	Define the ASA classification Discuss the clinical differences between the ASA scores			
The anaesthetist may present a patient as 'ASA 4'; the AA must understand the important clinical implications of this	Demonstrate ability to prepare anaesthetic room and theatre to provide individualised patient care, taking into account ASA scores			

Cont.

Box 6.5 *Continued*

1.2 Competency Aware of anaesthetic factors in the pre-operative clinical assessment of patients

Knowledge and skills	Indicators	Date performance criterion achieved	Trainee	Assessor
Basic clinical assessment of cardiovascular, respiratory, renal, neurological, haematological, hepatic, endocrine and GI systems with emphasis on factors which have a bearing on anaesthetic care	Use patient's records to recognise those pre-existing medical conditions which may adversely affect the patient during anaesthesia			
The AA should recognise important factors affecting anaesthesia (see the checklist-related competencies, 2.1 and 2.2) and know the more important clinical implications	Ensure anaesthetist and wider multidisciplinary team are aware of relevant pre-existing medical conditions			

ACKNOWLEDGEMENT

The authors would like to acknowledge the support of NHS Education Scotland in giving permission for the use of their material in this chapter.

NES PERIOPERATIVE WORKING PARTIES

A Route to Enhanced Competence (NES 2002)

Paul Wicker
Garry Bodsworth
Liz Gillies
Jill Ferbrache   Ann Molloy
Claire Lewsey   Jackie McHage
Jackie Leslie   Linda Dunion
Steve McIntosh   Christine Hughes
Christine Allan   Sue Johnston
Caroline McDonald   Liz Wood
Raymond Rose   Agnes Lafferty
Rosanne Robinson   Jackie McKendrick
Sue Johnstone

Core Competencies for Anaesthetic Assistants (NES 2008)

Heather Hosie   Frances Dodd
Dorothy Armstrong   Jill Ferbrache
Steve McIntosh   Carole Morley
John Hampson   May Hodgson
Claire Lewsey   Morag Gray
Sherran Milton   Ken Barker
Sue Hendry   Stuart Somerville
George Inglis   Alistair McDiarmid
Christine McPhee   Mary Glasgow

REFERENCES

Association of Anaesthetists of Great Britain and Ireland (AAGBI) (2005a) *The Anaesthesia Team*. AAGBI, London. www.aagbi.org/pdf/the_anaesthesia_team.pdf

Association of Anaesthetists of Great Britain and Ireland (AAGBI) (2005b). *Catastrophes in Anaesthetic Practice – dealing with the aftermath*. AAGBI, London. www.aagbi.org/pdf/catastrophes.pdf

Bevan, P. (1989) *Report on the Management and Utilisation of Operating Departments*. DHSS, London.

Bevan, P. (1994) Bevan on Bevan. *British Journal of Theatre Nursing* **4** (8), 5–6.

National Health Service Education Scotland (NES) (2002) *A Route to Enhanced Competence in Perioperative Practice*. NES, Scotland.

National Health Service Education Scotland (NES) (2008) *Core Competencies for Anaesthetic Assistants*. NES, Scotland.

NHS Quality Improvement Scotland (NHS QIS) (2003) *Anaesthesia: Care Before, During and After Anaesthesia Standards*. NHS QIS, Edinburgh. www.nhshealthquality.org/nhsqis/files/Anaesthesia.pdf

Wicker, P. & Strachan, R. (2001) Advancing perioperative care. *British Journal of Perioperative Nursing* **11** (1), 28–33.

FURTHER READING AND RESOURCES

Books

Barber, P. & Robertson, D. (2009) *Essentials of Pharmacology*. Open University Press, Maidenhead.

Clancy, J. McVicar, A.J. & Baird, N. (2002) *Perioperative Practice: Fundamentals of Homeostasis*. Routledge, London.

Gruendemann, B. & Fernsebner, B. (1995) *Comprehensive Perioperative Nursing (Vols. 1 and 2)*. Jones and Bartlett Publishers, London.

Hind, M. & Wicker, P. (eds) (2000) *Principles of Perioperative Practice*. Churchill Livingstone, Edinburgh.

Nightingale, K. (ed.) (1999) *Understanding Perioperative Nursing*. Arnold, London.

Palmer, R., Burns, S. & Bulman, C. (1994) *Reflective Practice in Nursing: The Growth of the Professional Practitioner*. Blackwell Scientific, Oxford.

Schober, J.E. & Hinchliff, S.M. (1995) *Towards Advanced Nursing Practice: Key Concepts for Health Care*. Edward Arnold, London.

Walsh, M. (1991) *Models in Clinical Nursing – The Way Forward*. Baillière Tindall, London.

Journals

AORN Journal
Journal of Perioperative Practice
Journal of Advanced Perioperative Care
Nursing Times
Technic – The Journal of Operating Department Practice

Professional guidelines

Association for Perioperative Practice (AfPP) (2009) *Standards and Recommendations for Safe Perioperative Practice*. AfPP, London.

College of Operating Department Practitioners (CODP) (2003) *Scope of Professional Practice*. CODP, London.

College of Operating Department Practitioners (CODP) (2006) *The Diploma in Higher Education in Operating Department Practice Curriculum Document*. CODP, London.

College of Operating Department Practitioners (CODP) (2009) *Standards, Recommendations and Guidance for Mentors and Practice Placements in Supporting Pre-registration Education in Operating Department Practice Provision*. CODP, London.

Difficult Airway Society (DAS) *Guidelines*. Reviewed and published annually. www.das.uk.com

Health Professions Council (HPC) (2004) *Standards of Conduct, performance and ethics*. HPC, London. www.hpc-uk.org/assets/documents/1000062CHPC034HPCA5_Standards_of_conduct_performance_and_ethics.pdf

The Perioperative Care Collaborative (2007) *Position Statement, Delegation: the Support Worker in the Scrub Role*. Association for Perioperative Practice, Harrogate.

The Perioperative Care Collaborative (2007) *Position Statement, Optimising the Role of the Perioperative Support Worker*. Association for Perioperative Practice, Harrogate.

The Perioperative Care Collaborative (2007) *Position Statement, The Role and Responsibilities of the Advanced Scrub Practitioner*. Association for Perioperative Practice, Harrogate.

Government documents

NHS Quality Improvement Scotland (NHS QIS) (2003) *Anaesthesia: Care Before, During and After Anaesthesia Standards*. NHS QIS, Edinburgh. www.nhshealthquality.org/nhsqis/files/Anaesthesia.pdf

NHS Quality Improvement Scotland (NHS QIS) (2005) *Clinical Governance and Risk Management: Achieving Safe, Effective, Patient-Focused Care – National Standards*. NHS QIS, Edinburgh. www.nhshealthquality.org/nhsqis/files/CGRM_CSF_Oct05.pdf

Scottish Medical and Scientific Advisory Committee (2002) *Anaesthetic Assistance: A Strategy for Training, Recruitment and Retention and the Promulgation of Safe Practice*. Edinburgh: Scottish Office, Edinburgh. www.scotland.gov.uk/Resource/Doc/47095/0013831.pdf

Scottish Executive (2000) *Adults with Incapacity (Scotland) Act*. www.scotland.gov.uk/Topics/Justice/Civil/16360/4927

Scottish Health Department (2001) *Decontamination of Surgical Instruments and Other Medical Devices*. www.show.scot.nhs.uk/sehd/publications/dsmid/dsimd-00.htm

www.hsedirect.com/ Health and safety website

www.ukonline.gov.uk Public face for various online government information

www.doh.gov.uk/ Department of Health website

www.hse.gov.uk Health and Safety website

www.doh.gov.uk/cjd/riskassessmentsi.htm Risk assessment of CJD and surgical instruments

www.official-documents.co.uk/ A database of official government documents

www.doh.gov.uk/nhs.htm Department of Health NHS site

www.doh.gov.uk/riskman.htm Controls assurance website

Websites

www.bioserve.latrobe.edu.au/vcebiol/cat1/aos2/u3aos21.html Introduction to homeostasis

www.nmap.ac.uk Guide to quality internet resources in nursing, midwifery and the allied health professions

www.baoms.org.uk/links.html Links and resources to educational web sites

www.watchtower.org/ The official site for Jehovah's Witnesses

www.linacre.org/ A Catholic healthcare ethics site

www.healthcentre.org.uk/hc/pages/ethics.htm A directory of healthcare ethics sites

www.nhsdirect.nhs.uk/ NHS Direct online

www.nhs.uk/ NHS home page

www.rhpeo.org/ Health promotion web site

www.eddesign.com/electrosafety/index.htm CONMED online education website for electrosurgery

www.uchsc.edu/sm/chs/ Interactive human simulation website

www.rnceus.com/index.html Online education and testing

www.ethicon.com Ethicon web site

www.regent.com Regent website

www.cochrane.org/ The Cochrane Library

www.chi.nhs.uk Commission for Health Improvement

www.hqs.org.uk Health Quality Service

www.kingsfund.org.uk The Kings Fund

www.gasnet.med.yale.edu GASNet

www.rah.sa.gov.au/periops/room.htm The recovery room

www.bads.co.uk The British Association of Day Surgery

www.baccn.org.uk The British Association of Critical Care Nurses

www.show.scot.nhs.uk/SIGN/index.html The Scottish Intercollegiate Guidelines Network

Professional associations

Association for Perioperative Practice www.afpp.org.uk

College of Operating Department Practitioners www.codp.org

Association of Anaesthetists www.aagbi.org/

Royal College of Anaesthetists www.rcoa.ac.uk

Preoperative Preparation of Perioperative Patients

7

Paul Wicker

LEARNING OUTCOMES

❏ Discuss the role of the practitioner in the *preoperative preparation* of patients.
❏ Discuss *preoperative assessment* and *care planning*.
❏ Identify ways to *reduce postoperative complications* through preoperative preparation.

INTRODUCTION

Good preparation of surgical patients improves their experience of surgery and anaesthesia and leads to positive outcomes. Perioperative practitioners are in a unique position to play a part in patient preparation because of their understanding of the perioperative environment and their ability to assess the individual needs of a patient for what is likely to be one of the most significant events of their life.

Although preoperative visiting is a useful tool for achieving this aim, there is little evidence that it is used widely (Williams 2002, Holmes 2005). Perhaps the hierarchical and segmented roles that practitioners adopt in anaesthetics, surgery and recovery do not fully align with the holistic needs of the patient. Further research may identify reasons for the lack of uptake of this role on a wide scale.

Some may argue, however, that it is possible to provide safe care to patients without any preoperative assessment by practitioners other than that gained in the few moments available in the anaesthetic room before induction. The routine delivery of care to patients, developed over years through experience, may be considered to be enough to ensure that suitable equipment is available and that practitioners follow the correct procedures and give the correct care. After all, situations such as this occur in every operating department, every day, do they not?

However, practitioners should be aware that surgeons, anaesthetists and other members of the perioperative team do not necessarily share the same priorities. For example, a surgeon may not see the need for a delay in the anaesthetic room while practitioners readjust the environment to the patient's individual needs. Members of the team should understand the implications of their own knowledge of the patient and share information useful for planning patient care. For example, sharing information about the patient's inability to extend an arm or their wish to keep dentures in position until the last possible minute may help with the overall preoperative preparation for surgery or anaesthesia. These principles have been encapsulated in the Surgical Safety Checklist, issued by the World Health Organization (WHO 2008) in an attempt to encourage the perioperative team to work together in preparing the patient for safer surgery (see Chapter 8 for a full discussion of this document). Many operating rooms have now added the Surgical Safety Checklist into the standard preoperative checklists for their department.

Planned preoperative visiting is important because lack of prior knowledge of the patient means that perioperative practitioners can only react to the patient's needs, rather than proactively prepare for them (Holmes 2005). For example, it would be better to prepare preoperative patients who have a needle phobia with topical anaesthetic cream, or to be prepared to provide distraction techniques, rather than be faced by a nervous and upset patient who suddenly finds out that he or she is about to be injected with a large needle. There is also little a practitioner can do in the confines of an anaesthetic room for a patient who suddenly voices worries about their dignity during surgery.

The patient is subject to many stressors that provoke anxiety (Welsh 2000), including, for example:

- threats to his or her sense of identity;
- fear of dying;
- fear of not awakening following anaesthesia;
- threat to body image caused by scars or deformation;

- fear of an unknown environment;
- financial worries.

The patient's anxiety could also increase because of problems such as a delay in surgery, change of anaesthetist, mistakes in documentation or lack of coordination of information. The practitioner is able to address some of these problems because of their involvement with the preoperative and postoperative care of the patient; and training in communication and interpersonal relationship issues.

Practitioners within the day surgery setting often carry out preoperative assessment and visiting as a necessary part of all patients' treatment. In this area, preassessment clinics enable the multidisciplinary team to find out which preoperative medical and nursing assessments need to be undertaken. Preassessment clinics are also used for elective patients; however, the involvement of perioperative practitioners is not as widespread.

This chapter is about taking the time to make the patient's experience safer, more comfortable and better informed than it would be otherwise. It includes a discussion of preoperative education, preoperative assessment, diagnostic screening and preoperative planning to prevent perioperative complications. In today's environment of increased accountability and increased awareness of patients' rights, it could be argued that preoperative preparation of patients is a fundamental role for the practitioner, and a fundamental right for the patient.

PREOPERATIVE PREPARATION

Preoperative education

Communication with perioperative patients is one of the essential skills that practitioners must develop. Research has long shown that informed patients are better prepared for surgery, experience the best outcomes from surgery and anaesthesia, and recover faster (Boore 1975, Hayward 1978). Effective communication between the ward staff and perioperative practitioners can help this process, especially when patients have specific needs, such as bariatric patients.

Skills involved in communication with patients are many and varied, and often only develop after years of experience. The roots of communication are in interpersonal experiences and relationships. Communication is open to many influences which can either improve or block it. An anxious patient is much less likely to voice his or her worries or share information about himself or herself than a relaxed patient. Most patients are not, of course, relaxed about their forthcoming surgery. It is therefore, a challenge to practitioners to identify and overcome the patient's normal reticence to share information. The patient's capacity to learn limits the information that he or she can absorb. Noise, discomfort, high levels of activities or other distractions affecting the surrounding environment can also reduce the information a patient absorbs (Dyke 2000). See Chapter 4 for further discussion about perioperative communication.

Practitioners can employ various teaching strategies to maximise patient education. For example, Schrecengost (2001) conducted a study to discover whether the use of humour in preoperative instruction affects patients' recall of this instruction. The study involving 50 patients compared the use of cartoons in a booklet used to teach patients about three postoperative pulmonary exercises. The results of this study were inconclusive; however, they implied that humour at worst was better than no education at all, and potentially could improve it. Humorous teaching strategies may promote open, flexible communication and allow patients to ask questions they otherwise may not ask and hear instructions they otherwise may not hear (Bellert 1989). Despite being inconclusive, this study supports the argument that patient information handed over in an informal and accessible way by perioperative practitioners may help this learning.

The traditional view of preoperative visiting in the ward on the day before surgery is not the only technique available for preoperative visiting (Holmes 2005). In fact, research shows that patients hold information better when given 2 or 3 weeks before their surgery (Nelson 1995). Practitioners achieve this in day surgery through preassessment clinics, or through specially arranged preoperative education sessions similar to antenatal classes provided by midwives.

Information leaflets are a useful and effective method of providing written information. Leaflets can be especially useful when giving specific information to the patient; for example, about patient-controlled analgesia or postoperative exercises.

Gaining information for intraoperative use

Another main aim for preoperative visiting is so that the practitioner can gain valuable information about the patient which he or she uses to help plan care. This role is important for various reasons. For example, the operating list gives little information about the patient's physical and mental status. If the medical notes are not available until the patient arrives in the operating department, the practitioner may obtain some information too late to be of use in planning care. For example, patients with Creutzfeldt–Jacob disease (CJD) need special precautions which practitioners can only fully carry out with correct planning and organisation of resources (McNeil 2004).

Also, elderly patients often present with various issues that may need special attention in both patient assessment and discharge planning – including, for example, lack of home support, non-compliance with drug regimes and concurrent medical conditions (Tappen *et al.* 2001). The practitioner can only carry out activities such as team briefings, preparation of disposable equipment and materials, and informing staff if there is enough time to do so. The alternative is a sudden flurry of activity as practitioners take emergency measures to try to ensure patient and staff safety – hardly reassuring for the patient or staff.

In emergencies, for example when preparing for trauma patients, preoperative visiting is a low priority because of time restraints and the patient's immediate needs. However, a trip to the accident and emergency department before the patient's arrival in the operating department may provide essential information about issues such as the patient's physical status, degree and location of injuries and mental status. Practitioners can use this information to prepare the right equipment and resources for the patient's admission to the operating department. This is important because quick and efficient treatment of trauma patients is one of the major factors involved in successful recovery from major injuries (Wilson *et al.* 2007).

The development of a relationship between the practitioner and the patient has to occur in a much shorter time-frame during emergencies. Practitioners need to identify problems and decide on solutions quickly; these are skills that practitioners develop through years of experience of emergency situations.

Informed consent

One of the major reasons that preoperative communication is so important is to support informed consent. The practitioner's role in this varies between NHS trusts, but in all situations the patient's right to a choice in their treatment is sacrosanct.

All actions carried out on the patient need his or her consent, otherwise the patient could claim to have been assaulted. Patients usually give consent either by implication, for example when a patient raises an arm to receive an injection, or verbally, for example when a patient agrees to receive a drug. However, some procedures are so dangerous, or the choices for the patient so complex, that it is necessary to record the act of consent. Most anaesthetic and surgical procedures fall into this category. The role of the practitioner is to ensure that the surgeon, anaesthetist or practitioner undertaking that particular task has obtained the informed consent. The practitioner is not usually responsible for obtaining written consent, only ensuring that it has been obtained. The policies and procedures of the hospital, underpinned by legal practices, guide the practitioner's role in ensuring patient safety.

Informed consent concerns the rights of the patient to be told of all the implications of the planned procedure and any possible alternatives. To be valid, consent has to be informed and voluntary, and come from a legally competent source. See Chapter 4 for further discussion on informed consent.

Discharge planning

Perioperative practitioners often carry out discharge planning, especially in day surgery units. In general surgical wards it is more often the responsibility of the surgical ward staff. Practitioners may forget that patients have a life outside hospital and the practitioner may overlook preparation for discharge during the early stages of the patient's treatment. If discharge planning is considered later, it may be difficult to make the necessary arrangements. With the increased use and sophistication of technology, the time patients stay in hospital has become much reduced. The need for discharge planning has therefore increased. Discharge planning should cover such areas as:

- postoperative drugs regimes;
- mobilisation exercises;
- pain relief;
- identifying and managing complications;
- dressing changes.

Community agencies, such as social services, district nurses, intermediate care teams, occupational therapists and community-based physiotherapists can provide support for such procedures.

PREOPERATIVE ASSESSMENT

Care planning
Practitioners have generally accepted the problem-solving approach as a suitable way of approaching the care of patients. This has been defined as 'the nursing process' and involves the following stages:

- assessment;
- diagnosis;
- goal setting;
- intervention;
- evaluation.

Care planning involves all these phases, and the literature explores various approaches to care planning.

Several models of care have been proposed as frameworks for developing approaches to patient care. The purpose of these models is to place the many different approaches to patient care within a more or less logical framework, which can help practitioners systematically deliver the care required. Each model of care focuses on a particular view of the patient's needs. For example, Roper Logan and Tierney stress the daily activities of living and their importance to normal patient life patterns, whereas Roy's model focuses on the patients' adaptation to their perioperative experiences (Roy 1976, Roy & McLeod 1981, Current Nursing 2009).

Practitioners can use an appropriate model of nursing to develop approaches to the delivery of the care that their patients need. These are usually formulated into care plans, which can then be used to plan and record individualised care. Perioperative care plans are usually standard documents which are individually completed for each patient. Accuracy and completeness of documentation is important for continuity of care and patient safety. The rest of this section will focus on assessing patients' needs as the root of all care planning.

The following areas of assessment were drawn from the stages of Roy's adaptation model:

- physiological assessment;
- psychosocial assessment:
  — self-concept;
  — role function;
  — interdependence;
  — contributing stimuli.

Assessment

Physiological assessment

Physiological assessment, according to Roy's model, looks at areas such as oxygenation, nutrition, elimination, activity and rest, protection, the senses, fluids and electrolytes, neurological and endocrine function.

Physiological assessment may involve areas of perioperative patient care, such as monitoring and assessing airways, intravenous fluids, mobilisation or pain. These areas are especially important for the perioperative practitioner in the recovery area. In the anaesthetic and operating rooms, these assessments are often within the role of the anaesthetist or surgeon. However, understanding the underlying physiological needs of the patient helps the practitioner to interpret the results from the various patient monitoring devices and to react proactively to changes in the patient's condition.

Psychosocial assessment
Assessment of the patient's psychosocial needs at this level involves the patient's self-concept, role function and interdependence. Practitioners often give the reason of 'lack of time' as a reason for not assessing the patient's psychosocial needs. However, experienced practitioners are often adept at assessing these needs during their other duties, so all is not lost even if the assessment does not happen during the preoperative care-planning stage. In other words, practitioners often see this area as being important and they may need to adopt innovative ways of assessing these needs before, during or after the patient's surgery or anaesthesia. Preoperative visiting allows the practitioner to undertake this assessment before the patient's arrival in the operating department, therefore reducing the need for immediate assessment of needs at a difficult time. It should also be remembered that lack of time is not seen in law as a valid reason for not taking appropriate and accepted steps for patient care and safety.

Roy's model identifies the following areas for assessment:

- self-concept;
- role function;
- interdependence;
- contributing stimuli.

Assessing self-concept focuses on how the patients view themselves and their self-esteem. This includes the physical self (such as appearance) and the personal self (such as characteristics, opinions, values and worth). This area includes the need to help patients maintain their dignity; sometimes this can only be achieved by speaking up for the patient when he or she cannot do it for himself or herself. Dignity and advocacy are discussed in Chapter 2. During preoperative assessment, this information is worth gathering to be able to plan preoperative teaching or information giving. For example, the feelings that patients experience when facing the challenges of facial surgery affect the way they perceive surgery and their behaviour in the anaesthetic room. Addressing this area is important because the patient's cooperation and understanding are important during his or her surgery.

This model also includes an assessment of the patient's spiritual needs. Many people are spiritual, and some choose to express this through their religion. Patients relate their spirituality to the way they view the world, their place in it, their self-worth or value to themselves and others, their views on life and death, and their relationships within society. The perioperative experience affects spirituality, and its impact varies from patient to patient. A practitioner must therefore be aware of how patients express their various spiritual needs, either through religion, personal beliefs or behaviours. In particular, knowledge of religions can make the patient's perioperative experience more effective and may help the practitioner to deliver effective patient-focused care.

Assessing the patient's role can help provide care later. Role function includes primary roles such as gender and age, secondary roles such as family and work, and tertiary roles such as interests and activities. Understanding these roles helps to avoid seeing the patient just as a 'patient' rather than as a holistic being with a life outside his or her current position. How often do practitioners get a surprise when they suddenly find out that their patient is a doctor, operating department practitioner or nurse; or discover too late that a partner died the previous year of the same condition?

Assessing interdependence involves exploring the patient's relationships with his or her family and friends, and support networks, and his or her relationship with the surgeon, anaesthetist and practitioners. There are various situations where this information may be important for planning and delivering care, for example:

- when considering discharge arrangements;
- family support in the anaesthetic room;
- informing family of the patient's return to recovery;
- support from partners during surgery, e.g. during caesarean section or local procedures.

The final area of assessment in Roy's model identifies the stimuli that produce normal or abnormal behaviours. Roy describes these as focal (the immediate or provoking factors), contextual (other stimuli affecting the patient's life) and residual (underlying stimuli which are not obvious). Such stimuli could include:

- concurrent illness;
- fear of surgery;
- impact of surgery on appearance;
- impact of surgery on role in society;
- change in physical abilities following surgery;
- anticipated positive changes;
- fear of anaesthesia;
- absence from work;
- family care worries;
- pet care worries;
- fear of needles;
- previous unvoiced unsatisfactory perioperative experiences.

CARE PATHWAYS

Care pathways have been in use for some years for surgical patients. The focus by all team members on the perioperative patient, and shared common aims and outcomes, can help identify an expected pathway for patient-care requirements within a cost-effective and efficient environment (Middleton & Roberts 2000).

A care pathway is a multidisciplinary approach to planning the patient's journey from admission to discharge. This plan guides and coordinates the patient's entire experience. It is especially effective in the more predictable situations, for example during minor surgery in otherwise healthy patients. Therefore, practitioners in day surgery find it especially useful.

Care pathways are potentially able to lessen duplication of care, and can also help to encourage cross-boundary interprofessional cooperation and communication. The use of these pathways does not reduce the need for individual care, however, since variations to the expected pathway occur in almost every patient. Patient care pathways should always therefore be flexible enough to allow the judgement of individual practitioners to come into play.

DIAGNOSTIC SCREENING

Diagnostic screening sets a baseline for assessment of changes to these measurements taken during anaesthesia or surgery and to ensure the patient receives the correct treatment. Recording of these measurements is common during surgery and so practitioners need to be familiar with normal levels so they can recognise deviations as they occur. Deviations from normal levels often require medical intervention or changes to therapy.

Observations range from standard tests and observations, such as blood pressure and pulse, to more specific and interventional tests such as blood tests and electrocardiograms (ECGs). Practitioners are often involved in the initial and continuing measurement of these observations.

Baseline observations

Chapter 1 discusses the physiological changes endured by the perioperative patient. Measuring these changes gives essential information which guides medical therapy. For example, there is often a preoperative rise in blood pressure because of stress, and a drop later because of the effects of anaesthetic drugs, hypovolaemia or surgery itself. Preoperative baseline observations normally include pulse, blood pressure, respiration and temperature. Practitioners often carry out routine urinalysis on patients because this simple test can help to identify many important conditions, such as diabetes and renal disease. During preoperative visits, the practitioner can ensure that patients have given consent for these procedures, that they understand the need for the tests and that they have been informed of any results, especially if abnormal.

Laboratory tests

Perioperative patients routinely undergo several blood tests. A full blood count (FBC) is carried out to exclude conditions such as anaemia. Patients usually have their blood cross-matched before major procedures, in case blood transfusion is required later, or if the risk is deemed to be small, then their blood is just grouped and saved. Patients undergoing minor procedures, such as day surgery patients, normally have their blood grouped and saved, but not cross-matched. Measuring blood urea and electrolyte levels (commonly known as U&Es) helps to exclude organ disease, for example diabetes or renal disease. Blood sugar is tested prior to surgery and results should be available prior to the patient entering the anaesthetic room.

PREOPERATIVE INVESTIGATIONS

Patients usually undergo several preoperative investigations. They are all designed to identify conditions that affect the patient perioperatively or to identify the need for surgery or other therapies. These investigations can guide the treatment required and help to plan the surgery and anaesthesia with greater accuracy and precision.

Radio-opaque dyes are used in various situations to outline the body passages or tubes and the flow of fluids through them.

Patients requiring surgery on the cardiovascular system or vascular system of organs such as the brain or renal system often undergo arteriograms and venograms. Blood vessels injected with a radio-opaque dye are viewed by x-ray or image intensifier to assess blood flow, blockages or abnormalities in vessel walls.

A barium swallow or enema allows the gastrointestinal tract to be viewed on an x-ray monitor in real-time and the images are then recorded for later use. An endoscopic retrograde pyelogram outlines the passages of the renal system while endoscopic retrograde cholangiopancreatography outlines the gall bladder and bile ducts. These tests can help to identify abnormalities in the bile ducts and tubes and the presence of renal or gallstones.

Diagnostic imaging involves investigations such as x-ray, ultrasound, computerised tomography (CT) and magnetic resonance imaging (MRI). Development of the latter three investigations has provided a more accurate and detailed view of the body than x-ray can provide. CT, MRI and ultrasound can provide three-dimensional views of the body and highlight organs that would be invisible to x-rays. These imaging techniques may be useful to identify conditions such as cancer or cerebral aneurysms.

Patients can undergo many more investigations and it is important they are aware of their purpose and the results. This will help to ensure compliance with the investigations and will also serve to contribute to the patient's understanding of the need for further interventions. Knowledge of the surgery and the possible perioperative implications of medical interventions will help the practitioner to work with medical staff to help the patient to understand the implications and possible alternatives to his or her surgery.

REDUCING POSTOPERATIVE COMPLICATIONS

Effective preoperative assessment, planning and patient preparation can help to prevent postoperative complications. This is achieved most effectively by involving the whole multidisciplinary team so that all are aware of the purpose of the various activities. Good teamwork such as this helps to address all aspects of patient care and avoids duplication of effort.

Respiratory care

Careful respiratory assessment can reduce the risk of postoperative chest infection. Common risk factors associated with postoperative chest infection include smoking and respiratory disease, especially in the elderly (Sweitzer 2008). To give effective care in relation to breathing, the practitioner will need to consider assessment in areas such as:

- baseline observations, including temperature;
- sputum and secretions;
- cardiovascular status;
- blood results;
- pulse oximetry;
- chest drains.

Stopping smoking preoperatively is usually of benefit, although it is usually too late to consider after admission to the hospital. However, under the right circumstances patients with respiratory problems may still benefit from education to alter future habits. Drug therapy for respiratory conditions will normally be started preoperatively, for example antibiotics or bronchial dilators. It is important that the patient understands the need to continue taking these drugs even during the immediate preoperative period. Preoperative respiratory care also involves educating the patient about the importance of postoperative coughing and breathing exercises and the need for good positioning when in bed.

A multidisciplinary approach to airway assessment and management is important because no technique of airway assessment has been proven to be 100% effective (Aitkenhead & Smith 2006); therefore, a team approach may help to identify all the predisposing factors. Neacsu (2002) proposes that preassessment practitioners are involved in airway assessment for difficult intubation and can support anaesthetists in this role. Neacsu states that an extensive airway assessment would reduce the risk of airway problems, achieve best airway management, release anaesthetists for more complex tasks and record information for audit. Important factors to consider include presence of thyroid disease, jaw protrusion, state of dentition, and head and neck distension. Difficult airway intubation equipment should always be made available and ready for use if required.

Joint stiffness

Patients with stiff joints will need particular care during surgery. For example, a stiff neck will make intubation difficult and may call for the use of flexible laryngoscopes. It will be difficult to place the patient in the lithotomy position if he or she has a stiff hip. Unintentionally forcing the patient's leg into an abnormal position could lead to further damage. A stiff arm may also be compromised by placing it on an arm board or at too obtuse an angle – placing strain on the brachial plexus. Assessment of joint stiffness is therefore important and preoperative exercises, as arranged by physiotherapists, may help to prepare the patient for surgery.

Urinary problems

Urinary tract infection is one of the most common infections for postoperative patients (Berger 2005) and can lead to discomfort, complications and prolonged postoperative recovery times.

Preoperatively, good catheter care is essential to prevent colonisation postoperatively. This will include educating the patient about self-care and stressing the need to maintain good fluid intake and following medical orders on fluid balance. Practitioners should follow normal sterile techniques during catheterisation in the operating department. The practitioner often inserts the urinary catheter following intubation to reduce the patient's discomfort. However, consent is still required and the patient should be informed of this procedure and consent acquired preoperatively. Care should also be taken postoperatively while the patient is recovering from anaesthesia since a confused patient could easily damage the urinary tract trying to remove the catheter forcibly. Maintaining postoperative fluid intake is important to prevent further urinary and renal problems, especially following surgery on the urinary tract.

Pressure sores

A pressure sore is an area of necrosis caused by excessive and prolonged pressure. The damage to the skin is initially caused by failure of the blood supply resulting in tissue hypoxia. Shearing forces or friction can then cause further mechanical damage to the weakened skin. The skin then blisters, breaks into open sores or develops areas of necrosis. Chapter 5 looks at a risk assessment approach to prevention and treatment of pressure sores.

Pressure sores result in extended stays and distress to patients (Schultz 2005). Although they are potentially preventable, they remain a problem, therefore early assessment of patients is essential to reduce their incidence.

Patients at risk include the elderly and those undergoing long surgical procedures; other factors include the presence of concurrent illness, those with reduced preoperative mobility and patients with poor general health and nutrition.

Pressure sores can occur anywhere the skin has pressure applied. They are therefore not only confined to common areas such as the sacrum or heels, but can also occur because of pressure caused by ill-fitting casts, table fittings pressing on the patient and poorly placed equipment. The operating table itself has also been blamed for avoidable pressure damage (Waterlow

1996, Scott 2000) because of the firm design of the mattress. The patient therefore requires constant vigilance to prevent harm.

The risk of developing pressure sores can be assessed using scales such as Waterlow (1985) or Norton (Norton *et al.* 1962). Scales such as these assess the risk factors for developing pressure sores, including age, gender, smoking history, nutritional status, mobility, build, medication, incontinence, existing vascular diseases and proposed duration of the surgical procedure. A high score is an indicator of the high potential for skin damage, therefore practitioners can carry out suitable preventive measures to protect the patient. The use of risk-assessment scales targets resources at patients who need them, and helps to prevent the overuse of resources where they are not required.

There is a vast array of pressure relieving devices available to patients and various techniques that practitioners should employ to reduce pressure sore development. Therefore, individual assessment of the patient is essential. For example, a patient at risk from pressure sores may need frequent changes of position during surgery. This may not be possible unless the practitioner raises awareness of the problem with the surgical team and special measures are taken before and during the surgical procedure. If moving the patient is not possible because of anaesthetic or surgical constraints, then the patient should be protected by using gel pads, careful positioning to prevent hotspots developing or by using low-pressure mattresses. Again, multidisciplinary involvement in the use of these devices is essential to gain the support of all members of the perioperative team.

Deep venous thrombosis (DVT)

Preoperative assessment can help to reduce the incidence of DVT: blood clots developing in the venous circulation of the legs as a result of clotting abnormalities. DVT is common, affecting between 15% and 40% of perioperative patients undergoing general surgery (Mood & Tang 2009). The result of DVT can be potentially fatal if it results in a pulmonary embolism. Three main contributing factors include endothelial damage to blood vessels; long periods of immobility which lead to venous stagnation; and concurrent medication which affects clotting mechanisms, for example the contraceptive pill. Other contributing factors also play a part in this condition, for example dehydration, pregnancy and nephritic syndrome (Arnold 2002a).

The more complex prophylactic treatments (e.g. anticoagulant therapy or intermittent pneumatic compression therapy [IPCT] such as Flowtron boots) should be aimed at patients at high risk from this condition. Therefore, risk assessment to identify high-risk patients is an important skill for perioperative practitioners to develop (Arnold 2002a). Preassessment or preoperative visiting provides the ideal time for DVT risks assessment.

DVT risks scales such as Autar (1996) improve risk assessment. The Autar assessment tool scores the patient for seven risk factors: age, build/body mass, mobility, trauma risk, disease, special risk and type of surgical intervention. One study (Quantrill 2001) places patients into low, medium or high-risk categories with treatment given accordingly:

- low risk – graduated compression stockings (GCS);
- moderate risk – GCS plus low-dose heparin;
- high risk – GCS, adjusted dose of heparin and IPCT.

In view of the effects of DVT, it would be wise to apply some basic precautions to all patients until good research can more clearly identify ways to assess the risk of DVT developing. In all patients, education about early mobilisation is important to help prevent postoperative DVT. It also appears that GCS may be the best way to provide generalised prophylaxis according to a Cochrane review (Amaragiri & Lees 2001). However, this study did point out that GCS worked best when used with other prophylaxis measures, and made no mention of problems that can occur when ill-fitting stockings are used. GCS may also not be appropriate for all patients, for example if ulcers are present. Most units now have protocols in place for DVT prophylaxis to help protect patients from this condition.

Preoperative assessment for DVT can also alert practitioners during the intraoperative period to high-risk patients (Arnold 2002a). The perioperative practitioner can use methods to decrease the factors contributing to DVT development and minimise the risk to the patient during surgery. For example:

- reduce endothelial damage by:
  — avoiding abnormal leg positioning;
  — avoiding extreme degrees of internal and external leg rotation (e.g. during orthopaedic surgery).
- increase venous return by:
  — performing passive limb exercises on the patient during long surgery;
  — being aware of the need to avoid excessive tourniquet pressures and extended periods of inflation;
  — preferentially placing the patient in a leg-up position wherever possible to encourage venous drainage (10% leg raise produces 30% better venous drainage [Thomas 1999]);
  — avoiding placing the patient in a limb-down position to reduce the risk of oedema developing in the lower limbs which could lead to venous stagnation and endothelial damage;
  — developing good techniques for applying and using GCS or IPCT.
- decrease hypercoagulability by educating patients about the benefits of complying with drug regimes involving:
  — heparin and warfarin or other anticoagulants;
  — antiplatelet drugs such as aspirin or dextran (Arnold 2002b).

Chapter 5 looks at a risk assessment approach to prevention and treatment of DVT.

Nausea and vomiting

Postoperative nausea and vomiting (PONV) is distressing for patients at best. At worst it could result in further illness such as aspiration of stomach contents into the lungs, leading to respiratory complications, damage to wound sites caused by straining and electrolyte imbalances caused by the loss of gastric acids. PONV occurs in around 20–30% of surgical patients (Arnold 2002c).

The medical treatment of PONV is based on the use of anti-emetics to antagonise the various neurotransmitter systems causing nausea and vomiting. These include drugs such as haloperidol, ondansetron, metoclopramide and cyclizine. Antiemetics are discussed in detail in Chapter 3. However, the variety of antiemetics available implies that no one of them is particularly good at its job (Arnold 2002c). The lack of a 'perfect' antiemetic means the role of the practitioner in assessing PONV and the use of non-medical approaches to treating PONV are especially important.

Various scoring tools are available to assess the patient's risk of developing PONV. Again, none of these is particularly accurate; however, they may prove useful in some situations.

Patients who are predisposed to PONV can be identified during preoperative assessment (Tramer 2003, Royston & Cox 2003). For example, a previous episode of PONV can highlight the need to include an antiemetic with the premedication or preoperative drug regime. Other risk factors include extreme anxiety and a history of seasickness. During preoperative assessment, patients can be informed of the possibility of PONV and the advantages of antiemetic therapy. Patient education is important as many patients believe that nausea and vomiting are inevitably associated with anaesthesia and do not necessarily know that it can be prevented.

Anxiety could be a contributory cause of PONV, although this is not certain. Common sense suggests however, that patient education about the incidence of PONV and how it can be prevented or treated can only help the patient during their postoperative care by reducing anxiety about this condition. Preoperative fasting may also affect PONV; this may be especially important to consider during emergency surgery when there may not have been time to prepare the patient properly.

Careful assessment of established PONV will also help ensure the patient receives prompt and effective treatment (Arnold 2002c) – once again patient education plays a part in this process. The practitioner could also play a part in prevention of PONV by exploring the incidence of this condition during postoperative care, in order to identify predisposing factors, efficacy of drug regimes or particular successful coping strategies by the patient. See Chapter 10 for further discussion on PONV.

Pain

The preoperative assessment of pain and education of patients in the use of preventive analgesia can help to reduce postoperative pain and associated problems (Mackrodt 2001). For example, many patients' perception of pain has been affected by previous experience or information from parents or friends. Some patients may therefore expect pain as a part of the surgical procedure and without education, may think that it is unavoidable. Misconception about addiction from using opiate analgesics may also prevent patients from taking full advantage of drug therapy available. Preoperative education of what to expect, the different approaches to pain treatment and the support available for the patient may therefore help to prepare the patient for managing their postoperative pain. Chapter 10 discusses postoperative pain relief.

Some hospitals have developed an acute pain service (APS). The main aim of this service is to educate patients and practitioners in all aspects of pain management (Mackrodt 2001). This service is normally led by anaesthetists with consultant nurses specialising in pain relief. The service often offers support for the preoperative and postoperative care of patients and can include help with patient-controlled analgesia, epidural infusions and other specialised areas of pain relief.

Patient-controlled analgesia (PCA) is a common method of giving analgesia and controlling pain. The technique involves the use of an analgesic infusion which is controlled by the patient using a hand-operated device. Because it involves patient involvement, the patient must be informed of its uses, advantages and disadvantages. It is a valuable way of controlling pain which involves patients in their own recovery, helping to support the patients to a full recovery. However, PCA may not work effectively if the patient is poorly educated and not well trained in its use. PCAs can also not be used in patients with arthritis or Alzheimer's disease. In these patient, epidural infusion may be used.

See Chapter 3 for further discussion on the pharmacology of analgesia and Chapter 10 for a discussion on postoperative analgesia.

Wound infection

Wound infection is a common complication and therefore it is important the practitioner takes any preoperative measures that help to reduce the risk of this condition. See Chapter 5 for a risk assessment approach to infection control.

Preoperative education about basic hygiene and cleanliness often points the way to good practice. For example, it may be necessary to bring beds into theatre, but if they are, it would make sense to ensure they are as clean as possible. The use of clean linen may also reduce the numbers of dead skin particles brought into theatre.

The need for preoperative skin preparation should be assessed preoperatively. For example, the patient may need occlusive dressings on open skin lesions. Patients with excess hair close to operative sites may need it removed using depilatory creams or shaving. Although this practice has come under much discussion in the literature, the need for shaving or hair removal is still open to question. If it is carried out, then it usually takes place in the anaesthetic room immediately prior to surgery.

CONCLUSION

Preoperative assessment and preparation is a necessary link in the chain for delivering holistic patient care. Practitioners can act as the patient's advocate and communicate relevant information to the rest of the perioperative team, helping to provide continuity of care.

Perioperative practitioners can be instrumental in providing patients with safe, positive surgical experiences and outcomes by focusing on patients as whole beings and not merely on their operative procedures, diseases or injuries. Effective patient education and preoperative assessment helps to prepare the patient effectively for their surgery and anaesthesia. Practitioners must use the small amount of time available preoperatively, to spend quality time interacting with patients so they are safe and feel cared for and secure during their perioperative experience.

REFERENCES
Aitkenhead, A. & Smith, G. (2006) *Textbook of Anaesthesia*, 5th edn. Elsevier Health Sciences, Edinburgh.

Amaragiri, S.V. & Lees, T.A. (2001) Elastic compression stockings for the prevention of deep vein thrombosis (Cochrane Review). In: *The Cochrane Library*, Issue 4. Update Software, Oxford.

Arnold, A. (2002a) DVT prophylaxis in the perioperative setting. Part 1. *British Journal of Perioperative Nursing* **12** (8), 294–297.

Arnold, A. (2002b) DVT prophylaxis in the perioperative setting. Part 2. *British Journal of Perioperative Nursing* **12** (9), 326–332.

Arnold, A. (2002c) Postoperative nausea and vomiting in the perioperative setting. *British Journal of Perioperative Nursing* **12** (1), 24–32.

Autar, R. (1996) Nursing assessment of clients at risk of deep venous thrombosis: the Autur DVT scale. *Journal of Advanced Nursing* **23** (4), 763–770.

Bellert, J.L. (1989) Humor: A therapeutic approach in oncology nursing. *Cancer Nursing* **12** (April), 65–70.

Berger, R. (2005) Bacteria of preoperative urinary tract infections contaminating the surgical fields and developing surgical site infections in urological operations. *The Journal of Urology* **174** (6), 2244.

Boore, J. (1975) *Prescription for Recovery*. RCN, London.

Current Nursing (2009) *Application of Roy's Adaptation Model in Nursing Practice*. http://currentnursing.com/nursing_theory/application_Roy's_adaptation_model.htm (accessed 7 June 2009).

Dyke, M. (2000) Perioperative communication. In: Hind, M. & Wicker, P. (eds) *Principles of Perioperative Practice*. Churchill Livingstone, Edinburgh.

Hayward, J. (1978) Information: A prescription against pain. *Royal College of Nursing Research Society Newsletter* Series **2** (5), 36–50.

Holmes, J. (2005) Preoperative visiting: Landmarks of the journey. *British Journal of Perioperative Nursing* **15** (10), 434-443.

Mackrodt, K. (2001) The role of an acute pain service. *British Journal of Perioperative Nursing* **11** (11), 492–497.

McNeil, M. (2004) Management of a CJD case Part 1 Preoperative organisation of the case. *British Journal of Perioperative Nursing* **14** (4), 164–170.

Middleton, S. & Roberts, A. (2000) *Integrated Care Pathways: A Practical Approach to Implementation*. Elsevier Health Sciences, London.

Mood, G. & Tang, W. (2009) *Perioperative DVT Prophylaxis*. http://emedicine.medscape.com/article/284371-overview (accessed 7 June 2009).

Neacsu, A. (2002) Predication of difficult intubation: A preassessment nurses' guide. *British Journal of Perioperative Nursing* **12** (7), 249–253.

Nelson, S. (1995) Preadmission clinics for thoracic surgery. *Nursing Times* **91** (15), 29–31.

Norton, D., McLaren, R. & Exton-Smith, A.N. (1962) *An Investigation of Geriatric Nursing Problems in Hospital*. National Corporation for the Care of Old People, London.

Quantrill, S. (2001) Deep vein thrombosis: Incidence and physiology. *British Journal of Perioperative Nursing* **11** (10), 442–451.

Roy, C. (1976) *Introduction to Nursing: An Adaptation Model*. Prentice Hall, Englewood Cliffs.

Roy, C. & McLeod, D. (1981) Theory of the person as an adaptive system. In: Roy, C. & Roberts, S.L. (eds) *Theory Construction in Nursing: An Adaptive Model*. Prentice Hall, Englewood Cliffs.

Royston D, Cox F (2003) Anaesthesia: the patient's point of view. *The Lancet* **362** (9396), 1648–1658.

Schrecengost, A. (2001) Do humorous preoperative teaching strategies work? *AORN Journal* **74** (5), 683.

Schultz, A. (2005) Predicting and preventing pressure ulcers in surgical patients. *AORN Journal* **81** (5), 986–1006.

Scott, E.M. (2000) The prevention of pressure ulcers in the operating department. *Journal of Wound Care* **8** (1), 18–21.

Sweitzer, B. (2008) *Handbook of Preoperative Assessment and Management*. Lippincott Williams & Wilkins, Philadelphia.

Tappen, R.M., Muzic, J. & Kennedy, P. (2001) Preoperative assessment and discharge planning for older adults undergoing ambulatory surgery. *AORN Journal* **73** (2), 464, 467, 469.

Thomas, S. (1999) Graduated compression stockings and the prevention of deep vein thrombosis (Part 2). *Journal of Wound Care* **8** (2), 93–95.

Tramer, M.R. (2003) The treatment of postoperative nausea and vomiting. *British Medical Journal (International edition)* **327** (7418), 762.

Waterlow, J. (1985) A risk assessment card. *Nursing Times* **81** (48), 49–55.

Waterlow, J. (1996) Operating table: The root of many pressure sores? *British Journal of Theatre Nursing* **6** (7), 19–21.

Welsh J (2000) Reducing patient stress in theatre. *British Journal of Perioperative Nursing* **10** (6), 321–327.

Wilson, W., Grande, C. & Hoyt, D. (2007) *Trauma: Emergency Resuscitation, Perioperative Anesthesia, Surgical Management, Vol I*. CRC Press, London.

Williams, M. (2002) Preoperative visiting – an urban myth? *British Journal of Perioperative Nursing* **12** (5), 168.

World Health Organization (WHO) (2008) *Surgical Safety Checklist*. http://www.who.int/patientsafety/safesurgery/en/ (accessed 11 August 2009).

Patient Care During Anaesthesia

8

Joy O'Neill

LEARNING OUTCOMES
❑ Understand *roles and responsibilities of the anaesthetic practitioner*.
❑ Identify *principles and techniques of* general *anaesthesia,* regional, local anaesthesia and sedation.
❑ Understand and recognise *safe use of anaesthetic equipment.*

INTRODUCTION
Anaesthesia can be administered via different methods. Each method should be considered, taking into account the patient's medical condition and age, ideal operating condition, patient comfort and choice. The different techniques are: general anaesthesia, regional anaesthesia, local anaesthesia and sedation. These methods, use of anaesthetic equipment and the roles and responsibilities of anaesthetic practitioners will be discussed in this chapter.

Anaesthetic practitioners, who may be nurses or operating department practitioners (ODPs), are integral to operating practice and safe, effective patient care. They have responsibilities to the patients and their colleagues to maintain safe practice in the operating room environment, and for their own professional development. Patients are at their most vulnerable during their perioperative journey.

It is important that the practitioner displays a professional, confident and caring attitude to patients during their perioperative journey. They should provide a safe environment for the patient undergoing general, regional or local anaesthesia, or sedation. The aim of the practitioner is to care for the patient during his or her perioperative journey, which includes:

- reception area where the anaesthetic practitioner greets the patient and checks the preoperative document;
- anaesthetic room where the anaesthetist establishes general anaesthesia, regional anaesthesia, local anaesthesia or sedation;
- operating room where the anaesthetist and anaesthetic practitioner maintain airway management and anaesthesia;
- recovery room where the recovery practitioner extubates and monitors patients until their condition is stable enough for the porter and ward nurse to escort them back to the ward.

This list does not include all the roles and responsibilities of the individual perioperative practitioners. These are described in the different chapters of the book.

Anaesthetic practitioners have a duty to maintain their professional competence and development in operating room practice. They undertake a competency-based training programme or a recognised university anaesthetic course before commencing anaesthetic practice. They should be aware of the specialised anaesthetic equipment, relevant anaesthetic drugs and safe positioning of the patient within the operating room environment to ensure a safe perioperative journey. Other responsibilities include maintaining the correct temperature and humidity in the individual operating room for the particular surgical procedures.

Assistance for the anaesthetist may be provided by ODPs or nurses. Whatever the background, the training for all anaesthetic assistants must comply fully with national standards (AAGBI 2005).

Anaesthetic equipment should be up to date, maintained regularly and the instruction manuals should be available and accessible. Equipment checks must be performed before an operating theatre session begins because a frequent cause of misadventure is the use of a machine which has not been checked properly, and which subsequently malfunctions. A thorough check of anaesthetic apparatus is an integral part of good practice; failure to check the anaesthetic equipment properly may amount to malpractice. The final pre-use check is the sole responsibility of the anaesthetist who is to use the machine (Aitkenhead *et al.* 2007).

- Careful preoperative assessment should be undertaken to identify risk factors such as concurrent disease, chronic medication, history of allergy or other untoward reactions to anaesthesia, and potential difficulties in tracheal intubation.
- Anaesthetic equipment must be maintained according to the manufacturer's recommendations and checked thoroughly before every operating room session, or when the equipment is changed during an operative session.
- The anaesthetic technique should be recognised as relevant for the individual patient and for the proposed type of surgery.
- The anaesthetist must always be present during anaesthesia.
- Appropriate monitoring, in accordance with national recommendations, should always be employed during anaesthesia and in the immediate recovery period. Alarms should be set at suitable levels and must not be disabled.
- All anaesthetists should be taught to manage common emergencies, such as failed intubation, anaphylaxis or malignant hyperthermia. It is advisable to have protocols available in every anaesthetising location to act as an *aide-memoire* for uncommon emergencies, and anaesthetists and operating room staff should rehearse emergency management regularly.
- The anaesthetist should keep careful records.

These issues are also applicable to anaesthetic practitioners in their practice within the operating room environment.

The roles and responsibilities of anaesthetic practitioners for the patient's perioperative journey are to:

- prepare and check relevant anaesthetic equipment and drugs;
- relieve the patient's anxiety by effective reassurance and communication throughout their perioperative journey (Mitchell 2005);
- undertake the preoperative check (Figure 8.1);
- locate any missing information or documentation before the start of the surgical procedure;

Checklist	Comments of ward nurse	Comments of anaesthetic practitioner
Consent form completed correctly		
Identification bracelet		
Notes, investigations, preoperative assessment		
Operation site if applicable		
Site: left, right, both		
Allergies (please note)		
Jewellery removed or taped		
Dentures removed		
Loose teeth, dental work		
Hearing aid or prosthesis removed		
Baseline observations (blood pressure, pulse, temperature, respirations, oxygen saturation)		
Ward urinalysis		
Blood sugar		
Weight		
Waterlow score		
Deep vein thrombosis (DVT) risk (high, medium, low)		
Anti-embolitic stockings/deep vein thrombosis (DVT) prophylaxis aid used		
Last menstrual period (LMP)		
Is there any chance of the patient being pregnant? Yes or no If yes, pregnostician performed? Yes or no		
Medication Drugs accompanying patient: Premedication: Time given: Prescribed drugs are:		
Nil by mouth from		
Interpreter required? If yes, booked for:		
Patient requests		
Patient accompanied by: Qualified nurse Student Health care worker Relative Other		

Fig. 8.1 Example of a preoperative checklist.

Checklist	Comments of ward nurse	Comments of anaesthetic practitioner
Additional information (e.g. identify if patient is nervous and reassure patient in the anaesthetic room)		
Signature by ward nurse	Date	Time
Signature by theatre practitioner	Date	Time

Fig. 8.1 *Continued.*

- assist the anaesthetist in the chosen anaesthesia;
- assist in the safe positioning of the patient, to prevent pressure damage;
- monitor the patient throughout anaesthesia ensuring homeostasis is regulated;
- complete effective and accurate documentation of patient's care;
- communicate effectively with the multidisciplinary operating room team.

The preoperative checklist

In 2002, the 55th World Health Assembly adopted a resolution calling to secure the safety of healthcare and monitoring systems. In May 2004, the 57th World Health Assembly approved the creation of an international alliance for improving patient safety and the World Alliance for Patient Safety was launched in October 2004. As part of this initiative, 'The Safe Surgery Saves Lives' programme was formed. For the first time, policy makers, surgical associations, anaesthesia societies and nurses from the entire world met to discuss and find pathways to reduce the adverse consequences of unsafe healthcare (WHO 2008).

The surgical safety checklist (Figure 8.2) was introduced to improve perioperative safety practice and to ensure the correct patient for the correct surgical procedure and effective communication between the perioperative team.

SURGICAL SAFETY CHECKLIST (FIRST EDITION)

World Health Organization

Before induction of anaesthesia ▶▶▶▶▶▶ Before skin incision ▶▶▶▶▶▶▶▶▶▶ Before patient leaves operating room

SIGN IN

☐ PATIENT HAS CONFIRMED
  • IDENTITY
  • SITE
  • PROCEDURE
  • CONSENT

☐ SITE MARKED/NOT APPLICABLE

☐ ANAESTHESIA SAFETY CHECK COMPLETED

☐ PULSE OXIMETER ON PATIENT AND FUNCTIONING

DOES PATIENT HAVE A:

KNOWN ALLERGY?
☐ NO
☐ YES

DIFFICULT AIRWAY/ASPIRATION RISK?
☐ NO
☐ YES, AND EQUIPMENT/ASSISTANCE AVAILABLE

RISK OF >500ML BLOOD LOSS
(7ML/KG IN CHILDREN)?
☐ NO
☐ YES, AND ADEQUATE INTRAVENOUS ACCESS
  AND FLUIDS PLANNED

TIME OUT

☐ CONFIRM ALL TEAM MEMBERS HAVE
  INTRODUCED THEMSELVES BY NAME AND
  ROLE

☐ SURGEON, ANAESTHESIA PROFESSIONAL
  AND NURSE VERBALLY CONFIRM
  • PATIENT
  • SITE
  • PROCEDURE

ANTICIPATED CRITICAL EVENTS

☐ SURGEON REVIEWS: WHAT ARE THE
  CRITICAL OR UNEXPECTED STEPS,
  OPERATIVE DURATION, ANTICIPATED
  BLOOD LOSS?

☐ ANAESTHESIA TEAM REVIEWS: ARE THERE
  ANY PATIENT-SPECIFIC CONCERNS?

☐ NURSING TEAM REVIEWS: HAS STERILITY
  (INCLUDING INDICATOR RESULTS) BEEN
  CONFIRMED? ARE THERE EQUIPMENT
  ISSUES OR ANY CONCERNS?

HAS ANTIBIOTIC PROPHYLAXIS BEEN GIVEN
WITHIN THE LAST 60 MINUTES?
☐ YES
☐ NOT APPLICABLE

IS ESSENTIAL IMAGING DISPLAYED?
☐ YES
☐ NOT APPLICABLE

SIGN OUT

NURSE VERBALLY CONFIRMS WITH THE
TEAM:

☐ THE NAME OF THE PROCEDURE RECORDED

☐ THAT INSTRUMENT, SPONGE AND NEEDLE
  COUNTS ARE CORRECT (OR NOT
  APPLICABLE)

☐ HOW THE SPECIMEN IS LABELLED
  (INCLUDING PATIENT NAME)

☐ WHETHER THERE ARE ANY EQUIPMENT
  PROBLEMS TO BE ADDRESSED

☐ SURGEON, ANAESTHESIA ARE PROFESSIONAL
  AND NURSE REVIEW THE KEY CONCERNS
  FOR RECOVERY AND MANAGEMENT
  OF THIS PATIENT

THIS CHECKLIST IS NOT INTENDED TO BE COMPREHENSIVE ADDITIONS AND MODIFICATIONS TO FIT LOCAL PRACTICE ARE ENCOURAGED.

Fig. 8.2 Surgical safety checklist, first edition (World Health Organization).

The National Patient Safety Agency (NPSA), in collaboration with a multi-professional expert reference group, has adapted the checklist for use in England and Wales. The goal is to strengthen the commitment of clinical staff to address safety issues in the surgical setting. This includes:

- improving anaesthetic safety practices;
- ensuring correct site surgery;
- avoiding surgical site infections;
- improving communication within the team.

Practitioners will incorporate this checklist within their existing patient checklist to improve patient safety within their theatre department.

The role of the operating room support worker is to assist anaesthetists and anaesthetic practitioners in the anaesthetic and operating rooms with patient positioning and during anaesthesia. They are known by different names in different hospitals but undertake the same responsibilities.

GENERAL ANAESTHESIA

General anaesthesia can be divided into three components: unconsciousness (hypnosis), pain relief (analgesia) and muscle relaxation. All anaesthetic drugs produce anaesthesia by their effect on the brain. Anaesthetic gases are inhaled and then must be transferred from the lungs to the circulation and finally to the brain to be effective (Morton 1997).

Anaesthetists identify the 'triad of anaesthesia' or 'balanced anaesthesia'. This incorporates unconsciousness, analgesia and relaxation (Figure 8.3).

Guedel's classic signs of anaesthesia are those seen in patients premedicated with morphine and atropine, and breathing ether in air. The clinical signs associated with anaesthesia produced by other inhalational agents follow a similar course, but the divisions between stages and planes are less precise.

- Stage 1 – stage of anaesthesia. This is seen when using nitrous oxide 50% in oxygen, as used in the technique of relative analgesia.

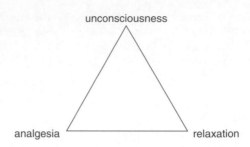

Fig. 8.3 Triad of anaesthesia.

- Stage 2 – stage of excitement. This is seen with inhalational induction, but is passed rapidly during intravenous induction. Respiration is erratic, breath-holding may occur, laryngeal and pharyngeal reflexes are active, and stimulation of pharynx and larynx (e.g. by insertion of a Guedel or laryngeal mask airway) may produce laryngeal spasm. The eyelash reflex is abolished in stage 2 but the eyelid reflex (resistance to elevation of eyelid) remains.
- Stage 3 – surgical anaesthesia. This deepens through four planes (in practice, three – light, medium, deep), with increasing concentration of anaesthetic drug. Respiration assumes a rhythmic pattern and the thorax component diminishes with depth of anaesthesia.
- Stage 4 – stage of impending respiratory and circulatory failure. Brainstem reflexes are depressed by the high anaesthetic concentration. Pupils are enlarged and unreactive. The patient should not be permitted to reach this stage. Withdrawal of the anaesthetic agents and administration of 100% oxygen lightens anaesthesia (Fell & Kirkbride 2007).

Airway management

The principal requirements of airway management in general anaesthesia are to:

- ensure a patent airway;
- deliver satisfactory ventilation:

— spontaneous – patients breathe themselves;
— mechanical or controlled – use of a ventilator and muscle relaxant and reversal drugs.
• monitor and record patients' physiological observations.

The aim of airway management is to secure and maintain a patient's airway. Induction of anaesthesia may cause the patient's soft palate and epiglottis to move towards the back wall of the pharynx. During inspiration, the walls of the pharynx can then collapse and obstruct the patient's airway.

Techniques that the anaesthetist or anaesthetic practitioner can use to secure a patent airway for patients with spontaneous breathing or ventilation are:

• head tilt – backward tilt of the head overcomes obstruction from the relaxed tongue. The manoeuvre stretches the muscles in the front of the neck and lifts the base of the tongue away from the posterior pharyngeal wall. Ideally the patient's head should be placed on a small pillow (Greaves *et al.* 2001);
• chin lift – the tongue is a muscle which is attached to the mandible and relief of the obstruction may be provided by lifting the chin (Greaves *et al.* 2001);
• head tilt and chin lift – the head tilt and chin lift technique is administered by placing one hand on the forehead and tilting the head backwards while using the fingers of the other hand to draw the chin upwards and open (Griffiths 1999);
• jaw thrust – provides an amplified effect of the chin lift. The technique involves lifting the mandible upwards and forward with the index, middle and ring fingers, and depressing the point of the chin slightly with the thumbs in order to open the mouth to allow air entry (Greaves *et al.* 2001). A jaw thrust manoeuvre is the technique of choice in the case of suspected cervical spine injury.

Anaesthetists can insert an oropharyngeal airway to maintain a patient's airway and to hold the tongue away from the posterior pharyngeal wall. It is inserted upside down and rotated 180° as it passes backwards into the mouth.

Nasopharyngeal airways are round, malleable plastic tubes, beveled at the pharyngeal end and flanged at the nasal end.

279

They lie along the floor of the nose and curve round into the pharynx. They are sized according to their internal diameter in millimeters and their length increases with the diameter. The correct size is estimated by comparing the airway diameter with that of the external nares (Gwinnut 2008).

If a nasopharyngeal airway (lubricated well) is inserted into the nostril, it is rotated gently into position. Nasopharyngeal airways are better tolerated than oropharyngeal airways in awake or lightly anaesthetised patients.

The anaesthetic practitioner can help the anaesthetist during these techniques by repositioning the patient's head on the pillow, by flattening or plumping up the pillow or by removing hair accessories to ensure the correct position of the patient's head. These techniques may be utilised within recovery care and this will be discussed in Chapter 10.

Spontaneous breathing
This may be observed in:

- patients with a face mask (with or without an airway adjunct) and a breathing circuit;
- patients with a laryngeal mask airway (LMA) and a breathing circuit;
- patients with an endotracheal tube (ET tube) and a breathing circuit.

Insertion of a laryngeal mask airway
The anaesthetist may insert an LMA and attach it to a breathing circuit to ensure that the patient breathes spontaneously throughout the surgical procedure. The role of the anaesthetic practitioner is outlined in Box 8.1.

Mechanical ventilation and tracheal intubation
Tracheal intubation is used to provide a secure and clear airway through which different modes of ventilation can be applied. It also protects the airway from blood, vomit and regurgitation. An ET tube is inserted through the mouth and into the trachea through the vocal cords with the aid of a laryngoscope.

Box 8.1   Role of the anaesthetic practitioner prior to and during the insertion of an LMA

Before the procedure, check:

- All piped and cylinder gases are flowing efficiently. Replace any cylinders, if necessary.
- The breathing circuit, with valve closed and open. Ensure the valve is open before use.
- Vaporisers are full and replenish if necessary.
- Suction is working and appropriate accessories are available.
- LMA.
- Induction equipment.
- Relevant drugs.
- All monitoring equipment
- An intravenous infusion is available (with or without a fluid warmer and extension with a three-way tap for administration of intravenous drugs).
- All equipment and anaesthetic machines in the anaesthetic room and operating room environment.
- All stock is available.

All equipment checked in accordance with AAGBI guidelines (2004, 2005a, 2007).
  When the patient is in the anaesthetic room:

- Reassure and communicate with the patient throughout procedure.
- Act as the patient's advocate.
- Attach all monitoring equipment and record observations before commencement of anaesthesia (a base reading).
- Maintain the patient's dignity at all times.
- Assist the anaesthetist in the venous cannulation of the patient.
- Attach a dressing to the venous cannula.
- Inform the anaesthetist of any allergies or medical conditions (arthritis, diabetes, etc) that the patient may have.

When the anaesthetist has administered the induction drugs the anaesthetic practitioner will:

- Pass the face mask and filter to the anaesthetist to pre-oxygenate the patient.
- Pass the lubricated LMA to the anaesthetist (and hold the patient's lower lip down for easy access).
- Pass the breathing circuit to the anaesthetist to attach to the filter.
- Inflate the cuff on the LMA until there is no obvious leak.
- Pass a catheter mount if necessary.
- Pass the tape or bandage to secure the LMA.
- Pass the tape for the eyes or eyegel to protect the eyes during the surgical procedure.

Cont.

> **Box 8.1** *Continued*
>
> Have available:
>
> • Muscle relaxants in case tracheal intubation is necessary.
> • Intubation equipment as described below.
>
> Be aware of the locality of all emergency equipment.

Preparation for induction and intubation procedure

The anaesthetic practitioner should check all relevant equipment for these procedures:

• the patient's trolley must have the facility of 'head down';
• monitoring equipment: heart rate, pulse, blood pressure, oxygen saturation, end tidal carbon dioxide, measurement of inhalation agent;
• relevant induction drugs;
• face mask, angled piece and filter;
• oral and nasal airway;
• laryngoscope with different blades and appropriate sized blades;
• ET tube, lubricating jelly and relevant size of breathing circuit (adult or paediatric);
• introducer or bougie for ET tube;
• catheter mount;
• syringe to inflate the ET tube cuff;
• suction equipment;
• stethoscope for the anaesthetist to check the correct position of the ET tube;
• bandage or tape to secure the ET tube.

The correct size of ET tube is selected and checked for the adult patient and a size smaller size is made available in case of emergency;

• for the female adult: a size 8.0, 7.5, 7.0 or 6.5;
• for the male adult: a size 9.0, 8.5, 8.0 or 7.5;
• for the paediatric patient the size of the tube is determined by the age and weight of the patient and this is discussed later in this chapter.

The role of the anaesthetic practitioner is outlined in Box 8.2.

Box 8.2   Role of the anaesthetic practitioner prior to and during intubation

Before the procedure check:

- All piped and cylinder gases are flowing efficiently. Replace any cylinders, if necessary.
- The breathing circuit, with valve closed and open, before the procedure. Ensure the valve is open before use.
- Vaporisers are full and replenish if necessary.
- Suction is working and appropriate accessories are available.
- Induction equipment.
- Relevant drugs.
- An intravenous infusion is available (with or without a fluid warmer and extension with a three-way tap for administration of intravenous drugs).
- All equipment and anaesthetic machines in the anaesthetic room and theatre.
- All stock is available.

All equipment checked in accordance with AAGBI guidelines (2005a).
  When the patient is in the anaesthetic room:

- Reassure and communicate with the patient throughout procedure.
- Attach all monitoring equipment and record observations before commencement of anaesthesia (a base reading).
- Maintain the patient's dignity at all times.
- Assist the anaesthetist in the venous cannulation of the patient.
- Attach a dressing to the venous cannula.
- Inform the anaesthetist of any allergies or medical conditions (arthritis, diabetes etc.) that the patient may have.

When the anaesthetist has administered the induction drugs:

- Pass the face mask and filter to the anaesthetist to pre-oxygenate the patient.
- Pass the laryngoscope – hold the patient's lower lip down for easy access of the laryngoscope. Have other laryngoscopes available as back-up.
- Pass the ET tube and after insertion inflate the cuff on the ET tube until there is no obvious leak.
- Pass the breathing circuit to the anaesthetist to attach to the filter.
- Pass a catheter mount if necessary.
- Pass the tape or bandage to secure the ET tube.
- Pass the tape for the eyes or eye gel to protect the eyes during the surgical procedure.

Have available:

- Suction equipment and suction catheters (ready under the patient's pillow for easy access).

Cont.

Box 8.2 *Continued*

- Relevant size of oropharygeal airway.
- A bougie. The anaesthetist may have difficulty when inserting the ET tube.
- A stethoscope for the anaesthetist to check the correct position of the ET tube.

Be aware:

- Cricoid pressure may be necessary to ensure tracheal intubation is successful.
- Where to find all emergency equipment.

The anaesthetist may connect the patient to the ventilator in the anaesthetic room or after transfer on to the operating table.

Rapid sequence induction (RSI)

This procedure is applied in emergency surgical procedures when the patient has a full stomach, in patients who have a hiatus hernia or with patients prone to reflux and therefore at risk of aspiration of the gastric contents into the lungs. It is the same procedure as tracheal intubation with cricoid pressure. The patient is pre-oxygenated for 3–5 minutes to maximise oxygen reserves and elimination of nitrogen. This reduces the risk of hypoxia and ensures oxygenation of the lungs in difficult intubation or airway obstruction. The ET tube is inserted by the anaesthetist. If any problems arise, he or she reapplies the face mask to manually ventilate the patient and to ensure reoxygenation of the lungs and will attempt intubation again. The intubation procedure is as previously described in Box 8.2.

Cricoid pressure (Sellick's manoeuvre)

The unconscious patient, during tracheal intubation, is at risk from regurgitation or aspiration of stomach contents. Cricoid pressure can relieve these problems by occluding the oesophagus between the cricoid cartilage (ring) and the vertebral column (Figure 8.4). The anaesthetist discusses this procedure with the patient at their preoperative visit.

Cricoid pressure, (Sellick's manoeuvre) is applied by an assistant from the beginning of induction until confirmation of ET

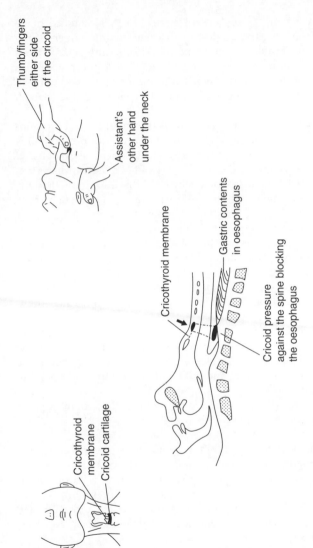

Fig. 8.4 Position for cricoid pressure.

tube placement. It entails displacement of the cricoid cartilage against the vertebral bodies. In this manner, the lumen of the oesophagus is ablated, while the complete nature of the cricoid cartilage maintains the tracheal lumen. Cricoid pressure is contraindicated with active vomiting (risk of oesophageal rupture), cervical spine fracture and laryngeal fracture (Barash *et al.* 2007).

To perform cricoid pressure correctly, the thumb and forefinger press the cricoid cartilage firmly in a posterior position, thus compressing the oesophagus between the cricoid cartilage and the vertebral column. Because the cricoid cartilage forms a ring, the tracheal lumen is not distorted. It is important that the assistant can identify the cricoid cartilage, as compression of the thyroid cartilage distorts laryngeal anatomy and may render tracheal intubation very difficult (Turner 2007).

Cricoid pressure is a technical skill that requires constructive education using measured techniques with continual practice and monitoring of skill level (Hein & Owen 2005).

Cricoid pressure can be performed by the assistant either one handed or two handed. Practitioners should follow their training method or local policy.

Practitioners may use the dominant hand to perform cricoid pressure and the non-dominant hand to support the neck. If the practitioner performs single-hand cricoid pressure, he or she will use the dominant hand only and not use the other hand to support the neck.

When anaesthetic practitioners or operating room support workers perform cricoid pressure, they:

- inform the patient that they are going to apply pressure as the anaesthetist administers the induction drugs and commences intubation. They support the patient's neck with one hand and with the other hand apply the cricoid pressure;
- maintain the correct pressure throughout the procedure (10 Newtons until the patient is unconscious and 30 Newtons thereafter);
- do not remove this pressure until the anaesthetist is satisfied the ET tube is in the correct position and anaesthesia is established.

• remove the cricoid pressure on instructions from the anaesthetist if the patient actively vomits. Vomiting may rupture the oesophagus if the cricoid pressure is not released.

During this procedure, preparation is the key and all anaesthetic personnel need to be aware of their responsibilities and the safety of the patient. Anaesthetists do not ask for cricoid pressure during the tracheal intubation procedure if the patient is actively vomiting.

Cricoid pressure should not be confused with optimal external laryngeal manipulation (OELM) or backward upward right pressure (BURP) on the thyroid cartilage, which is used to improve visualisation of the vocal cords when intubating (Knill 1993). BURP is performed by an assistant and moves the larynx to the right whilst the tongue is displaced to the left by the laryngoscope blade. These are techniques employed to improve visualisation of the vocal cords and do not protect the lungs from regurgitation (Hein & Owen 2005).

Awake intubation

This technique is used principally if the anaesthetist suspects a difficult airway management problem such as difficult intubation. The patient is awake during the intubation and is breathing spontaneously and therefore is able to manage his or her own airway until the ET tube is securely in position. The anaesthetist can then administer induction drugs to maintain anaesthesia and ventilation of the patient.

A fibre-optic laryngoscope can be used during an awake intubation procedure. Before the procedure, the anaesthetic practitioner or anaesthetist can thread the ET tube onto the scope ready for intubation.

Awake intubation is used to check the patient's airway anatomy (nose, larynx and trachea), for confirmation of the correct insertion of the ET tube, to evaluate trauma or the signs of infection. The patient's posterior pharynx is sprayed with local anaesthetic to minimise the gag reflex and other airway reflexes when the fibre-optic laryngoscope is inserted.

The fibre-optic laryngoscope is inserted gently into the anaesthetised nostril and advanced towards the nasopharnyx. The scope is then advanced through the tracheal tube and the pharynx and laryngeal aperture. As maximal vocal cord abduction occurs during inspiration, the scope is advanced slowly in small steps coordinated with inspiration. Even with a good upper airway anaesthesia, entry into the larynx results frequently in a violent cough. After passing through the larynx the position of the scope is confirmed by visual recognition of the tracheal rings and the ET is railroaded over the scope into the trachea. Position is again confirmed by seeing the tracheal rings and the scope is removed (Turner 2007).

After use the anaesthetic practitioner cleans and sterilises the laryngoscope following local policy guidelines. The role of the anaesthetic practitioner in this procedure is outlined in Box 8.3.

Complications of tracheal intubation

The Difficult Airway Society issued Guidelines for Difficult Intubation in 2007 and Recommendations for Practice in 2009 (Difficult Airway Society 2009).

Difficult intubation

The difficult airway algorithm of the American Society of Anesthesiologists (ASA) was developed to guide clinicians in the management of the patient who is either predicted to have a difficult airway or whose airway cannot be adequately managed after induction of anaesthesia (ASA 1993).

The difficult airway represents a complex interaction between patient factors, clinical setting and the skills of the practitioner (ASA 2003).

Difficult tracheal intubation can be related to the inability to visualise the glottic opening or those procedures requiring multiple and/or unsuccessful attempts to place the ET. Reasons for these are many, including, but not limited to, upper airway oedema, trauma, airway anomalies, obesity, limited neck mobility or limited opening of the mouth (Adams 2009).

Occasionally the anaesthetist may have difficulty in the tracheal intubation procedure because of the patient's anatomy or pathology. Cormack & Lehane (1984) classified difficult airways based on the view obtained at laryngoscopy:

Box 8.3   Role of the anaesthetic practitioner prior to and during the awake intubation procedure

Prepare:

- Fibre-optic laryngoscope, bite guard and light source (battery or mains).
- Reinforced or oral ET tube (6.0/7.0).
- Difficult intubation tray.
- Local anaesthetic throat spray.
- Nasal spray.
- Oral and nasal airways
- Syringe, needles, kwill and normal saline.
- Assorted types of LMAs.
- Manujet.
- Suction tubing.
- Nasal oxygen.
- Vomit bowl.
- Tape to secure the ET tube.
- A stethoscope available for the anaesthetist to check the position of the ET tube.

During the procedure:

- Reassure and communicate with the patient.
- Attach all monitoring equipment and record observations before the start of the anaesthetic to have a base reading.
- Assist the anaesthetist in the venous cannulation of the patient.
- Attach a dressing to the intravenous cannula.
- Have available an intravenous infusion (with or without a fluid warmer and extension with a three-way tap for administration of intravenous drugs) for the anaesthetist.

Have:

- Relevant induction drugs.
- A breathing circuit.
- Suction ready for use.
- Emergency equipment to hand.

- Grade 1 – most of the glottis is visible and there should be no difficulty;
- Grade 2 – if only the posterior aspect of the glottis is visible then there may be slight difficulty. Light pressure on the larynx will nearly always bring at least the arytenoids into view, if not the vocal cords.
- Grade 3 – if no part of the glottis can be seen, only the epiglottis, then there may be fairly severe difficulty.

- Grade 4 – if not even the epiglottis can be exposed, then intubation may be impossible except by alternative methods (Gwinnutt 2008).

Other anatomical issues may be observed, such as patient limited head extension and difficulty in opening of the mouth, restricted neck movements, tracheal stenosis or deviation that might produce a difficult intubation procedure.

Anaesthetic practitioners will prepare the standard equipment for tracheal intubation but, in addition, have all laryngoscopes, including the McCoy and short-handle laryngoscopes, the fibre-optic laryngoscope and cricothyroid needle set, available during the procedure.

The anaesthetists can use either a bougie or an introducer:

- a bougie aids the insertion of the ET tube. The anaesthetist inserts the bougie through the larynx and vocal cords under direct vision or blind. The anaesthetic practitioner passes the ET tube over the bougie and the anaesthetist feeds the tube through the vocal cords. The anaesthetic practitioner removes the bougie on the instructions of the anaesthetist whilst the anaesthetist holds the ET tube in position;
- an introducer or stylet can alter the shape of the ET tube. The anaesthetic practitioner inserts the appropriate type (introducer or stylet) into the selected ET tube and ensures it does not protrude beyond the distal end of the tube as this might cause damage to the larynx. The anaesthetic practitioner removes the introducer on the instructions of the anaesthetist after correct insertion of the ET tube.

Failed intubation

The anaesthetist will attempt to oxygenate the patient by any means necessary. He or she will try to insert an oropharyngeal airway and oxygenate the patient with 100% oxygen. He or she will:

- request help from other anaesthetists;
- ask for cricoid pressure and try to intubate the patient with a size 6 ET tube;
- insert an LMA;

Box 8.4

(a) Role of the anaesthetic practitioner during a cricothyroidotomy procedure using a needle

- Assist the anaesthetist in the procedure.
- Prepare a cricothyroidotomy needle.
- Have the venturi injector device to provide a high pressure oxygen source through the cricothyroidotomy needle (50 psi pressure).
- Have available an intravenous infusion (with or without a fluid warmer and extension with a three-way tap for administration of intravenous drugs) for the anaesthetist.
- Pass tape to secure the needle.

Have:

- Suction ready for use.
- Emergency equipment to hand.

(b) Role of the anaesthetic practitioner during a surgical cricothyroidotomy procedure using an ET tube

- Assist the anaesthetist in the procedure.
- Prepare the ET tube or tracheostomy tube.
- Have a syringe for inflation of tube.
- Have a breathing circuit to attach to the ET tube or tracheostomy tube.
- Have available an intravenous infusion (with or without a fluid warmer and extension with a three-way tap for administration of intravenous drugs) for the anaesthetist.
- Pass tape or bandage available to secure the tube.

Have:

- Suction ready for use.
- Emergency equipment to hand.

- wake the patient and undertake a regional anaesthetic technique;
- undertake an awake intubation;
- attempt a needle cricothyroidotomy. Complications of this procedure are pneumothorax, surgical emphysema and problems with exhalation. The role of the anaesthetic practitioner in this procedure is outlined in Box 8.4. Figure 8.5 shows the equipment used;
- postpone the surgery.

Laryngospasm

Laryngospasm occurs as a result of a foreign body (e.g. oral or nasal airway), saliva, blood or vomitus touching the glottis, or

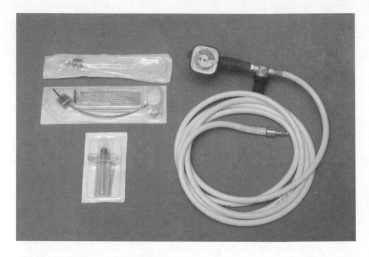

Fig. 8.5 Cricothyroid equipment.

even a light plane of anaesthesia. Obstruction to mask ventilation may be caused by laryngospasm with a reflex closure of the vocal cords. Hypoxia as well as non-cardiogenic pulmonary oedema can result if there is continued spontaneous ventilation against closed vocal cords. Treatment includes removal of the offending stimulus (if it can be identified), continuous positive airway pressure, deepening of the anaesthetic state and use of a rapid-acting muscle relaxant (Barash *et al.* 2007).

The laryngeal muscles contract and occlude the glottis. The anaesthetist will use appropriate suction, administer 100% oxygen and deepen the anaesthesia to relieve it or administer a muscle relaxant and ventilate the patient.

Aspiration of gastric contents

Patients with a history of hiatus hernia, acid reflux or other intra-abdominal pathology that may cause the possibility of aspiration of gastric contents at intubation are identified. In this case the anaesthetist will carry out a rapid sequence induction (RSI) procedure. He or she will advise the anaesthetic practitioner or operating room support worker of the need to undertake cricoid pressure during the RSI procedure. Complications of aspiration are bronchospasm, acute (adult) respiratory distress syndrome (ARDS), sepsis and eventually death.

Bronchospasm

General anaesthesia may alter airway resistance by influencing bronchomotor tone, lung volumes and bronchial secretions. Patients with increased airway reactivity from recent respiratory infection, asthma, atopy or smoking are more susceptible to bronchospasm during anaesthesia. It may be precipitated by the rapid introduction of a pungent anaesthetic agent, the insertion of an artificial airway during light anaesthesia, stimulation of the carina or bronchi by a tracheal tube or by drugs causing beta-blockade or release of histamine (Hardman 2007).

Bronchospasm is temporary narrowing of the bronchi and any irritants present can cause this. The anaesthetist will administer 100% oxygen to the patient and, if necessary, administer bronchodilator drugs.

Bronchospasm may occur during anaesthesia due to:

- surgical stimulation;
- presence of airway or tracheal tube;
- pharyngeal/laryngeal/bronchial secretions or blood;
- aspiration of gastric contents;
- anaphylaxis or anaphylactoid reaction;
- pulmonary oedema.

It is particularly likely in patients with asthma or chronic obstructive airway disease (COAD), and if anaesthesia is inadequate, the features observed are wheezing, reduced movement of the reservoir bag, increased expiratory time and increased airway pressure.

Treatment is of the primary cause, increased inspired concentration of volatile anaesthetic agent or salbutamol or adrenaline (epinephrine) (Yentis *et al.* 2001).

The anaesthetist will use appropriate suction, administer 100% oxygen, maintain the airway and reposition the ET tube if necessary.

Acute (adult) respiratory distress syndrome (ARDS)
ARDS is a syndrome when the alveoli become inflamed, causing them to fill up with liquid and then they collapse. Gas exchange ceases and the body becomes starved of oxygen. Mechanical ventilation is necessary.

Other induction complications

Anaphylaxis
Anaphylaxis is an exaggerated response to a drug or foreign substance.

Anaphylactic reactions are mediated by immunoglobulin E (IgE) antibodies causing massive degranulation of mast cells in sensitised individuals. Activation of mast cells releases histamine and serotonin, with systemic kinin activation. This leads to rapid vasodilation, a fall in systemic vascular resistance (SVR), hypotension, severe bronchospasm, hypoxia and hypercapnia. Prompt treatment with oxygen, fluids, adrenaline (epinephrine), hydrocortisone and an antihistamine is required. The anaesthetist will stop giving the trigger substance (Anderson 2003).

Anaphylaxis (type 1 hypersensitivity) is an IgE-mediated reaction to an antigen. Antibodies bind to mast cells, which degranulate, releasing the chemical mediators of anaphylaxis. These include histamine, prostaglandins, platelet-activating factor (PAF) and leucotrienes. The signs produced by the action of these mediators of anaphylaxis are urticaria, cutaneous flushing, bronchospasm, hypotension, arrhythmia and cardiac arrest. Anaphylaxis has been reported in patients without apparent previous exposure to the specific antigen, probably because of cross-reactivity. This is particularly true of reactions to muscle relaxants; cosmetics and some foods contain structurally similar compounds (Hardman 2007).

Latex is emerging as one of the most important causes of anaphylaxis during anaesthesia and surgery (see Chapter 5, page 206).

Hypotension and tachycardia are identified by observation of the patient's physiological readings. The anaesthetist will stop all administration of anaesthetic drugs, will administer 100% oxygen and maintain the airway, and give emergency drugs as

Box 8.5   Role of the anaesthetic practitioner during an anaphylactic attack

Assist the anaesthetist:

- Provide appropriate emergency drugs (oxygen and appropriate dosage of adrenaline [epinephrine]).
- Prepare an intravenous infusion.
- Record all physiological readings.
- Record all relevant care.

Have available:

- Resuscitation equipment.

Undertake cardiopulmonary resuscitation if necessary.

---

necessary. The role of the anaesthetic practitioner in this instance is outlined in Box 8.5.

Malignant hyperpyrexia
This is a rare inherited disorder in which there is a release of abnormally high concentrations of calcium from the sarcoplasmic reticulum, causing increased muscle activity and metabolism. Excess heat production causes a rise in core temperature of a least 2° C/hour. It is triggered by exposure to the inhalational anaesthetic agents and suxamethonium. The incidence is between 1:10,000 and 1:40,000 anaesthetised patients (Gwinnutt 2008).

Increased end tidal carbon dioxide and tachycardia are observed from the physiological recordings. The anaesthetist will stop all administration of anaesthetic drugs and volatile agents, will administer 100% oxygen, maintain the airway and administer dantrolene and sodium bicarbonate intravenously. The role of the anaesthetic practitioner in this instance is outlined in Box 8.6.

ANAESTHETIC EQUIPMENT

Face masks
These are available in black rubber or transparent plastic (single use) and in different sizes (Figure 8.6). Their design aims to fit

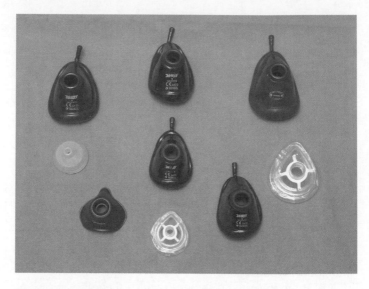

Fig. 8.6 Face masks.

Box 8.6 Role of the anaesthetic practitioner during malignant hyperpyrexia

Assist the anaesthetist:

- Provide dantrolene and intravenous infusions including sodium bicarbonate.
- Provide ice packs to reduce the patient's temperature.
- Record all physiological readings.
- Prepare any relevant equipment for further treatment, e.g. arterial and central venous pressure.

Have available:

- Resuscitation equipment.

---

the patient's face without any leaks (the anaesthetic team can observe any secretions through a transparent mask). The air-filled cuff of the mask helps to minimise the mask's pressure on the patient's face. Suitable sizes should be available for the patient. An angle piece and an airway filter fits onto the face mask, and a catheter mount and the breathing system fits onto the airway filter.

Airway filter/humidifier

Dry anaesthetic gases can cause damage to the cells lining the respiratory tract, impairing ciliary function. This increases the patient's susceptibility to respiratory tract infection. A decrease in body temperature occurs as the respiratory tract humidifies the dry gases.

Airway filter humidifiers are single use and prevent the spread of infection from the patient into the breathing circuit or ventilator.

Characteristics of the ideal humidifier are:

- capable of providing adequate levels of humidification;
- low resistance to flow and low dead space;
- provides microbiological protection to the patient;
- maintenance of body temperature;
- safe and convenient to use;
- economical.

Heat and moisture exchanger (HME) humidifiers are compact, inexpensive and effective for most clinical situations. Their efficiency is gauged by the proportion of heat and moisture returned to the patient. Adequate humidification is achieved with a relative humidity of 60–70%. Inspired gases are warmed to temperatures of between 29 and 34° C (Al Shaikh & Stacey 2007).

Catheter mount

The catheter mount is a corrugated disposable tubing (single use), which may have a concertina design. It lessens the transmission of accidental movements and allows adjustment of the breathing system to the ET tube. Its length contributes to the apparatus dead space.

Laryngeal mask airways (LMA® airways)

The LMA, invented by Brain in 1981, is a general-purpose airway that fills a niche between the face mask and ET tube, both in anatomical location and degree of invasiveness. It sits with its tip in the hypopharynx at the interface between the

gastrointestinal and respiratory tracts, and here it forms a circumferential low-pressure seal around the glottis. This has the
advantages of maintaining the gas flow through the upper
airway and providing direct access to the glottis without loss of
airway control. The LMA® airway allows the administration of
gases through a minimally stimulating airway (Intavent 1999).

The advantages over the ET tube include avoidance of laryngoscopy, less invasion of the respiratory tract, avoidance of the
risks of endobronchial or oesophageal intubation and less
trauma to local tissues. The main disadvantage of the LMA®
airway compared with the ET tube is that air leakage and gastric
insufflation are more likely. It also does not secure the airway
as effectively as an ET tube and airway obstruction at the glottic
and subglottic level cannot be prevented (Intavent 1999).

Anaesthetists insert LMA® airways for general anaesthesia
when the patient breathes spontaneously throughout the surgical procedure. The LMA® airway is lubricated by the anaesthetic practitioner just before insertion so that the lubricant does
not dry out. It is only necessary to lubricate the back of the
mask. If the front of the LMA® airway is lubricated, globules
of lubricant may block the tube, especially in children, or the
patient may inhale the lubricant after insertion, causing laryngeal spasm or coughing.

The LMA® airway has an inflatable silicone ring and cuff.
When the cuff is inflated by the anaesthetic practitioner, the
mask fills the space around and behind the larynx. This ensures
a tight seal and no detection of any leak. The LMA® airway is
secured by using either bandage or tape. Different sizes of the
various LMA® airways are available for patients of all ages. It
is essential to check the laryngeal mask before use.

Consultant anaesthetists (because they are experienced) may
use an LMA® airway in the tracheal intubation procedure in
the place of an ET tube. The anaesthetic practitioner should
always have an ET tube available in case of inadequate
ventilation.

Standard LMA® airway

The original LMA® airway (or classic LMA® airway) is a reusable device requiring sterilisation between each patient, but

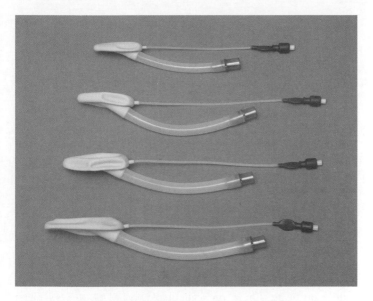

Fig. 8.7 Standard laryngeal masks.

recent concerns about the possible risk of prion disease transmission have resulted in increasing use of disposable versions
(Gwinnutt 2008).

The LMA® airway is made of medical grade silicone rubber;
it is latex free. It may be disposable or reusable (in which case
it is sterilised by steam autoclaving). It consists of a flexible
curved opening into the lumen at the distal end of a small ellip-
tical mask that has an inflatable outer rim (Figure 8.7).

Reinforced LMA

This LMA® airway design is ideal for use in surgery to the
head, neck and upper torso where the standard LMA® airway
would either interfere with the surgical field or occlude or be
displaced by the surgeon. It is crush proof and kink-free, but
not bite proof because of a stainless steel wire spiral in its wall.
The tube can be moved during surgery without loss of the cuff's
seal against the larynx. The breathing system can easily be

connected at any angle from the mouth. A throat pack can be used if requested by the anaesthetist. It has a smaller internal diameter and longer length than the standard version, causing an increase in flow resistance. This makes its use with spontaneous ventilation with prolonged periods less suitable (Al Shaikh & Stacey 2007).

Disposable LMA® airway
This has similar properties to the standard LMA® airway, but is more rigid and has a thicker cuff than the reusable LMA® airway.

Intubating LMA® airway
This has better intubation characteristics than the standard LMA® airway. It consists of an anatomically curved, short, wide-bore, stainless steel tube sheathed in silicone, which bonds to an LMA® airway and a guiding handle. It has a single moveable epiglottic elevator bar, a guiding V-shaped ramp and can allow up to an 8-mm tracheal tube. The LMA® airway has a dedicated straight-cuffed silicone tracheal tube with a soft bevelled tip (Gwinnutt 2008).

This type of LMA® airway does not protect against aspiration of gastric contents (Al Shaikh & Stacey 2007).

Proseal LMA® airway
The proseal LMA® airway is designed to conform to the contours of the hypopharynx, with its lumen facing the laryngeal opening. The mask has a main cuff that seals around the laryngeal opening and a rear cuff helps increase the seal. Attached to the mask is an inflation line terminating in a pilot balloon and valve for mask inflation and deflation. A removable introducer tool is available to aid insertion of the LMA® airway to avoid placing a finger in the mouth on insertion (Intavent 1999).

The proseal has an additional posterior cuff to improve the seal between mask and larynx, and reduce leak when the patient is ventilated. It also has a secondary tube to allow drainage of gastric contents (Gwinnutt 2008).

I-gel LMA® airway

This is the latest development which uses a solid, highly malleable gel-like material contoured to fit the perilaryngeal anatomy in place of the traditional inflatable cuff. It is single use (Gwinnutt 2008).

Intubating laryngeal mask (ILM)

This is a modification of the LMA® airway in which the mask part is almost unchanged; however, a shorter, wider metal tube with a 90' bend in it with a handle replaces the flexible tube. It is inserted using a similar technique to that for a standard LMA® airway, but by holding the handle rather than using the index finger as a guide. A specially designed reinforced, cuffed tracheal tube can then be inserted which will almost pass into the trachea, due to the shape and position of the ILM. Once it has been confirmed that the tube lies in the trachea, the ILM can either be left *in situ* or removed (Gwinnut 2008).

Cleaning and sterilisation

Practitioners need to follow their policies for cleaning and sterilisation of their reusable LMA® airways. Many theatre departments use disposable LMA® airways in their practice.

Pre-use tests of LMA® airways

- Test 1: Examine the interior of the tube to ensure it is free from blockage or loose particles. Then flex the tube to increase its curvature. Kinking of the tube should not occur when it bends around 180°. Do not bend beyond 180° in order to avoid permanent damage to the tube.
- Test 2: The tube should be transparent so any fluids or contaminants within it are readily obvious. Discoloration of the tube usually indicates considerable use beyond the warranty use (40 uses), and hinders the ability to detect potential airway problems. Ensure the connector has a secure fit.
- Test 3: Examine the opening in the mask to ensure integrity of the mask open bars. The spaces between the bars must be free from any particulate matter.
- Test 4: Deflate the mask cuff to a high vacuum so the cuff walls are tightly flat against each other. Remove the syringe

from the syringe port with a rapid twisting action. Now examine the cuff walls to ensure they remain tightly flattened against each other. Gradual inflation suggests there is a faulty valve or a leaking cuff.

- Test 5: Inflate the cuff from complete vacuum as follows: size 1–7 ml, size 2–10 ml, size 2.5–14 ml, size 3–20 ml, size 4–30 ml, size 5–40 ml. If no leak is apparent, inflate 50% more air into the cuff and again check for leaks. There should not be uneven bulging of the cuff, either end or on one or other of the sides (Intavent 1999).

Equipment for tracheal intubation

Other equipment for tracheal intubation includes face masks, airway filter and catheter mount, which have been described earlier for spontaneous breathing.

Laryngoscope

The anaesthetist uses the laryngoscope to examine the larynx and to aid insertion of the ET tube. It consists of a handle and a blade. The handle contains the power source, batteries and the blade, which has a light carrier with a bulb. The electrical current flows from the battery to the bulb through an insulated contact at the top of the handle. When the laryngoscope blade is opened, the light comes on and it is ready for use. When the blade is closed, the light switches off. The bulb illuminates the larynx. The relevant size of blade is used for the individual patient.

Each laryngoscope is checked by the anaesthetic practitioner prior to use. Failure of the batteries or light bulb can cause a delay in intubation, a worry for the anaesthetist and anaesthetic practitioner and a danger to the patient's care. Usually two laryngoscopes are available with different size blades (4 and 3), for intubation of female and male adults. The second laryngoscope is available as back-up in case the light or batteries fail.

The McCoy laryngoscope is based on the standard MacIntosh blade but has a hinged tip (Figure 8.8). When the lever on the handle is pressed, the tip of the blade bends forward and this improves the view of the larynx. This laryngoscope is used in the difficult intubation procedure.

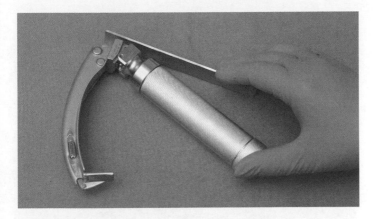

Fig. 8.8 McCoy laryngoscope.

Anaesthetic practitioners should be familiar with the identified laryngoscope and blades, and the other different types available in their operating departments.

Practitioners need to follow their policies for cleaning and sterilisation of their laryngoscope blades. Disposable laryngoscopes and blades may be used by anaesthetists.

After use the laryngoscope blade is cleaned following local policy, for example:

- the blade is detached and the light carrier is removed;
- the blade is cleaned and sent to the Hospital Sterilisation and Disinfectant Unit (HSDU);
- a new blade is attached to the handle and the light is checked ready for the next patient.

The light carrier or batteries are changed if the light does not work. Standard precautions are followed during the cleaning procedure. If the policy is to use disposable laryngoscope blade covers, the anaesthetic practitioner will dispose of the laryngoscope blade cover and attach a new one.

Fibre-optic laryngoscope
The laryngoscope consists of an eye piece and insertion tube (Figure 8.9). A light source and suction is necessary for these

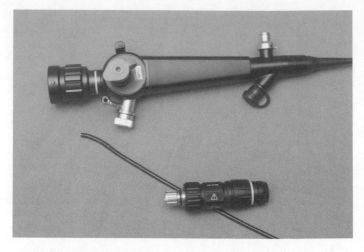

Fig. 8.9 Fibre-optic laryngoscope.

procedures. Anaesthetic practitioners and anaesthetists should take care with the preparation and use of the instrument because the optic fibres are delicate and easily damaged.

ET tube

ET tubes provide a safe way of securing the patient's airway. They are plastic and transparent for reduction of trauma and easy view of secretions (Figure 8.10). They are for single use, and they have a radio-opaque line running along their length to enable easy identification of anatomical position on chest x-rays.

The usual size for a female adult patient is 7–8 mm and for a male adult is 8–9 mm. The anaesthetist decides on the choice of size for paediatric patients depending on the weight and size of the patient. Some anaesthetists prefer their ET tubes cut and some prefer to insert them uncut. Anaesthetists observe the desired length of the ET tube on the outside of the patient's mouth. Anaesthetic practitioners should ensure the connection (cut or uncut) at the end of the ET tube is secure. There are

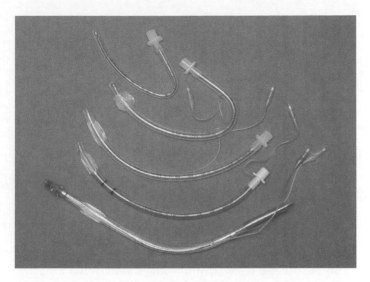

Fig. 8.10 Endotracheal tubes. From top to bottom: Ring–Adair–Elwyn (RAE) tube, RAE tube (cuffed), Lo-pro tube, microlaryngotracheal (MLT) tube, endobronchial tube.

marks on the ET tubes which signify the internal diameter (mm) and the length of the tube (cm).

There is a risk of advancing the tube into one of the main bronchi, usually the right side, if the anaesthetist inserts the tube too far. Correct choice of the ET tube size is essential to minimise the risk of trauma of the larynx.

The ET tube may have a cuff which the anaesthetic practitioner inflates and this provides an airtight seal between the ET tube and trachea. This protects the patient's airway from aspiration of gastric fluid and allows the efficient ventilation during intermittent positive pressure ventilation (IPPV). Non-cuffed ET tubes are used for paediatric anaesthesia under the age of 11 as cuffed tubes may damage the patient's larynx and trachea.

There are different types of tubes and sizes (adult and paediatric) used in anaesthesia:

- oral – these are made of plastic and have a gentle curve to ease insertion. Adult tubes have a cuff to provide an air-tight fit;
- Ring–Adair–Elwyn (RAE) – RAE tubes have a preformed shape to fit the mouth or nose without kinking. They have a bend located just as the tube emerges so the tube connections to the breathing system are at the level of the chin or forehead and they do not interfere with surgical access;
- reinforced (armoured) – reinforced tubes are plastic or silicone. They are thicker and contain a spiral of metal wire or tough nylon. This prevents kinking and occlusion of the tube when the head or neck rotates or flexes during surgery. Anaesthetic practitioners cannot cut this tube so there can be a risk of bronchial intubation. There are markers just above the cuff to advise the anaesthetist of the correct position of the tube;
- laser – these tubes are used for laser surgery on the larynx or trachea. They are designed to withstand the effect of carbon dioxide and other laser beams, avoiding the risk of fire or damage to the tracheal tube. They have a flexible steel body. Reflected beams from the tube are defocused to reduce the accidental laser strikes to healthy tissues. Some designs have two cuffs to ensure a tracheal seal should the upper cuff be damaged by the laser. An air-filled cuff, hit by the laser beam, may ignite and so it is recommended that the cuffs are filled with saline instead of air (Al Shaikh & Stacey 2007). The anaesthetic practitioner covers the patient's eyes with damp gauze swabs and padding during the surgical procedure;
- endobronchial or double lumen tubes – during thoracic surgery there is a need to deflate one lung. This offers the surgeon easier and better surgical access. Either a right- or left-hand tube is selected to allow the patient to be ventilated via that specific lung during access to the adjacent chest cavity;
- Montandon – the tube allows the anaesthetist to ventilate a patient through laryngectomy access. It has a curve at one end to ensure easy access;
- Tracheostomy – these are plastic or metal tubes (curved) that the anaesthetist usually inserts through the second, third or fourth tracheal cartilage rings. They are used for:

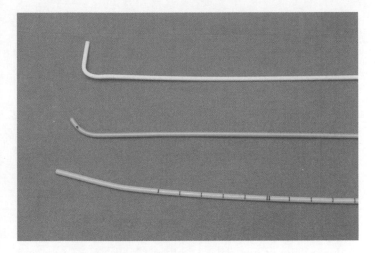

Fig. 8.11 Introducer with bougie.

— long-term IPPV;
— avoidance of an upper airway obstruction that cannot be bypassed with an oral or nasal tracheal tube;
— maintenance of the airway after the laryngectomy surgical procedure;
— control of excessive bronchial secretions, particularly for patients with reduced consciousness over a long period.

Introducer
Anaesthetists may use this to alter the shape of the ET tube and to aid them in a difficult intubation procedure. Figure 8.11 shows an introducer and bougie.

Bougie
A bougie can be used in a difficult intubation procedure. This can be a single-use item or be sterilised following local policy. There are a range of different sizes available for adult and paediatric patients.

If it is not possible to see the larynx in the tracheal intubation procedure, the anaesthetist will pass and insert the bougie

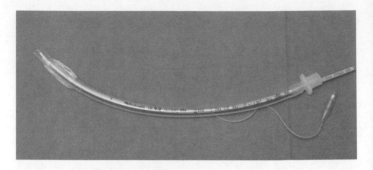

Fig. 8.12 Bougie within an endotracheal tube.

blindly through the vocal cords. The anaesthetic practitioner threads the ET tube on to the bougie and the anaesthetist pushes it down into position. The anaesthetist holds the ET tube and the anaesthetic practitioner removes the bougie once the ET tube is in position.

Figure 8.12 illustrates a bougie within an ET tube.

Oropharyngeal airway

Airways are available in different sizes for adult and paediatric patients. They are inserted through the mouth into the oropharynx above the tongue to protect the airway. They may be required to prevent obstruction caused by the tongue or collapse of the pharynx in the patient without a tracheal tube. There are different sizes for adult and paediatric patients (Figure 8.13).

An airway should never be inserted if the patient has epiglottitis because of the risk that total airway obstruction may be precipitated (Illingworth & Simpson 1994).

Nasopharyngeal airway

These airways are inserted through the nose into the nasopharynx. Care must be taken with insertion. They are contraindicated in patients who are anticoagulated, patients with basilar skull fractures, patients with nasal infections and deformities, as well as in children (because of the risk of epistaxis).

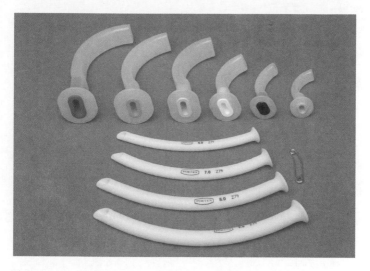

Fig. 8.13 Oropharyngeal and nasopharyngeal airways.

Their role is to provide a patent airway between the nostril and laryngeal opening. These airways are available in different sizes for adult and paediatric patients (Figure 8.13).

Ryles tube (nasogastric tube)

A Ryles tube can be inserted through the nasopharnyx, down the oesophagus into the stomach to allow emptying of the liquid contents of the stomach before or during the surgical procedure. The ET tube may be inserted before the Ryles tube or afterwards, depending on the preference of the anaesthetist. The anaesthetist will need Magill forceps and a laryngoscope available for insertion. The role of the anaesthetic practitioner is described in Box 8.7.

Magill forceps

Magill forceps are used when the anaesthetist inserts a Ryles tube or a throat pack, or for the removal of foreign body or bodies from the oropharynx and larynx. There are suitable sizes for the adult and paediatric patient (Figure 8.14).

Box 8.7   Role of the anaesthetic practitioner during the insertion of a Ryles tube

Assist the anaesthetist:

- Select the correct size of tube. Have a smaller and larger size available.
- Pass the lubricated Ryles tube to the anaesthetist.
- Pass the laryngoscope to the anaesthetist.
- Pass the Magill forceps to the anaesthetist to help position the Ryles tube.
- Have suction ready for use.

After insertion:

- Attach a bag to the end of the Ryles tube. Do not forget to close the valve on the end of the bag to prevent leakage. The bag has markings on to identify the quantity of the contents of the bag.
- Secure the Ryles tube to the nose with a nasal dressing.
- Clean the Magill forceps following local policy and then send them to HSDU for sterilisation.

The anaesthetist will not insert a Ryles tube for patients with:

- Head injuries.
- Fracture of the base of the skull.

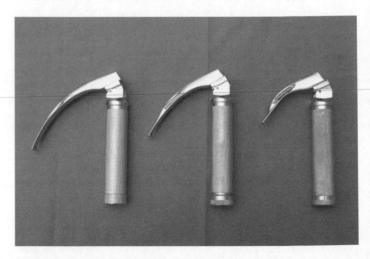

Fig. 8.14   Magill laryngoscope.

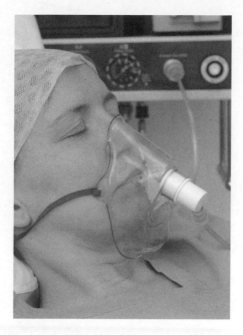

Fig. 8.15 Patient with oxygen mask.

Oxygen mask

Patients can receive oxygen from a mask which attaches via tubing to the cylinder or piped gas fitting (Figure 8.15). A venturi mask delivers different concentrations of oxygen and anaesthetic; recovery practitioners use this mask when they need to deliver a specific concentration of oxygen to the patient. Different colour attachments represent different concentrations of oxygen. Masks are available for delivering 24%, 28%, 31%, 40%, 50% or 60% of oxygen.

These are used when it is important to deliver a precise concentration of oxygen, unaffected by the patient's ventilatory pattern, for example patients with chronic obstructive pulmonary disease (COPD) and carbon dioxide retention. These masks work on the principle of high airflow oxygen enrichment.

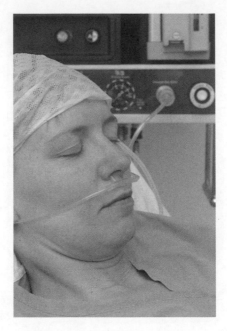

Fig. 8.16 Patient with nasal cannula.

Oxygen is fed into a venturi that entrains a much greater but constant flow of air. The total flow into the mask may be as high as 45 L/min. The high gas flow has two effects: it meets the patient's peak inspiratory flow, reducing volume of air drawn in around the mask, and flushes expiratory gas, reducing rebreathing (Gwinnutt 2008).

Nasal cannula

The nasal cannula delivers 2–4 litres of oxygen per minute to the patient. There are two prongs that fit inside the nose and the tubing attaches to the oxygen cylinder or piped oxygen (Figure 8.16). There is the potential for trauma to the nasal cavity by the dry airflow; however, humidified oxygen can help to reduce this.

MAINTENANCE AND EMERGENCE FROM ANAESTHESIA

Anaesthesia is maintained by the anaesthetist by two methods:

- anaesthesia with inhalational agents and oxygen;
- anaesthesia with total intravenous anaesthesia (TIVA).

Other drugs that may be administered throughout the anaesthesia are:

- analgesics;
- muscle relaxants;
- antiemetics;
- antibiotics;
- anticholinergics;
- antipressors;
- antidisarrythmias;
- emergency drugs.

These drugs are discussed in further detail in Chapter 3.

The anaesthetic practitioner will also ensure that the following effective care is given to the patient:

- patient monitoring;
- fluid management;
- temperature management: operating room temperature and humidity control, intravenous fluids and warming blankets;
- deep vein thrombosis (DVT) prophylaxis;
- pressure area care;
- documentation.

The role of the anaesthetic practitioner is summarised in Box 8.8 and the documentation completed in the operating room during the maintenance of anaesthesia is summarised in Figure 8.17.

REGIONAL ANAESTHESIA

Regional anaesthetic techniques may be used alone or in combination with sedation or general anaesthesia, depending on the individual requirements of the patient. Preservation of consciousness is often considered to be a significant advantage of regional anaesthesia. Of major benefit to all patients is the quality of early postoperative analgesia, which may be

Box 8.8 Role of the anaesthetic practitioner during the maintenance and emergence from anaesthesia in the operating room

- A safe transfer of the patient onto the operating table.
- All attachments (intravenous infusion, catheter, etc) are contained during transfer.
- Patient is comfortable and the use of relevant accessories to prevent any nerve or tissue injuries.
- Attachment of all patient monitoring devices to the monitoring machine.
- All patient physiological recordings are within normal limits.
- Use of warming blankets and temperature probes (following local policies) to prevent the occurrence of hypothermia.
- Availability of relevant intravenous infusions or blood throughout the surgical procedure.
- Availability of any further equipment or anaesthetic requirements for the anaesthetist.
- Availability of the relevant trolley, using an aseptic technique, for any further required procedures.
- Availability of relevant pain management equipment and documentation.
- Completion of documentation for the establishment of anaesthesia and patient care throughout the surgical procedure.
- Locality of emergency equipment and daily checks for immediate use.

Have:

- Reversal drugs available for the anaesthetist.
- Suction equipment available.
- Syringe available to deflate the ET tube cuff if appropriate.
- Patient's facemask, oxygen cylinder and breathing circuit available to transfer the patient from the operating room to the recovery area.
- Scissors to cut the bandage securing the ET tube.

Give:

- An effective handover to the recovery practitioner of the patient's care in the operating room (anaesthesia, intravenous drugs, surgical procedure, method of pain management, drains, catheters, etc and any issues from the preoperative checklist [allergies, loose teeth, hearing aid, etc]).

Ensure:

- Recovery practitioner is satisfied with handover and patient's condition.
- Transfer of any postoperative management equipment into the recovery area. The anaesthetist may start pain management in the anaesthetic room or operating room.
- Patient's monitoring equipment is connected to the recovery monitor.

Relevant equipment checked and available (Sign)
Ensure check list corresponds to theatre list (Sign)
Monitor and assess patient throughout induction and surgical procedure:

Induction	**Perioperative**
Oxygen saturation	Oxygen saturation
ECG, Heart rate	ECG, Heart rate
Non-invasive blood pressure	Non-invasive blood pressure
Arterial blood pressure	Arterial blood pressure
Central venous pressure	Central venous pressure
Respirations	Respirations
Temperature	Temperature
Other	Other

Transfer patient to operating table as per local policy
Patient's position:
Aids used to minimise potential risk of pressure or nerve damage:
Temperature maintained by:
Ensure diathermy or tourniquet is applied and used as per local policy
Diathermy site: Site checked postoperatively:
Tourniquet site: Tourniquet on: Tourniquet off:
Assess viability of existing intravenous access Assist in and perform in intravenous cannulation Cannula site: Cannula size:
Record intravenous fluids given and expiry date:
Record urological fluid regime Record initial urine output if catheterised Preoperatively: Postoperatively:
Additional information (for example note of allergies, loose teeth, etc.) Any inhalers with patient: Application of flowtron boots: Waterlow score: Blood sugar result and time if appropriate:
Anaesthetic practitioner signature: Print name:

Fig. 8.17 Outline of a patient care plan.

prolonged by using catheter techniques either centrally or peripherally (Coventry 2007).

Regional anaesthetic techniques

These techniques produce analgesia in a specific part of the body. A local anaesthetic is injected near suitable nerves to achieve regional anaesthesia of the chosen area. The chosen local anaesthetic is injected at or near the nerves of the surgical site and it temporarily interrupts sensory nerve impulses during manipulation of sensitive tissues.

Regional anaesthetic techniques decrease intraoperative stimuli and diminish the stress response to surgical trauma. Regional anaesthesia reduces the stress response and increases the blood flow, which can have benefits for wound healing and diseases such as thrombophlebitis. It can reduce pain intraoperatively and postoperatively.

The patient can solely have a regional anaesthetic for the surgical procedure and will be awake or lightly sedated. In addition the patient may receive oxygen via a nasal cannula or mask. The regional anaesthetic may also be supplemented (for pain management postoperatively) with a general anaesthetic.

The anaesthetic practitioner communicates with, supports and reassures the patient during delivery of regional anaesthesia. The patient's correct position is maintained by the anaesthetic practitioner as this is essential for the anaesthetist to achieve the procedure successfully.

There are different types of regional anaesthesia. The most common are spinal and epidural.

Spinal

Spinal anaesthesia, also referred to as an intrathecal block, causes desensitisation of spinal ganglia and motor roots. A local anaesthetic is injected into the lumbar intrathecal space. The local anaesthetic blocks conduction in the spinal nerve roots and dorsal ganglia. Paralysis and analgesia occur below the level of the injection.

During spinal anaesthesia the anaesthetist selects and injects the local anaesthetic drug into the cerebrospinal fluid (CSF) within the subarachnoid space to produce motor, sensory and

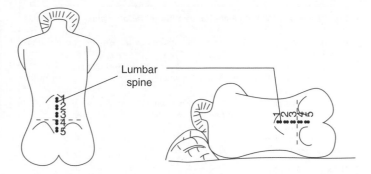

Fig. 8.18 Positioning for spinal anaesthesia.

autonomic blockade by bathing the nerve roots as they leave the spinal cords. This injection will anaesthetise the spinal nerves, resulting in analgesic properties, muscular relaxation and sympathetic blockade. The drug diffuses into the CSF around the ganglia and nerves before it is absorbed into the bloodstream. This technique is used in lower abdominal, inguinal, perineal and obstetric surgical procedures.

Spinal anaesthesia is administered with the patient either in the sitting position (patient is awake), or in the lateral position (patient is awake or anaesthetised; Figure 8.18). The patient flexes his or her spine for easier access for the anaesthetist to undertake this procedure. The circulating practitioner supports the patient throughout the procedure, maintaining the optimum position, and gives reassurance throughout. Figure 8.19 illustrates the position of the injection site within the spine.

Box 8.9 details a checklist for the preparation of the spinal anaesthesia equipment before the procedure.

Epidural

The local anaesthetic is injected into the extradural space (epidural space; Figure 8.20). The results are similar to a spinal anaesthetic. However, during an epidural, the local anaesthetic is injected into the potential space immediately outside the dura mater and this permeates the fatty areolar tissue, contacting the nerves as they transverse into the epidural space. The epidural

---

Box 8.9 Role of the anaesthetic practitioner before spinal anaesthesia

- Utilises an aseptic technique to prepare the relevant trolley and equipment.
- Relevant size of sterile gown and gloves for the anaesthetist.
- Prepares the preferred skin cleansing solution.
- Relevant drape.
- Relevant syringes for local anaesthetic (skin and spinal).
- Relevant needles and filter needle.
- Normal saline.
- Relevant dressing.
- Documentation labels.

Before the procedure:

- Applies all monitoring equipment.
- Reassures the patient.
- Helps to position the patient correctly before the procedure.
- Maintains the dignity of the patient throughout the procedure.
- Communicates and reassures the patient throughout the procedure.
- Documents physiological recordings throughout the procedure.
- Ensures preparation of the relevant intravenous infusion with a warming coil.

Have:

- All relevant monitoring available. Record all physiological readings.
- Nasal cannula or oxygen mask available.
- Tracheal intubation equipment available.
- Relevant drugs available.
- Emergency equipment available.

---

space lies between the vertebral ligaments and the dura mater of the spinal cord. An injection into the epidural space affects the spinal nerves and causes anaesthesia along these nerves (dermatomes; Figure 8.21).

By virtue of its great versatility, epidural anaesthesia is probably the most widely used regional technique in the UK. It may be used for procedures from the neck downwards and the duration of analgesia can be tailored to meet the needs of surgery and postoperative pain relief by using a catheter system (Coventry 2007).

It can be used for surgery for the lower limbs, perineum, pelvis, abdomen and thorax.

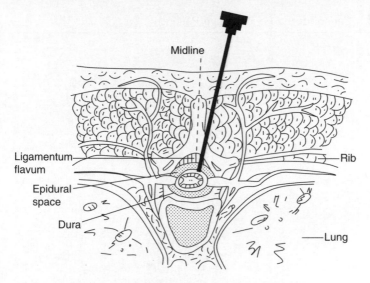

Fig. 8.19 Position of needle within the spine for spinal anaesthesia.

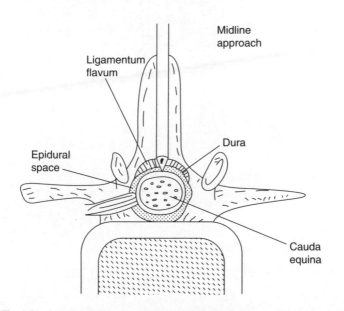

Fig. 8.20 Lumbar epidural anaesthesia – midline approach.

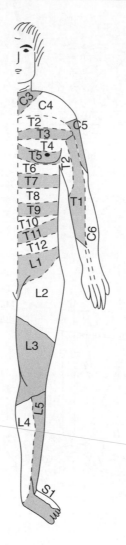

Fig. 8.21 Dermatomes.

A continuous local anaesthetic agent infusion is commenced in the operating room for postoperative analgesia. A test dose of local anaesthetic is injected to ensure the infusion catheter is correctly in place before the catheter is secured with a dressing. Normal saline is injected into the epidural space through the epidural needle and the epidural tubing is flushed for the epidural infusion. Normal saline can be differentiated from CSF as the latter will be at body temperature and not as cold as the normal saline.

Preparation of equipment for an epidural by an anaesthetic practitioner important for the anaesthetist is outlined in Box 8.10.

Contraindications for a spinal
These are:

- patient refusal;
- infection at the site of injection;
- hypovolaemia;
- indeterminate neurological disease;
- severe coagulaopathy;
- increased intercranial pressure (Hadzic 2007).

Complications and side effects of a spinal anaesthetic
Spinal anaesthesia is a common procedure but the anaesthetic practitioner must be aware of the risks associated with it:

- toxicity;
- higher volume;
- less predictable block;
- less dense block.

High or total spinal
This can occur if the anaesthetist injects an excessive quantity of local anaesthetic into the subarachnoid space. The block can increase upwards, causing a high block and the side effect of hypotension. The recovery team may observe the patient having difficulty in breathing. To assist the patient's breathing both preoperatively and postoperatively, the anaesthetist may

---

Box 8.10 Role of the anaesthetic practitioner before an epidural procedure

- An aseptic technique to prepare the relevant trolley and equipment.
- Relevant size of sterile gown and gloves for the anaesthetist.
- Skin cleansing solution.
- Relevant drape.
- Epidural pack (Tuohy needle, catheter, filter). The catheter allows the topping up of the epidural local anaesthetic.
- Relevant syringes and needles for local anaesthetic (skin).
- Normal saline for flush of epidural tubing and filter.
- Relevant dressings.
- Documentation labels.
- Equipment for the epidural infusion:
    — infusion bag – relevant infusion local anaesthetic and opiate (e.g. bupivacaine and fentanyl);
    — infusion pump with fully charged batteries;
    — infusion set;
    — documentation labels.

Before the procedure:

- Communicates and reassures the patient throughout the procedure.
- Helps to position the patient in the relevant position.
- Maintains the dignity of the patient throughout the procedure.

Have:

- All relevant monitoring available. Record all physiological readings.
- Intravenous infusion with warming coil.
- Nasal cannula or oxygen mask available.
- Tracheal intubation equipment available.
- Relevant drugs available.
- Emergency equipment available.

---

intubate the patient. He or she may also treat the hypotension with the appropriate drug.

Headache

Postdural puncture headache is a common complication of spinal anaesthesia. The headache is characteristically mild or absent when the patient is supine but head elevation rapidly leads to severe fronto-occipital headache, which again improves on returning to supine position. The headache is believed to result from the loss of CSF through the meningeal needle hole, resulting in decreased buoyant support for the brain.

If the headache persists, an epidural blood patch is performed. An epidural blood patch is inserted to form a clot over the meningeal hole, thereby preventing further CSF leakage while the meningeal rent heals. Ten to 20 ml of autologous blood is aseptically injected into the epidural space at or near to the interspace at which the meningeal puncture occurred (Hadzic 2007).

Contraindications for an epidural
These are:

- patient refusal;
- severe uncorrected hypovolaemia (Hadzic 2007).

Side effects of an epidural

Dural puncture
If the epidural needle punctures the dura, the anaesthetist may give a spinal by accident. Leakage of CSF will occur from the epidural needle.

Side effects of a spinal and epidural anaesthetic

Hypotension
It is essential to monitor the patient during this procedure. Hypotension can arise because of the use of the local anaesthetic. The appropriate drug should be available to reverse the hypotension. Intravenous infusion can increase the circulatory volume.

Infection
To prevent an infection, the anaesthetic practitioner will set up the relevant spinal or epidural trolley utilising an aseptic technique. Anaesthetists do not undertake these procedures if there are any problems with an underlying infection or clotting.

323

High block
When a high block occurs, anaesthetists will sit the patient up and monitor the patient's physiological recordings. To relieve the patient's breathing both preoperatively and postoperatively, the anaesthetist may intubate the patient. Hypotension may also be treated with appropriate drugs.

Urinary retention
The patient may have problems urinating after these procedures. The surgeon may catheterise the patient to alleviate this preoperatively or postoperatively.

Other problems of regional anaesthesia are failure of the blocks, nausea and vomiting, respiratory depression, toxic reactions, pneumothorax or neurological damage.

Combined spinal–epidural anaesthesia (CSEA)
This is a useful technique by which a spinal block and an epidural catheter are placed simultaneously. This technique is popular because it combines the rapid onset, dense block of spinal anaesthesia with the flexibility afforded by an epidural catheter. The technique is easily performed by first placing a standard epidural needle in the epidural space and then inserting an appropriately sized spinal needle through the shaft of the epidural needle into the subarachnoid space.

The desired local anaesthetic is injected into the subarachnoid space, the spinal needle removed and a catheter placed into the epidural space via the epidural needle. The catheter can then be used to extend the height or duration of the intraoperative block or can be used to provide postoperative epidural analgesia (Hadzic 2007).

Use of regional techniques
For all regional techniques the anaesthetist will secure venous access before the start of the regional anaesthetic procedure. The anaesthetic team monitors the patient throughout the regional anaesthetic within the anaesthetic room and operating room environments. If the patient is awake throughout the surgical procedure, anaesthetic practitioners will fit a nasal cannula or

oxygen mask onto the patient and they will support and observe the patient during the surgical procedure.

If the regional anaesthetic is not effective or if any complications occur, the anaesthetist may consider a general anaesthetic. The anaesthetic practitioner will have tracheal intubation and resuscitation equipment ready for this event.

Resuscitation equipment, including oxygen, a means of ventilating the patient, suction and drugs must be available. The anaesthetic practitioner must be aware of potential side effects and must monitor the patient for these both during the procedure and following its completion (Shields & Werder 2002).

Factors to consider with regional anaesthesia are listed in Box 8.11.

LOCAL ANAESTHESIA, LOCAL INFILTRATION AND NERVE BLOCKS

Local infiltration is a technique that surgeons or anaesthetists use to block a nerve to produce local anaesthesia. The local anaesthetic diffuses into the cell membrane to produce this effect. Efficacy depends on the degree of myelination, size of nerve and the position of the fibre within the nerve. Infiltration of the local anaesthetic will act on the sensory nerve ending.

Anaesthetists and surgeons use a local anaesthetic for many reasons:

- complete anaesthetic for minor surgery;
- the patient has a medical condition which prevents the anaesthetist administering a general anaesthetic;
- preference of the patient, anaesthetist or surgeon;
- local infiltration for pain management after an invasive procedure.

Local field block

Anaesthetists or surgeons can inject a local anaesthetic subcutaneously to produce a local field block. This allows the surgeon to perform minor surgery, such as removal of lumps and bumps after injecting a local anaesthetic into the relevant site to freeze the surgical procedure area. A local anaesthetic can also be injected with a vasoconstrictor (adrenaline [epinephrine]),

---

Box 8.11   Factors to consider with regional anaesthesia

Level of insertion
- Cervical;
- Thoracic;
- Lumbar;
- Caudal.

Choice of drug/dosage
Local anaesthetic
- Bupivacaine or lidocaine.

Opioid
- Fentanyl.
- Diamorphine.

Considerations before procedure
- Patient choice/cooperation.
- Abnormalities of spinal cord.
- Coagulopathy.
- Vascular disorders.
- Skin infection.
- Raised intracranial pressure.
- Hypvolaemia.

Infusion/rate of infusion
- Continuous infusion.
- Intermittent boluses.

Monitoring
- ECG.
- Pulse oximeter.
- Blood pressure.
- Respiration.
- Level of block.
- Temperature.
- Oxygen administration if applicable.

Treatment
- Drugs (e.g. vasopressors, anti-emetics, emergency IV infusion)
- Resuscitation equipment

which can increase the speed of action of the local anaesthetic by local vasoconstriction. The latter can never be used in nasal, digit or penile surgery.

Local infiltration

Surgeons use a local anaesthetic to infiltrate a surgical wound subcutaneously (before or after suturing the skin) for postoperative pain management of a surgical procedure in coordination with other methods.

Local nerve block

A local anaesthetic can be injected into nerve plexuses (brachial, lumbar, cervical), a major or a minor nerve to produce local anaesthesia for intraoperative and postoperative pain management for a surgical procedure. Major nerves (e.g. femoral or sciatic) and minor nerves (e.g. ulnar or digital) are examples of nerve blocks that the anaesthetist might perform.

The anaesthetic practitioner will prepare and check all relevant equipment before the procedure, described in Box 8.12.

Topical anaesthesia

Anaesthetists may request a topical cream (e.g. Emla) for paediatric patients before they perform venous cannulation. This cream desensitises the skin and aids pain management for this procedure. This cream can also be used for adult patients who have a needle phobia. It is preferable that the ward staff apply this an hour before the anaesthetic for it to be effective. Practitioners should remove the cream immediately prior to the venflon being inserted by the anaesthetist.

SEDATION

Sedative drugs may be administered during a regional or local anaesthetic. Surgeons may use them during an endoscopy procedure. Sedative drugs can reduce the patient's anxiety and produce sleep. They can produce airway problems and hypotension so the appropriate oxygen and reversal drug should be available.

Baseline monitoring is required with intravenous access (McMillan 2008)

Box 8.12   Role of the anaesthetic practitioner for a local nerve block procedure

- An aseptic technique to prepare the relevant trolley and equipment.
- Relevant size of sterile gown and gloves for the anaesthetist.
- Skin cleansing solution.
- Relevant drape.
- Relevant size of nerve block needle.
- Relevant syringes and needles for local anaesthetic (skin and nerve block).
- Normal saline.
- Relevant dressings.
- Intravenous infusion with warming coil.

Before the procedure:

- Helps to position the patient in the relevant position.
- Communicates and reassures the patient throughout the procedure
- Maintains the dignity of the patient throughout the procedure.

Have:

- All relevant monitoring available. Records all physiological readings.
- Nasal cannula or oxygen mask available.
- Tracheal intubation equipment available.
- Relevant drugs available.
- Emergency equipment available.

The anaesthetic practitioner will prepare and check all relevant equipment before the procedure, described in Box 8.13.

THE PAEDIATRIC PATIENT

The practitioner must remember that the paediatric patient can be a neonate, a small child or an adolescent. It is important to reassure, support and involve the paediatric patient and parent or carer in the reception area and anaesthetic room.

According to Meeseri *et al.* (2004), the induction for surgery is a stressful time for both child and family. Donnelly (2005) argues that a young child's emotional development is immature and that the presence of a parent or carer will provide reassurance to maintain the child's sense of security.

Mallet & Dougherty (2001) state that paediatric patients have special communication needs within the operating room envi-

---

Box 8.13   Role of the anaesthetic practitioner during sedation

- Reassure and communicate with the patient throughout the procedure.
- Attach all monitoring equipment and record observations.
- Assist the anaesthetist or surgeon in the venous cannulation of the patient.
- Attach a dressing to the venous cannula.
- Ensure an intravenous infusion is available if required.
- Have a nasal cannula available.
- Measure the level of consciousness of the patient.

Have available:

- Reversal of the sedative drug.
- A face mask and filter.
- Tracheal intubation equipment.
- Suction equipment and suction catheters.
- Relevant size of oropharyngeal airway.
- A gum elastic bougie. Anaesthetists may have difficulty when they insert the ET tube.
- A stethoscope for anaesthetists to check the correct position of the ET tube.
- Emergency equipment.

---

ronment. They have the same anxieties as adult patients but are unable to articulate them as well. The anaesthetic practitioner needs to involve the parents of the patient in the preoperative care and promote security and comfort in the anaesthetic room for the patient and the parent(s) or carer(s). Anaesthetic practitioners may use distraction techniques during the care of the patient, especially during the intravenous cannulation and induction of the patient.

When a child undergoes anaesthesia, the anaesthetist must be assisted by staff (ODPs/assistants/anaesthetic nurses who have specific paediatric skills and training) (AAGBI 2005a). Paediatric anaesthesia can present many challenges to the anaesthesia team, both anatomically and physiologically. Children are not small adults, they are unique in that the conditions they present with are often exclusive to them (Hardcastle 2007).

The differences in anatomy and physiology between children, especially infants, and adults have important consequences in many aspects of anaesthesia (De Melo 2007). The technical behavioural issues due to immaturity may make induction of anaesthesia more challenging in the child compared to the adult (Mellor 2004).

Occasionally the patient will need to have an inhalational gas induction as, when deemed, it is too distressing for the patient to undergo venous cannulation. The anaesthetic practitioner can help to relax the patient and parent and can ensure that the induction procedure is as comfortable as possible. Keeping calm and confident can help the patient, the anaesthetist and the parent.

A full range of monitoring devices, paediatric anaesthetic equipment and disposable items for general and regional anaesthesia should be available in theatres and all areas where children are anaesthetised. This should include all sizes and ages (Bristol Royal Infirmary Report 2001).

Monitoring of the patient is essential before and during induction of anaesthesia as the paediatric patient's condition can deteriorate more quickly than an adult's. Therefore, before commencing induction of the paediatric patient, the anaesthetic practitioner must prepare two laryngoscopes, suction apparatus, a range of ET tubes, LMAs and masks. (preparation is the same as for an adult patient). Clear facemasks are the choice of most anaesthetists as the patient's colour and secretions can be checked during the intubation procedure.

There are important considerations with regard to airway management as indicated by the Association of Anaesthetists of Great Britain and Ireland (AAGBI 1998). It suggests that there are some special features peculiar to the paediatric airway. Children have a relatively large head, short neck, a prominent occiput and a relatively large tongue. The larynx is high and anterior and the epiglottis is long and U-shaped. Furthermore, infants breathe mainly through their nasal airway, although their nostrils are small and easily obstructed.

Anaesthesia is commonly induced in children and infants by means of a gaseous induction via a facemask with a volatile agent. Inhalational induction is preferred by some children who fear the insertion of an intravenous cannula, are needle phobic, have had a psychologically traumatic experience in the past with intravenous induction or prefer this method of induction (Hardcastle 2007).

Box 8.14   Recommended endotracheal tube sizes (Rusy &
Usleva 1998)

Internal diameter

Age	Size of tube
Premature	2.5–3.00 mm
Neonate–6 months	3.0–3.5 mm
6 months–1 year	3.5–4.00 mm
1–2 years	4.0–5.0 mm
>2 years	Use the formula 4 + (age + 4)

Length in cm
(Age in years + 2) + 12

An inhalational induction is often used in babies and small infants because of difficulties obtaining venous access (Bagshaw & Stack 1999).

With regards to the preparation of airway management, the anaesthetic practitioner must consider the size and weight of the paediatric patient. The size of the ET tube is critical, as one that is too large will exert pressure on the internal surface of the cricoid cartilage resulting in oedema. This could lead to airway obstruction when positive pressure is applied to it. Box 8.14 provides details of the recommended size of ET tube to use, depending on the patient's age.

The anaesthetic practitioner selects the size of the ET tube according to the width and length of the trachea. The anaesthetist uses an uncuffed ET tube in the paediatric patient under 11 years of age. This allows for a slight space around the exterior circumference. Soft tissue at the narrowest level of the cricoid cartilage located just below the vocal cords forms a loose seal around the tube.

Preparation for intubation

Anaesthetic practitioners should check all relevant equipment for this procedure as for the adult procedure.

Infants and neonates are at an increased risk of developing hypothermia because of their increased ratio of body surface to body mass. Infants also are unable to shiver to generate heat in response to hypothermia (Day 2006, Kempainen & Brunette 2004).

Perioperative thermal management is critical in decreasing morbidity and, thus, accurate measurement of body temperature is necessary for timely detection and management of temperature disturbances.

Rusy & Usaleva (1998) advocate that measures should be taken by the anaesthetic practitioner to reduce hypothermia, including: warming the environment, using warming devices and blankets, warming inspired gases and intravenous fluids.

THE PREGNANT PATIENT: CAESAREAN SECTION

Anatomical and physiological changes during pregnancy result in the pregnant patient being at greater risk from airway problems and difficult and failed intubation than a non-pregnant patient (Kuczkowski 2003). These difficulties can be due to capillary engorgement of the respiratory mucosa, predisposing upper airways to trauma, bleeding and obstruction.

There are three main anaesthetic techniques for a caesarean section: general, epidural or spinal anaesthesia. The latter two can be performed together (CSEA) (Gwinnutt 2008).

The anaesthetic practitioner therefore must have all airway and resuscitation equipment available before induction of a general anaesthetic or for the regional techniques of epidural, spinal or combined spinal–epidural.

Aortocaval compression

From mid-pregnancy the enlarging uterus compresses both the inferior vena cava and the lower aorta when the patient lies supine. Compression of the inferior vena cava reduces venous return to the heart, leading to a fall in pre-load and cardiac output. The fall in blood pressure may be severe enough for the mother to lose consciousness. Compression of the aorta may lead to a reduction in uteroplacental and renal blood flow. During the last trimester, maternal kidney function is markedly lower in the supine than in the lateral position. Furthermore, fetal transplacental gas exchange may be compromised. For these reasons no woman should lie supine in late pregnancy.

Most unanaesthetised women are capable of compensating for the resultant decrease in stroke volume by increasing systemic vascular resistance and heart rate. Blood from the lower limbs may return through the paravertebral and azygos systems.

General anaesthesia, subarachnoid and epidural blocks abolish the sympathetic response and increase the risk of supine hypotension. During caesarean section and for other situations requiring a supine position, the uterus should be displaced (usually to the left) by placing a rigid wedge under the hip and/ or tilting the table (UK Anaesthesia 2009).

Mendelson's syndrome

Airway management is compromised with the physiological changes to the gastrointestinal system.

In the later stages of pregnancy there is an increased risk of regurgitation and acid aspiration which could lead to Mendelson's syndrome (chemical pneumonia) (Smith 2006 cited in Nunney 2008). The risk of Mendelson's syndrome results from weakness of the gastro-oesophageal sphincter (Popat & Simpson 2002).

Gastro-oesophageal reflux and delayed gastric emptying are features of pregnancy and therefore the risk of aspiration is taken into consideration at intubation. Anaesthetists administer sodium citrate before induction. If anaesthetists undertake induction, the anaesthetic practitioner applies cricoid pressure to prevent the regurgitation of gastric contents into the pharynx.

The anaesthetic practitioner attaches routine monitoring equipment as hypertension is one of the frequent complications of pregnancy. It is important that the patient's physiological readings are checked and recorded frequently.

The AAGBI (2005b) state that parturients requiring anaesthesia have the right to the same standards of perioperative care as all surgical patients, including anaesthetic assistance. In the UK, anaesthetic assistance may be provided by an ODP or registered nurse. Whatever their background, the training for all anaesthetic assistants must comply with current qualification standards (AAGBI 2005b).

THE ELDERLY PATIENT

Surgical risk increases with age, and complications are poorly tolerated by the elderly patient. Although surgical risk is significant, careful preoperative assessment, risk assessment and intraoperative management offer the patient the best possible outcome.

Obtaining vascular access may be more difficult in the elderly patient because his or her veins may be fragile, making it difficult to place monitoring devices and for the administration of intravenous drugs, fluids and blood products. Arthritic changes could make patient intubation and operative positioning difficult and these aspects need particular consideration by the anaesthetic practitioner.

The provision of active warming devices and anti-pressure sore apparatus is mandatory for the elderly. In the elderly, maintenance of body temperature is essential. Elderly patients may be unable to increase their metabolic rate to counteract heat loss. Shivering may increase oxygen demand above respiratory capacity. Conservation of heat by the use of active warm air systems, by warming intravenous fluids and by operating, where possible, in a warm ambient environment all help to maintain body temperature and aid recovery.

Most pressure sores develop within the first 24 four hours following surgery. Pressure sores prolong hospital stay, delay essential rehabilitation and may produce sepsis which can be fatal. Preventative measures are especially important during prolonged operations and may be compounded by periods of hypotension with poor skin perfusion. Adequate equipment in both operating theatre and recovery areas for the prevention of skin damage must be provided and maintained (AAGBI 2001).

Older patients are particularly prone to the development of hypothermia. This is primarily because older persons lose heat more rapidly than younger persons because of decreased fat and muscle mass. In addition, changes in vascular tone in the older adult inhibit vasoconstriction and thus decrease heat production. Furthermore, general anaesthesia or major regional anaesthesia impair thermoregulatory mechanisms of an older person to a greater extent those of a younger person (AORN 2009 cited in Hegarty *et al.* 2009).

In the induction of anaesthesia, arm–brain circulation time is increased and induction agent dose requirements are drastically reduced. Decreased cardiac output means that circulation time for drugs and anaesthetic agents used is longer.

The number of elderly patients presenting for anaesthesia and surgery has increased exponentially in recent years. Regional anaesthesia is frequently used in elderly patients undergoing surgery. Although the type of anaesthesia (general *versus* regional anaesthesia) has no substantial effect on perioperative morbidity and mortality in any age group; it intuitively makes sense that elderly patients would benefit from regional anaesthesia because they remain minimally sedated throughout the procedures and awaken with excellent postoperative pain control. However, a multitude of factors influence the outcome, such as the type, duration and invasiveness of the operation, co-existing medical and mental status of the patient and the skill and expertise of the anaesthetist and surgeon. These factors make it difficult to decide if and when one technique is equivocally better than another. Thus, it is more important to optimise the overall management of the patient during the perioperative period and, in most cases, it is the quality of the anaesthetic administered rather than the type of anaesthetic which is most important. Sedatives used for regional anaesthesia in the elderly should be short acting, easy to administer, have a low adverse effect profile and high safety margin (Tsui *et al.* 2004).

Anaesthetic practitioners need to give adequate time for the elderly patient to answer questions and ensure that they understand the practitioner's communication. They should be vigilant in the positioning of elderly patients as they may have frail skin and correct positioning is important to prevent damage on pressure areas such as heels, sacrum and elbows. They should use appropriate thermoregulation equipment to conserve the patient's temperature and decrease the possibility of hypothermia. Care must be taken when moving the patient's limbs as the patient may suffer from degenerative conditions such as arthritis or osteoporosis.

CONCLUSION

To deliver and maintain effective patient care in their anaesthetic practice, practitioners must be aware of their roles and responsibilities and provide efficient collaboration within the multiprofessional team of the operating department.

REFERENCES

Adams, S.A. (2009) *Difficult Airways: Always Have a Plan B.* www.rtmagazine.com/issues/articles/2009_03_01.asp

Aitkenhead, A.R., Smith, G. & Mushambi, M.C. (2007) Anaesthetic apparatus. In: Aitkenhead, A.R., & Smith, G. & Rowbotham, D.J. (2007) *Textbook of Anaesthesia*, 5th edn. Churchill Livingstone, Edinburgh, pp 220–264.

Al Shaikh, B. & Stacey, S. (2007) *Essentials of Anaesthetic Equipment*, 3rd edn. Churchill Livingstone Elsevier, Edinburgh.

American Association of Anesthesiologists (ASA) (1993) Practice guidelines for the management of the difficult airway. A report by the ASA Task Force on Management of the Difficult Airway. *Anesthesiology* **78**, 597.

American Association of Anesthesiologists (ASA) (2003) Practice Guidelines for Management of the Difficult Airway. An Updated Report by the American Society of Anesthesiologists' Task Force on Management of the Difficult Airway. *Anesthesiology* **98**, 1269–1277.

American Operating Room Nurses (AORN) (2009) *Recommended Practices for the Prevention of Unplanned Perioperative Hypothermia in Perioperative Standards and Recommended Practices.* AORN, Denver.

Anderson, I.G. (2003) *Care of the Critically Ill Surgical Patient.* Hodder & Arnold, London.

Association of Anaesthetists of Great Britain and Ireland (AAGBI) (1998) *Paediatric Surgery Standards of Care.* AAGBI, London.

Association of Anaesthetists of Great Britain and Ireland (AAGBI) (2001) *Anaesthesia and Peri-Operative Care of the Elderly.* AAGBI, London.

Association of Anaesthetists of Great Britain and Ireland (AAGBI) (2004) *Checking Anaesthetic Equipment 3.* AAGBI, London.

Association of Anaesthetists of Great Britain and Ireland (AAGBI) (2005a) *The Anaesthesia Team.* AAGBI, London.

Association of Anaesthetists of Great Britain and Ireland (AAGBI) (2005b) *Obstetric Anaesthetists Association/AAGBI Guidelines for Obstetric Services.* Revised Edition. AAGBI, London.

Association of Anaesthetists of Great Britain and Ireland (AAGBI) (2007) *Recommendations for Standards of Monitoring During Anaesthesia and Recovery*, 4th edn. AAGBI, London.

Bagshaw, O.N.T. & Stack, S.G. (1999) A comparison of halothane and isoflurane for gaseous induction of anaesthesia in infants. *Paediatric Anaesthesia* **9**, 25–29.

Barash, B.G., Cullen, B.F. & Stoelting, R.K. (2007) *Clinical Anaesthesia*, 5th edn. Lippincott Williams Wilkins, Philadelphia.

Bristol Royal Infirmary Report (2001) *Learning From Bristol; The Report of the Public Enquiry into Children's Heart Surgery at the Bristol Royal Infirmary 1984–1995.* The Stationery Office, London. www.dh.gov.uk/assetrOOT/04/05/94/79/0459479.pdf

Cormack, R.S. & Lehane, J. (1984) Difficult tracheal intubation in obstetrics. *Anaesthesia* **39**, 1105.

Coventry, D.M. (2007) Local anaesthetic techniques. In: Aitkenhead, A.R., Rowbotham, D.J. & Smith, G. (eds) *Textbook of Anaesthesia*, 5th edn. Churchill Livingstone, Edinburgh, pp 315–344.

Day, M.P. (2006) Hypothermia: A hazard for all seasons. *Nursing* **36** (12 pt 1), 44–47.

De Melo, E. (2007) Paediatric anaesthesia and intensive care. In: Aitkenhead, A.R., Rowbotham, D.J. & Smith, G. (eds) *Textbook of Anaesthesia*, 5th edn. Churchill Livingstone, Edinburgh, pp 653–670.

Difficult Airway Society (2009) www.guideline.gov.summary/summary.aspx?doc_id=6183&nbr=0039882&string=tube

Donnelly, J. (2005) Care of children and adolescents. In: Woodhead, K. & Wicker, P. (eds) (2007) *A Textbook of Perioperative Care*. Elsevier, London, pp 267–283.

Fell, D. & Kirkbride, D. (2007) The practical conduct of anaesthesia. In: Aitkenhead, A.R., Rowbotham, D.J. & Smith, G. (eds) *Textbook of Anaesthesia*, 5th edn. Churchill Livingstone, Edinburgh, pp 297–314.

Greaves, I., Hodgetts, T. & Porter, K. (2001) *A Texbook for Paramedics*. W.B. Saunders, London.

Griffiths, R.V. (1999) Anaesthesia: airway management. *British Journal of Nursing* **9** (10), 480–484.

Gwinnutt, C. (2008) *Clinical Anaesthesia*, 3rd edn. John Wiley & Sons Ltd, Oxford.

Hadzic, A. (2007) *Textbook of Regional Anesthesia and Acute Pain Management*. McGraw Hill, New York.

Hardcastle, T. (2007) Intravenous induction versus inhalation induction for general anaesthesia in paediatrics. In: Smith, B., Rawling, P., Wicker, P. & Jones, C. (eds) *Core Topics in Operating Department Practice. Anaesthesia and Critical Care*. Cambridge University Press, Cambridge, pp 102–109.

Hardman, J.G. (2007) Complications during anaesthesia. In: Aitkenhead, A.R. & Smith, G. & Rowbotham, D.J. (eds) *Textbook of Anaesthesia*, 5th edn. Churchill Livingstone, Edinburgh, pp 367–399.

Hegarty, J., Walsh, E., Burton, A., Murphy, S., O'Gorman, F. & McPolin, G. (2009) Nurses' knowledge of inadvertent hypothermia. *AORN Journal* **89** (4), 701–713.

Hein, C. & Owen, H. (2005) The effective application of cricoid pressure. *Journal of Emergency Primary Health Care* **3** (1–2), Article No 990101.

Illingworth, K.A. & Simpson, K.H. (1994) *Anaesthesia and Analgesia in Emergency Medicine*. Oxford University Press, New York.

Intavent (1999) *Anaesthesia: LMA. Instructions for Use*, 4th edn. Intavent Research Ltd., Coalville, Leicestershire.

Kempainen, R.R. & Brunette, D.D. (2004) The evaluation and management of accidental hypothermia. *Plastic Surgery Respiratory Care* **49** (2), 192–205.

Knill, R.L. (1993) Difficult laryngoscopy made easy with a 'BURP'. *Canadian Journal of Anesthesiology* **40**, 279–282.

Kuczkowski, K.M. (2003) Airway problems and new solutions for the obstetric patient. *Journal of Clinical Anaesthesia* **15**, 552–563.

Mallet, J. & Dougherty, L. (2001) *The Royal Marsden Hospital: Manual of Nursing Procedures*, 5th edn. Blackwell Science, London.

McMillan, R. (2008) Day surgery. In: Woodhead, K. & Wicker, P. (eds) *A Textbook of Perioperative Care*. Churchill Livingstone Elsevier, Edinburgh, pp 199–220.

Meeseri, A., Caprilli, S. & Busconi, P. (2004) Anaesthesia induction in children: A psychological evaluation of the efficiency of parents' presence. *Paediatric Anaesthesia* **14**, 551–556.

Mellor, J. (2004) Induction of anaesthesia in paediatric patients. *Update in Anaesthesia* **18** (8), 1. www.nda.ox.ac.uk/wfsa/html/ul8/ul08_01.

Mitchell, M.J. (2005) *Anxiety Management in Adult Day Surgery. A Nursing Perspective*. Whurr, London.

Morgan, G.E. & Mikhail, M.S. (1996) *Clinical Anaesthesiology*. McGraw-Hill, New York.

Morton, N.S. (1997) *Assisting the Anaesthetist*. Oxford University Press, Oxford.

Nunney, R. (ed) (2008) Providing perioperative care for pregnant women. *Nursing Standard* **22** (47), 40–44.

Popat, M. & Simpson, P.J. (2002) *Understanding Anaesthesia*, 4th edn. Butterworth Heinemann, Oxford.

Rusy, L. & Usaleva, E. (1998) *Paediatric Anaesthesia Review*. www.nda.ox.ac.uk/wfsa/html/u08/u08_003.htm

Shields, L. & Werder, H. (2002) *Perioperative Nursing*. Greenwich Medical Media, London.

Tsui, B.C.H., Wagner, A. & Finucane, B. (2004) Regional anaesthesia in the elderly: A clinical guide. *Drugs and Aging* **21** (14), 895–910.

Turner, D.A.B. (2007) Emergency anaesthesia. In: Aitkenhead, A.R., Smith, G. & Rowbotham, D.J. (eds) *Textbook of Anaesthesia*, 5th edn. Churchill Livingstone, Edinburgh, pp 540–553.

UK Anaesthesia (2009) *Anatomical & Physiological Changes in Pregnancy Relevant to Anaesthesia*. www.frca.co.uk

Visser, L. (2001) *Epidural Anaesthesia*. www.nda.ox.ac.uk/wfsa/html/u13/u/311-01.ht#epid

Yentis, S.M., Hirsch, N.P. & Smith, G.B. (2001) *Anaesthesia & Intensive Care: A-Z An Encycopaedia of Principles and Practice*, 2nd edn. Butterworth-Heinemann, Oxford.

World Health Organization (WHO) *Surgical Safety Checklist* www.who.int/patientsafety/safesurgery/…checklist/…index.html

Patient Care During Surgery

9

Paul Wicker and Adele Nightingale

LEARNING OUTCOMES

❏ Discuss the *role of the scrub and circulating practitioner* in the surgical team.

❏ Discuss the *key clinical skills and knowledge* required in the following areas of care:

infection control in the operating room;

positioning the patient;

surgical skills – managing recordable items, haemostasis and wound management.

INTRODUCTION

The perioperative team must provide a holistic approach to the evidence-based, safe and effective care of the patient. The team must achieve this in the short time available while the patient undergoes his or her anaesthesia and surgery.

The scrub practitioner works within the perioperative team to provide care and clinical expertise to help the surgical procedure to progress smoothly and efficiently. Because of this, the role of the scrub practitioner merits special considerations. As part of the more holistic perioperative role, the scrub practitioner is central to the patient's treatment. The work of the scrub practitioner can make the difference between a smooth, efficient procedure and a procedure fraught with delays, frustrations and errors (Taylor & Campbell 1999a). Specific roles include providing supplies to surgeons and assistants undertaking the surgery, managing instruments and medical devices, and providing skilled help to the surgeon with the surgical procedure.

The circulating practitioner is responsible for supporting the surgical team and providing skilled care and support for the patient. This includes, for example, positioning of the patient, protecting the patient from pressure damage, keeping the patient safe from harm during long procedures and safe transfer to and from the reception and recovery areas.

Chapter 3 describes how to improve care by preparing the patient and the perioperative team for this experience. Chapter 6 describes in detail the competencies required of scrub and circulating practitioners. This chapter discusses the underpinning skills and knowledge in three particular areas of care:

- infection control in the operating room;
- positioning the patient;
- surgical skills – managing recordable items and haemostasis, and wound management.

INFECTION CONTROL IN THE PERIOPERATIVE ENVIRONMENT

The control of infection in the perioperative environment is one of the most important roles for practitioners. Some 75% of nosocomial (hospital acquired) infections occur in surgical patients. Most postoperative infections arise from the patient's own flora and the commonest sites of infection include the urinary tract, respiratory tract and blood (septicaemia) (Surgical Tutor 2005a) (Table 9.1). Other common sites of infection include wounds and areas of the body involved in the surgery.

Practitioners must therefore be aware of potential sources of contamination and measures that they can take to prevent or reduce perioperative infection. Hand washing is the single most important measure for preventing nosocomial infections (Doebbeling *et al*. 1992, Fell 2000, Pinney 2000).

Standard precautions

'Standard precautions' is the term used to describe an approach to infection control which offers protection for individuals against contamination from all sources, whether or not they carry a known infection risk (Wicker 1991, Pearson 2000, Gruendemann & Magnum 2001, Beesley & Pirie 2005). It

Table 9.1 Common sites of perioperative infection.

Infection	Common causes	Prevention
Urinary tract (40%)	Urinary catheterisation, renal disease	Aseptic technique, hand washing
Respiratory tract (15%)	By-passing respiratory defence systems, e.g. ET tubes, oral airways. Aspiration of stomach contents	Prophylactic antibiotics, aseptic technique, patient education on coughing and breathing exercises
Bacteraemia (5%)	Infection of the blood often caused by contaminated intravenous lines, catheters and other invasive devices	Aseptic technique, regular changing of catheters and lines, checking solutions before infusing
Other (40%)	Wound and surgical sites	Aseptic technique, careful instrument management, good draping techniques, good surgical techniques

involves assessing the risk of contamination by any blood and body fluids (organic matter) and providing protection against it.

Practising standard precautions involves confining and controlling spillages of contamination, and providing a barrier between the contamination and the practitioner. Following standard precautions helps to ensure the safety of practitioners and patients. Confining and controlling spillages includes such measures as:

- wiping up blood spillages immediately rather than waiting to the end of the case;
- decontaminating spillages with suitable solutions;
- using suction with lavage to prevent spillages on the floor;
- soaking excess lavage with packs and disposing of these safely;
- using suitable drapes for containing spillages when anticipating large amounts of fluid;
- changing contaminated clothing immediately;

- providing protection from contamination for practitioners involves using protective clothing – this includes surgical masks, hats, gloves, shoes, gowns and goggles.

It is the employer's responsibility to provide personal protective equipment (PPE). If PPE is provided, practitioners have a responsibility to use it. PPE can provide different levels of protection. For example, a simple paper mask may offer some protection against splashing to the face, whereas high filtration surgical masks can offer hours of protection against fluid splashes and inhalation of aerosols or surgical smoke. Surgical masks are also used to provide protection to the patient from micro-organisms expelled from the mouth and nose of the surgical team (AfPP 2007). The quality of surgical gowns also differs widely, from simple cotton gowns to high-tech gowns which are impermeable to any fluid.

Similarly, some surgical procedures carry more risk of contamination than others. For example, removing a sebaceous cyst on the hand carries much less risk of contamination than a hemiarthroplasty of the hip joint, where the risk of contamination by blood and aerosols is much higher (MHRA 2003).

The ability to assess the risk of contamination is therefore a key skill for the perioperative practitioner. Risk assessment is a measure of the perceived likelihood of something happening and the impact if it does happen. The Association for Perioperative Practice (AfPP)'s *Risk and Quality Management System* (AfPP 2006) offers guidelines on the risk assessment of clinical situations, including identifying best practice. This tool uses standards, assessment of criteria to meet the standard and allocation of a score to help practitioners assess risk.

Practitioners do not always need such a detailed risk assessment if the practitioner understands the features of the clinical situation, the appropriate standards of practice and the criteria that must be met. For example, a scrub practitioner may identify a high risk of glove perforation and inhalation of aerosols from pulse lavage during a major orthopaedic case. The relevant standards include protection from contamination, so the practitioner should use a high-filtration face mask and visor, waterproof barrier gown and double gloves. Similarly, a circulating practitioner who needs to clean potentially contaminated operating room furniture, following the removal of a sebaceous cyst, may decide that gloves are sufficient. The standard in both situations is identical – protection from contamination – but the risk assessment has shown the way to different practices which are equally safe. The ability to undertake such assessments is one which experienced practitioners develop through continual professional development and learning from experience.

Sources of perioperative contamination

The spread of contamination occurs when organisms move from one area to another. If the organisms infect a human being, then disease can occur. Continued vigilance and following the principles of standard precautions is essential to reduce the possibility of infection from contamination.

Operating departments normally provide a low infection risk environment for patient care. However, the biggest infection source is from people, and often clinical requirements and operational demands increase infection risk. For example, the need to perform extended surgery increases infection risk because of exposed instruments, increased possibility of contamination and exposure of the wound site. However, the patient's well-being may be dependent on the successful completion of the surgery, regardless of the time taken. Similarly the constant opening of doors to and from the anaesthetic or disposal room may disturb ventilation systems, but may be essential to carry out clinical procedures safely and efficiently (Line 2003).

Potential problems in infection control in the operating department include:

- staff;
- patients;
- ventilation systems;
- equipment;
- surgical gowns and drapes.

Staff

The process of the surgical scrub, gloving and gowning aims to reduce the risk of transferring organisms from the surgical team to the patient's open wound. The scrub procedure and antimicrobial solution used are important to reduce skin flora as far as possible (Beesley & Pirie 2005).

However, despite the surgical scrub, even thorough hand washing does not permanently reduce the number of microorganisms on the skin – organisms from deep within skin pores reappear on the skin surface in 10–20 minutes. Therefore, practitioners must also wear sterile surgical gloves to help reduce the risk of contamination. Several makes of surgical glove are available, but all aim to reduce organisms spreading to and from the patient (Fell 2000, Pinney 2000). Gloves should be discarded after each procedure or contact with a patient, or when they are visibly contaminated (AfPP 2007).

The use of masks in the operating room remains controversial (Lipp & Edwards 2002). However, the use of masks within the operating department is recommended. Masks filter bacteria and can reduce the number of organisms inhaled or given off into the operating room atmosphere. They also provide a physical barrier to contamination from the blood or body fluids of the patient. However, there are several issues associated with masks which make them less effective. For example:

- removing the mask transfers organisms on to the hands; therefore, masks should be removed using the ties only and discarded in an appropriate receptacle, and hands washed;
- masks become ineffective when wet; in this case they should be removed at the earliest time possible and disposed of appropriately;
- contaminated air can easily escape from badly fitting masks; the nose and mouth should be covered by the mask, it should fit the contours of the face and be securely fastened (AfPP 2007).

Poor compliance with mask wearing can occur when practitioners do not understand the need for reducing infection or the features of the mask (Pearson 2000). For example, practitioners should be aware that standard masks do not always protect users against inhaling surgical smoke and laser plume, especially if they are badly fitting.

Table 9.2 Normal body flora.

Body area	Normal flora
Skin	*Staphylococcus aureus, Streptoccoccus pyogenes*, methicillin-resistant *Staph. aureus* (MRSA)
Oral cavity	Staphylococci, streptococci and anaerobes
Nasopharynx	Staphylococci, streptococci, *Haemophilus* and anaerobes
Large bowel	Gram-negative rods (e.g. *Escherichia coli, Enterobacter*), enterococci and anaerobes *Clostridium*
Urinary tract	Normally sterile

The practitioner should always use a mask for protection against contamination:

- when the operating room does not have plenum air ventilation, because aerosols are not removed efficiently by normal ventilation systems;
- when assisting during surgical procedures where there is a risk of contamination, splashing or inhalation of droplets or other foreign bodies, or when the practitioner is close enough to the surgical site to be exposed to contamination from splashing by blood or body fluids;
- when frequently opening operating room doors (as this reduces the efficiency of the ventilation system).

Patients

Normal bacterial flora live in the nose, groin, armpit, gut, skin and hair of everybody (Table 9.2). They are part of the human body's ecosystem and are conducive to life. Organisms may become pathogenic when they move out of their normal area on the body to an open wound. For example, healthy people's noses often contain *Staphylococcus aureus*, which can cause wound infection. Organisms normally resident in the gut can cause wound and other infections, and good surgical technique is essential to prevent their transfer to other areas of the body. Prophylactic antibiotics can help to reduce the possibility of

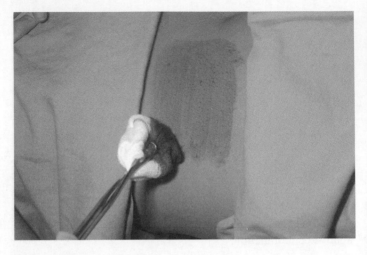

Fig. 9.1 Patient skin preparation.

infection when a surgical procedure has a known high infection risk (NICE 2008).

Practitioners use a wide range of antimicrobial solutions to reduce the risk of skin organisms infecting wounds. Despite these precautions, normal surgical activities may still transfer organisms from exposed areas of the patient's skin to the wound area. Practitioners still require good aseptic technique to reduce the risk of cross-infection (Gruendemann & Magnum 2001).

Historically, preoperative skin preparation sometimes took place on the ward; nowadays skin preparation is undertaken within the operating department. Figure 9.1 illustrates the typical surgical preparation of the patient's skin. The purpose of skin preparation is to remove visible contaminants and to reduce levels of naturally occurring skin flora, potentially reducing the risk of surgical site infection. Immediately prior to incision the skin should be prepared using an antiseptic preparation (AfPP 2007, NICE 2008).

Skin shaving helps to keep hair away from the wound site and is most effective at reducing wound infection when per-

Table 9.3 Skin preparation solutions.

Solution	Actions
70% Isopropyl alcohol	Acts by denaturing proteins. Bactericidal and short acting. Effective against Gram-positive and Gram-negative organisms, fungicidal and virucidal
0.5% Chlorhexidine	Quaternary ammonium compound which acts by disrupting the bacterial cell wall. Bactericidal but does not kill spore-forming organisms. It is persistent and has a long duration of action (up to 6 hours). More effective against Gram-positive organisms
70% Povidone-iodine	Acts by oxidation and substitution of free iodine. Bactericidal and active against spore-forming organisms. Effective against both Gram-positive and Gram-negative organisms. Rapidly inactivated by organic material such as blood and body tissues

formed immediately before surgery. Infection rate increases from 1% to 5% if performed more than 12 hours before surgery, because of organisms moving from deeper levels of the skin to the surface, and because of the damage to skin caused by shaving. Razors should not be used as it has been found that they increase the risk of surgical site infection as abrasions can cause colonisation, which can lead to wound infection. Clippers or depilatory creams have been found to reduce infection rates, thus reducing surgical site infection (Tanner *et al*. 2006). However, NICE (2008) suggests that, if hair removal is necessary, electrical clippers with a single-use disposable head should be used on the day of surgery.

Skin preparation solutions
There are several skin preparation solutions available with the commonest being alcoholic or aqueous iodine solutions and clear or coloured alcohol-based chlorhexidine solution (Surgical Tutor 2005b) (Table 9.3). Povodine-iodine or chlorhexidine are the most suitable (NICE 2008). Choice of solution is dependent on factors such as surgical likes and dislikes, the presence of allergies and the condition of the skin, and whether the

procedure requires electrosurgery or laser often influences choice of solution. For example, alcohol-based solutions may ignite through heating by electrosurgery or laser beams, causing patient burns. Therefore, skin prep should be allowed to dry by evaporation and pooling should be avoided. Patient skin sensitivity to these lotions can sometimes cause a chemical burn or irritation which resembles an electrosurgery burn, especially when associated with pooling of solutions underneath the electrosurgery return electrode.

Ventilation systems

The cleanest areas in the operating room should be the surgical site and instrument table. Although aseptic technique and appropriately used prophylactic antibiotics can reduce wound infection, suitable ventilation can reduce bacterial contamination of these areas.

Panels in the operating room ceiling provide large volumes of clean air filtered over the surgical site. Infectious particles shed by the operating team therefore move away from the operating table toward the margins of the room. Normal ventilation systems provide air changes at a rate of 20 per hour. Laminar flow provides 300 air changes per hour; these systems are commonplace in orthopaedic theatres. This is due to the increased risk of infection during bone surgery or following the insertion of a prosthesis.

Ventilation systems provide airflow out of the operating room. Maintaining the pressure gradient is a problem when windows or doors are left open, resulting in air moving in and out of the operating room. Doors and windows should therefore be closed, apart from necessary use, while the surgical site is open (Beesley & Pirie 2005).

The surgical team is a potential reservoir of infection because people shed potentially infectious particles of sloughed skin. However, with proper ventilation, such shedding should not pose an infection risk to patients.

Equipment

Practitioners should keep equipment outside the operating room as far as possible, given the requirements for the surgical procedure. Storage of equipment within the operating room is not advisable because it may provide a surface for dust, lint and other potential sources of contamination. However, it may be necessary if storage space is lacking externally. Equipment stored in the operating room should be kept away from clinical activities and, if possible, under cover or in a cupboard. Using plastic covers for delicate or sensitive equipment protects it from contamination and risk of damage. However, these covers can also become contaminated and when removed transfer their contamination to a practitioner's hands. Bacteria and viruses can live for significant lengths of time if surrounded by contamination from blood or body fluids, and so may cause cross-infection by contaminating practitioners working with the same equipment later (Line 2003).

Applying the principles of standard precautions to equipment ensures its protection from contamination, but if it does become contaminated, then the practitioner should control it through immediate cleaning and removal of the contaminant. The most effective way of cleaning such equipment is normally using a disposable single-use lint-free cloth with a suitable hospital detergent. Disinfectants are at best ineffectual, because they require prolonged contact times to be effective, and at worst could damage equipment (Gruendemann & Fernsebner 1995, Department of Health 2009). If used, they must be used in the correct concentrations following manufactures instructions or local infections control policies, labeled and stored safely according to Control of Substances Hazardous to Health (COSHH) regulations (AfPP 2007)

Equipment brought into the operating room is also a risk if local decontamination procedures have not been followed. There are many examples of equipment sharing between areas; for example, instrument trays from storage areas or x-ray machines and clinical monitors transferred from another operating room. Effective cleaning policies with good documentation may help to reduce incidents of cross-contamination.

Equipment leaving the operating room also poses a potential problem for staff transferring and repairing the equipment. Documented evidence of cleaning verifies that this has taken place before the equipment leaves the clinical area. On return, equipment should be effectively cleaned prior to entering the clinical area.

Local instrument reprocessing

During litigation, a trust may have to prove that its instruments did not cause infection, rather than the patient having to prove that they did. A decontamination survey conducted by NHS Estates in September 2000 (NHS Estates 2000) identified major concerns with the local reprocessing of instruments. As a result, reprocessing within the operating room has reduced following the implementation of safer alternative methods. The survey also found that many of the smaller reprocessing units were inadequate; as a result they were closed and the work moved to larger purpose-built sterile supply departments (Line 2003).

There are several advantages to reprocessing surgical items locally. These include quicker turnaround, especially where there are limited numbers of instruments; local control over expensive and fragile equipment; and reduced chance of losing equipment in the system. However, there are also significant problems with local reprocessing. For example, equipment must be clean to sterilise it effectively, yet it is difficult to clean equipment or instruments with lumens and, unlike larger ster-ilising units, few operating rooms have adequate competency-based training programmes and quality assurance systems associated with cleaning by practitioners. Therefore nowadays, instruments are sent to on- or off-site theatre sterile supplies units (TSSUs). In these areas instruments are decontaminated according to manufactures' instructions, and processed and sterilised using a validated automated process; this facilitates the tracking and traceability of instruments. The latter allow the decontamination process to be tracked and also identification of patients whom the instrument set has been used on in the event of potential exposure risk.

Surgical gowns and drapes

Surgical gowns and drapes should carry the CE mark as they are classed as medical devices and should conform to the European standard EN13795: 'surgical drapes, gowns and clean airsuits, used as medical devices, for patients, clinical staff and

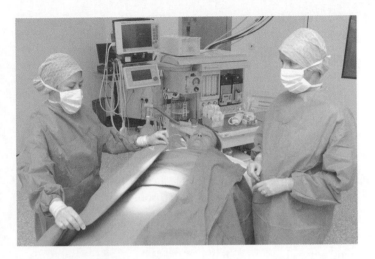

Fig. 9.2 Surgical draping of a patient.

equipment' (AfPP 2007). They are subject to legally binding minimum standards in areas such as microbial penetration, tensile strength, linting and permeability to fluids. Surgical gowns and drapes are either reusable or single use.

Figure 9.2 shows the surgical draping of a patient.

Reusable gowns and drapes
Polycotton is one of the most widely used materials for reusable gowns because it is cheap and easy to produce, comfortable to wear, permeable to perspiration and durable in use. However, polycotton is also permeable to bacteria and fluids which can be a problem during major procedures. Traditional cotton or polyester cotton gowns and drapes do not offer a high enough level of protection to perioperative staff or patients from infective agents nor do they have any barrier properties in the absence of special measures, such as repeated impregnation with hydrophobic agents (Graff *et al*. 2001, MHRA 2003). Drapes made from a special blend of cotton and polycotton are available which are coated with a fluid-repellent flurocarbon

treatment (AfPP 2007). As this repellent reduces after a number of washes, excellent standardized and validated reprocessing procedures must be established to record integrity of the material.

Because of these limits, other reusable materials have developed which offer better protection from contamination, while being comfortable to the wearer. A wide range of materials are available which are predominantly 'non-woven'. These range from single-layer hydrophobic material to fully impermeable materials.

Many hospital-run laundry departments have closed, which affects fast processing and safe transport of large amounts of contaminated material. For these reasons, many trusts use single-use materials as an economic and safe way of providing surgical drapes and gowns (Line 2003).

Single-use gowns and drapes
As a result of the increased focus on quality and risk assessment, single-use materials are now the materials of choice in most situations and are available from several manufacturers. They also take several different forms, including single-layer and multilayer materials and plastic materials. All try to provide properties similar to or better than reusable materials, for example resistance to bacterial penetration, wetting and tearing, and increased comfort and durability in use. Manufacturers are usually responsible for sterility and fitness for purpose of single-use gowns. The trust may see this as an advantage if litigation raises questions of sterility or wound infection. Single use eliminates the concern regarding effectiveness of the barrier due to reprocessing and gives consistency. In the transitional period of moving from reusable to single use, practitioners may be offered training as the draping technique with single-use drapes is considered to be different.

The single-use against multi-use materials argument is complex and involves financial, environmental and risk-assessment factors. However, as standards of use rise, it is likely that single-use drapes and gowns will continue to be popular (Beesley & Pirie 2005).

POSITIONING THE PATIENT

The ability to position a patient safely and effectively for surgery can take many years to develop and is an essential skill for the safe care of patients. The practitioner must be able to display and apply safe principles of surgical positioning for anaesthetised patients. This involves consideration in such areas as positioning unconscious patients, understanding the physiological effects of surgical positioning, considering surgical, anaesthetic and patient-related factors when positioning the patient, and managing potential problems of patient positioning.

Careful positioning of the surgical patient helps to provide surgical access to carry out the surgical procedure. Therefore, practitioners place patients in a large variety of positions, many of which are potentially dangerous, uncomfortable or painful.

At the same time, there are many other considerations apart from the need for surgical access. For example, the anaesthetist must be able to gain access to the patient's airway, even, for example, when undergoing surgery to the head, which would normally exclude non-sterile personnel from the area. The anaesthetist will also need access to other anaesthetic equipment such as intravenous lines, monitors and catheters.

Practitioners must also consider the patient's dignity. If the patient is awake, unnecessary exposure can cause embarrassment and increase anxiety. As well as being unpleasant for the patient, this can lead to anger, frustration, disempowerment and justifiably result in non-cooperation. If the patient is anaesthetised, it is the responsibility of the perioperative team to maintain the patient's dignity. Treating the unconscious patient as less than human, also dehumanises the perioperative team. The team may develop a lack of respect for the patient which can make members of the team less concerned about the patient's well-being.

Preparation and planning is the key to effective and safe positioning techniques. Prior to positioning the patient, a moving and handling risk assessment should have been undertaken, as this may reduce the risk of injury to staff or the patient. A methodical approach using the TILE (Task, Individual, Load and Environment) format could be used (AfPP 2007). This format considers the safe transfer, positioning, prepping, and moving and handling of patients and equipment. The practitioner should position the operating table in the best position within the operating room. This will involve considering such issues as position of the anaesthetist and anaesthetic equipment, lighting, space for surgical instrument trays and access for x-ray machines. All table fittings should be available before the patient enters the operating room. This involves discussing requirements with the surgeon and anaesthetist and agreeing the best position to adopt for the patient.

It is essential to adopt a team approach to position the patient safely and effectively. A coordinated approach is necessary to avoid damage by sudden jerky movements of limbs, or abnormal twisting or torsion of parts of the patient's body. At the same time, practitioners should ensure that they adopt a slow, careful and ergonomical approach to moving the patient (Clarke & Jones 1998).

Various positioning aids help to achieve and maintain the patient's position. Patient positioning devices help to support or position the patient's limbs or back when in a lateral position. Laminectomy frames support the patient in a modified prone position, which encourages the gap between vertebrae to open for lumbar laminectomies. Limbs can be flexed against posts fixed to the table; for example, when undertaking an arthroscopy or for supporting the patient from the front in the lateral position. Placing kidney elevators beneath the patient's iliac crest while in the lateral position causes the operative area between the 12th rib and the iliac crest to lift. Gel pads have various uses for supporting and protecting bony prominences and limbs. Stabilising the head is especially important because of the potential risk to the airway and the neck. Various positioning aids are available for the head, including the 'doughnut' or ring, sandbags or gel pads (Gruendemann & Fernsebner 1995).

Physiological effects of positioning

Poor positioning can have a detrimental effect on the well-being of the patient. Optimal positioning will limit interference with the circulatory, respiratory and musculoskeletal systems. It is imperative that the circulatory system is not compromised and that adequate tissue perfusion is maintained at all times. Failure to do so may cause lasting damage to the tissues or limbs. Where possible the patient's position should remain neutral, without excessive flexion.

Obstructing the flow of blood, for example in the legs, can also increase the incidence of damage to blood vessels, resulting in such conditions as thrombophlebitis and deep vein thrombosis.

Neurological complications include damage to the brachial plexus, for example when extending the shoulder for long periods of time. Any prolonged pressure or stretching of nerves has the potential to damage the nerves, potentially leading to nerve palsies (Davy & Ince 2000).

During positioning, several other factors affect the patient and which practitioners must also consider. For example, maintaining normal body alignment helps to prevent nerve damage, circulation deficits and skin damage. Padding or protective devices, such as low-pressure mattresses or intermittent pressure pneumatic devices, may help protect the patient (Taylor & Campbell 1999b).

Other safety considerations include the use of padded safety straps and upholding acceptable staffing levels. Preventing pooling of skin prep solutions around equipment helps to avoid the risk of potential skin damage or inflammation of alcohol-based solutions. The patient should not be in contact with grounded metal objects, which may cause problems with electrosurgery burns (see Chapters 2 and 5). Practitioners should protect catheters and intravenous cannulae from stretching, pulling or unintentional removal. Preoperative assessment of patients may identify risks such as obesity, low bodyweight, potential for skin damage, incontinence, stiff joints and other physical conditions which may affect positioning.

Postoperative evaluation of the patient's response to positioning is an important part of patient care. Erythema or changes in skin integrity at bony prominences and pressure areas may be signs of lasting pressure damage and pressure sore development. There may be evidence of strained muscles or ligaments if the patient complains of stiff or aching limbs or joints.

Box 9.1   Potential complications of surgical positioning

- Peripheral nerve injuries.
- Skin injuries.
- Eye or ear injuries.
- Finger injuries.
- Ligament damage.
- Cardiovascular effects.
- Venous air embolism.
- Respiratory effects.

Excessive damage may result in instability or dislocation of joints or altered range of motion. Compressed or injured nerves can display themselves through numbness or tingling.

The practitioner should record, in the patient's medical notes or perioperative care plan, the position, details of equipment used and any signs or symptoms of harm suffered by positioning, and the patient should be told of any potential injuries (Box 9.1).

Common surgical positions

There are four common surgical positions for the patient – supine, lithotomy, prone and lateral. Several variations of these four positions have developed to address local requirements.

Supine position

The supine position and its variants are common positions for surgery. The patient lies on the back, with arms on arm boards at a 90° angle or less to the body (Figure 9.3). Alternatively, the arms may remain parallel to the body and held in place by padded armrests to prevent ulnar nerve damage. A small pillow or pad may stabilise the head and prevent neck strain. Legs should be parallel and uncrossed to prevent pressure on calf muscles and compression of circulation. Padding helps to avoid pressure damage to areas such as the sacrum, heels, elbows and bony prominences.

Backache and neckache are common problems associated with this position. Neckache can occur following extreme or prolonged neck rotation; therefore, the head should be placed

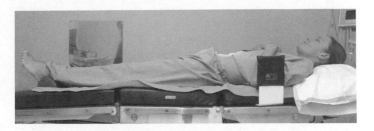

Fig. 9.3 Supine position.

in a neutral position. Backache can occur because of prolonged tension in the sacrolumbar region. This occurs because of flattening of the vertebrae as the paraspinal muscles relax under the influence of muscle relaxants and other anaesthetic drugs. Placing a small support in the space beneath the small of the back reduces this condition by helping to support the normal lumbar curve (Gruendemann & Fernsebner 1995).

Trendelenburg's position involves lowering the head and raising the feet. The downwards angle should not be excessive and is limited to a maximum of 20° (AfPP 2007). Only friction stops the patient from sliding off the table, therefore it is advisable to use a non-slip mattress. Reverse Trendelenburg involves a head-up and foot-down position. A footboard can prevent the patient sliding down the table and helps to prevent foot drop or plantar flexion.

Arms need special consideration in any of these positions. The anaesthetic team needs access to peripheral lines and to the upper arm for blood pressure readings. The surgical team needs unobstructed access to the surgical site. The common positions for arms are parallel to the body, across the chest or on arm boards at an angle to body according to the procedures taking place.

When placed on arm boards, there are several considerations for the practitioner. The angle of the arm to the body must be a maximum of 90°, ideally with the palms turned upwards. Hyperabduction of the arm results in stretching of subclavian and axillary blood vessels, resulting in thrombosis and vessel wall damage, and stretching of the brachial plexus, ulnar nerve and other superficial nerves in the arm.

Severe hypotension can result from this position, especially if the patient is pregnant. This occurs because of pressure on the vena cava, which reduces venous return and cardiac output. It is caused by the weight of the internal organs or the fetus. Tilting the patient 15°, preferably left lateral, reduces pressure on the vena cavae. This can be achieved either by tilting the table or by placing pillows or a wedge underneath the patient (Hind & Wicker 2000).

Patients adopt a highly modified supine position if they need treatment on a traction table. The traction table places fractured legs into traction while undergoing internal fixation. An image intensifier displays the fracture in real-time using x-rays, and the large C-arm of this machine must have access close to the site of surgery. The patient is normally supine and the unaffected leg abducted to 90° at the hip and knee. A well-padded perineal post attached to the table braces against the perineum. Stretching the leg through fittings at the foot of the table applies traction to reduce the fracture to its normal alignment. Flexing and abducting the arm on the unaffected side across the chest helps C-arm access. The practitioner must watch carefully for potential complications since this position is so extreme and can place great stress on the patient's body if wrongly carried out.

Prone position

The patient adopts this position for surgery on the dorsal surface. The patient is anaesthetised in the supine position and then practitioners roll the patient over into the face-down position, ensuring spinal alignment is maintained. Several practitioners should help in this procedure because of the danger of twisting limbs or compromising the airway. The operating surgeon should take ultimate responsibility for the safe positioning of the patient and should take an active role. The patient's arms are rotated simultaneously and symmetrically through their normal range of movement to rest beside the head (Figure 9.4), or left at the side of the body. The head is protected from abnormal movement and the eyes and ears padded to prevent pressure damage. Specifically designed blocks, pads or

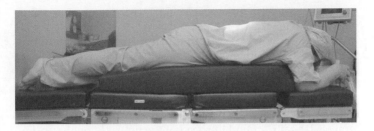

Fig. 9.4 Prone position with arms by the head.

pillows placed under the chest and hip regions ease breathing by allowing expansion of the diaphragm. A pad placed under the lower legs and ankles also helps to prevent foot drop.

When adopting this position for laminectomies or surgery on the spine, using a frame can stabilise the spine and open the laminar arches for easier surgical access.

There are several variations to this position including, for example, the jackknife, knee–chest and prone sitting positions, used for specialised neurosurgical or proctological procedures.

Lateral position

Patients adopt this position for lateral surgical access during procedures such as hip arthroplasty, kidney surgery and some chest surgery (Taylor & Campbell 1999b). The patient is anaesthetised supine and then turned on the side. This procedure needs several practitioners to perform safely. Supporting the head on a pillow, and the torso with supports or posts, helps to keep spinal alignment. Placing a pillow between the legs relieves the pressure of the upper leg on the lower leg and flexing both legs slightly helps to improve stability.

Bringing the lower shoulder forward slightly or positioning a pressure-relieving device under the axilla relieves pressure on the brachial plexus, and the lower arm is either placed on an arm board or flexed to rest beside the patient's head. The upper arm often rests on a raised arm board or a carter braine support and is placed above the head whilst maintaining a neutral position away from the surgical field. Protecting pressure points with padding reduces the risk of harm.

A special rest may be placed under the patient's hip for procedures on the kidney. This 'kidney rest' elevates the space between the 12th rib and the iliac crest, exposing the surgical area. Flexing the table at this point increases the angulation of the patient's body.

The peroneal nerve leaves the posterior aspect of the knee and travels laterally around the head of the fibula. Enough padding of the lateral knee is therefore essential because it is susceptible to pressure in this area because of the weight of the leg on the operating table.

Lithotomy position

Patients adopt the lithotomy position for gynaecological and lower bowel surgery. This is a highly unnatural position which therefore carries with it risks because of stretching and pressure on nerves, joints and tendons.

From the supine position, practitioners simultaneously raise the patient's legs, flex the hips and knees, abduct and externally rotate the thighs, and place the feet in stirrups attached to poles. Lithotomy stirrups are now available in a power-assisted variety, which allows the practitioners to easily and safely manoeuver the legs without having to physically lift the legs into position. Surgical access to the patient's perineal area is achieved by removing the end of the table.

The arms are either placed over the abdomen or crossed over on the chest, and in either case secured using armrests. To help venous access, one arm may be placed on an arm board at less than a 90° angle to the body.

When placing the patient in this position, practitioners must raise and lower both legs simultaneously to prevent leg and back strain. Practitioners must also take care to ensure the legs can move through the required range, especially where movement is compromised, for example when the patient has had a hip replacement. Pressure should be avoided on areas such as the inner leg from the posts and on the feet from the stirrups. This position also restricts breathing to a degree because of increased pressure of the viscera on the diaphragm (Beesley & Pirie 2005).

Lloyd-Davies stirrups can be used in place of lithotomy poles to offer popliteal and ankle support. Using these stirrups during prolonged procedures reduces the risk of pressure damage to the legs.

SURGICAL SKILLS

The scrub practitioner role is challenging but satisfying. The role challenges practitioners to use their knowledge of anatomy and surgical technique in the direct treatment of the patient's condition. Here, on the operating table, is where the focus of the patient's care resides. The whole point of the surgical patient's admission is to undergo a surgical procedure and it is here, at the operating table, that the scrub practitioner can engage directly in the patient's return to health. The experienced scrub practitioner can make the difference between a procedure that progresses slowly, with many delays, to one which is smooth and efficient.

To achieve this aim, the scrub practitioner calls on many competencies, such as those discussed in Chapter 6. Three areas of perioperative care which the scrub practitioner must develop competence in are:

- managing recordable items;
- haemostasis;
- wound closure, dressings and drains.

Managing recordable items

Managing items used during a surgical procedure is one of the core roles of the scrub practitioner (AfPP 2007) and remains an area of high risk if policies and procedures are not implemented. All items used in a procedure are accountable and some, for example swabs and instruments, are also recordable. There are many different approaches to this procedure and many different items that need recording; therefore, practitioners need to be fully aware of local policies and procedures.

The purpose of counting and recording items is to avoid retaining any in the patient's wound. A retained swab or instrument is a potential source of infection and can interfere with the anatomy of the wound area, leading to bleeding, loss of function or pain. The potential for psychological damage to the patient is also high because of worry about the error and its future implications. The patient will also need to undergo more surgery to remove the item and face the extra risks which this poses.

Errors in managing surgical items have often resulted in litigation (Woodhead 2005, WHO 2009). The patient may claim that the surgical team has been negligent in its duties and can often claim damages for loss of earning, pain, psychological and physiological stress and inconvenience. Patients may sue the hospital directly, with members of the surgical team involved in the blame for any errors. All members of the team, not just the surgeon, are accountable for this check. The practitioner's role is to make the surgeon aware of the status of the surgical items. Any act (e.g. carrying out a false check) or omission (e.g. failing to tell the surgeon of an incorrect count) may leave the practitioner open to the charge of negligence (Beesley & Pirie 2005, HPC 2008, NMC 2008).

Every item used during surgery is accountable at every stage of surgery. Most items are also recordable on the swab board or perioperative care record. Recordable items include, for example:

- swabs;
- muslin packs;
- pledgets;
- instruments;
- sutures;
- blades;
- bulldog clips;
- tapes or slings;
- electrosurgery tips;
- neuro patties.

The operating department should have a policy that specifies which items are recordable, and the documentation, counting and recording procedures (AfPP 2007).

Principles for managing recordable items

Practitioners must count recordable items for every surgical procedure to improve patient safety and reduce the risk of items left accidentally in the wound. This also includes minor cases when there is little possibility of loss, since a lost item may interfere with a count for a following case.

The scrub practitioner decides when the checks take place, which can include:

- before the surgical procedure;
- on receiving extra packs of swabs or other items;
- at the closure of a body cavity such as the stomach;
- at the start of wound closure;
- at the start of skin closure;
- following completion of the case.

The circulating practitioner records items on the count board, in the intraoperative record (computer or otherwise) and on the tray list. The count board is usually a large white-board which displays the recordable items used during the surgical procedure. Since the practitioner wipes the count board clean after every case, an intraoperative record and tray list provide permanent documentary evidence of the counts. The scrub and circulating practitioners should count aloud and in unison and record items together. One of these two practitioners should be a qualified and experienced member of the team. The practitioners should check the instrument tray on opening and before first use of the instruments. Instruments that come in several parts should have each part independently identified. The scrub practitioner must be satisfied that every item is complete, and there are no missing parts, before use.

There are various ways of recording recordable item checks in the operating room. In most procedures, the count board has swabs, packs, sutures and blades marked before the case starts. During a procedure practitioners count used items, weigh them to estimate blood loss and store them safely near the count board.

Practitioners also mark the outcome of each count on the intraoperative care record and sign them. Removing all opened (used and unused) recordable items from the operating room at the end of the procedure helps to prevent errors in future counts.

The scrub and circulating practitioner sign their names in the relevant area of the operating record and on the perioperative care plan to show completion of a correct count and to accept accountability for the procedure. The scrub practitioner's responsibility is to tell the surgeon of the outcome of an incorrect count, while it is the surgeon's responsibility to decide what to do about unaccounted items. As part of the World Health Organization (WHO) surgical safety checklist (2009) the checking and verification that all instruments, swabs and sharps are correct is part of the 'sign out' phase (NPSA 2009).

Many operating theatre suites now have electronic means of recording a patient's perioperative journey, for example ORMIS (operating room information management system). This type of system offers a number of management systems, one of which captures the patient's perioperative journey. This allows for the creation of care plans and the documentation of swab, sharps and instrument checks. If these systems are introduced into the theatre suite, it is important that all members of the perioperative team have had competency-based training.

See Chapter 4 for further discussion on documentation.

Incorrect counts must be recorded and corrective action taken where possible. The surgeon will decide whether to continue the closure, to look inside the wound for the item or to wait until the item is found. Practitioners may check the patient, drapes, rubbish bags, linen bags, floor, specimens and swab bags at this stage. Swabs and other items can often be found in unexpected places, for example having fallen down inside boots, under the operating table or stuck to the soles of a staff member's shoes.

The surgeon may arrange for an x-ray to find out whether the missing item may be inside the patient. The surgeon will not necessarily order an x-ray if there is no possibility of the missing item being inside the patient, and this decision should be recorded in the patient's notes. It is the surgeon's decision whether to carry on with closure even if the scrub practitioner reports the item is still missing. The scrub practitioner should record missing items in the operating register and an incident form must be completed.

Surgical haemostasis

The scrub practitioner should understand the principles of surgical haemostasis to assist the operating surgeon effectively and to promote the smooth progress of the surgical procedure.

Surgical haemostasis is a complex subject which requires knowledge of anatomy and physiology as well as surgical procedures. For example, the techniques used for haemostasis of capillary bed bleeding are different from haemostasis of large blood vessels. Similarly, blood vessels can be temporarily or permanently occluded with slings, ties, tapes, tourniquets or sutures. When electrosurgery is used, a whole raft of instruments and techniques can be used, especially when the bleeding is deep within the body, or the procedure is carried out with a laparoscope.

Arterial bleeding

Arterial bleeding can be identified because of the bright red colour of the oxygenated blood, the spurting action as the heart pumps it out of the damaged vessel; and the force with which it is pumped out of the vessel.

Major arterial bleeding can be serious because of the potential for high blood loss in a short time. For example, surgeons must control bleeding quickly during a ruptured aortic aneurysm or the patient may only have minutes to live. Often the only way to stop major arterial bleeds is to clamp the damaged vessel and then repair it using a suture or graft.

Direct pressure or ligation often controls minor arterial bleeds.

Venous bleeding

Venous bleeding can be identified by the dark red colour of the blood, the low-pressure release of the blood from the vessel and the turgid way in which the bleeding occurs (compared with the high pressure of arterial bleeds).

Major venous bleeding can be serious but is more easily controlled than major arterial bleeding. Nonetheless, major venous

bleeds can occur over large areas of tissue, arising spontaneously from damaged tissue. Venous bleeding can also be insidu-
ous in onset, perhaps not making its presence known for hours
after surgery has finished, lulling practitioners into a false sense
of security.

Cutting through veins, venules or capillaries often causes
minor venous bleeds. The usual course of action is to tie the
vessel or coagulate it with electrosurgery. If the bleeding is
coming from a capillary bed, such as the gall bladder bed, then
electrosurgery using fulguration or spray settings, or pharmacological coagulation using collagen or gelatin sponges may be
the methods of choice.

Haemostasis procedures

The first stage in treating perioperative bleeding problems is
evaluation of the bleeding source. The method of haemostasis
then has to be determined. The experienced practitioner can
contribute to this process by anticipating the surgeon's needs.
Some of the criteria for consideration include those in Table 9.4.

Instruments used for haemostasis

Haemostatic instruments are either permanent or temporary.
The surgeon uses temporary haemostats when the role of the
vessel will be required following the procedure, for example
when temporarily occluding a carotid artery to allow surgery
to take place. Permanent haemostats lead to complete vessel
occlusion and permanent loss of function. These are used where
the vessel itself is not required, or the part of the body which
the vessel serves is either removed or becomes non-functional,
for example during bowel resection.

Temporary haemostats include:

- bulldog clips – these small spring-loaded clips are used
  widely in vascular surgery. They gently pinch the vessel,
  occluding it. When removed, normal blood flow resumes;
- ringed vascular clamps – these are similar in shape to artery
  forceps but with specialised tips which are atraumatic to
  vessels. They are available in various sizes, shapes, angles and
  curves;

Table 9.4 Considerations for deciding the method of haemostasis.

Factor affecting mode of haemostasis	Issues for consideration	Implications for the scrub practitioner
Arterial or venous source	• Major or minor artery bleed? • Serious or minor blood loss anticipated? • In venous bleeding is it a general ooze or specific vein damage?	• Ligation of artery using suture, ligature, clips or electrosurgery • Repair of major blood vessel may be required • Pharmacological methods may be used to control venous oozes
Size of vessel	• Is it small enough for electrosurgery? • Are there fine ligatures available?	• Clamping of the vessel using artery forceps • Different methods of presenting ligatures
Accessibility of vessel	• Is it superficial or deep? • Can tapes or ties be passed underneath the blood vessel? • Does the ligature need to be mounted on artery forceps to pass under the vessel?	• Long and/or short artery forceps may be required • Tapes or loops may be used to stabilise the blood vessel • Long electrosurgery instruments may be required
Adjoining tissues	• Are the adjoining tissues likely to be damaged during haemostasis?	• Bipolar electrosurgery may be used where pinpoint electrosurgery is required (e.g. brain tissue) • The vessel may need to be dissected away from sensitive tissues
Permanent or temporary haemostasis required	• Is it essential to preserve the role of the vessel? • Can the vessel be removed without compromising the circulation to the area?	• Vascular clamps may be required • Tourniquets may be required (finger or limb)
Absorbable or non-absorbable suture required	• Does the vessel need long-term ligation? • Is the vessel superficial?	• Large blood vessels often require non-absorbable sutures (e.g. high saphenous ligation and suturing of bowel perforations)

- tourniquets – these vary from small finger or glove tourniquets, to large major limb pneumatic tourniquets;
- vessel loops – these are flexible plastic slings which manipulate and stabilise blood vessels during vascular surgery and provide haemostasis when wrapped around the vessel and pulled tight.

Permanent haemostats include:

- ligatures – these consist of a piece of thread, made from various natural and synthetic materials, which is tied around an anatomical structure, normally using artery forceps; general-purpose removable clamps used for most sizes of blood vessels;
- vascular staples – these are metal staples, applied using special clamps. They are left in position and body tissue surrounds them during the healing process;
- vascular glue – methylacrylate glue bonds tissue edges together;
- electrosurgery – this is possibly the most common way of providing haemostasis and every operating room has an electrosurgical generator as a basic item of equipment. Chapter 2 discusses this device;
- laser – this can provide haemostasis. Chapter 2 also contains a discussion of this device.

All surgical specialities use ligatures (ties) free-hand, dispensed from a reel, attached to artery forceps or used with a suture to transfix blood vessels. The basic technique of vessel ligation is to clamp the end of a cut vessel with artery forceps and then place a tie around the vessel under the clamp, knot it and remove the clamp. This set routine can become quick and effective when the surgeon and practitioner learn to work together in harmony. Alternative methods include passing ties underneath the vessel using artery forceps or angled clamps and tying the vessel in continuity before dividing it.

Pharmacological agents
Various pharmacological agents provide haemostasis and are especially useful where surgeons cannot use ties or sutures.

These include collagen or gelatin sponges, such as Spongistan, and may be used, for example, in the nose, on bone ends, oozing vascular surfaces such as the gall bladder bed and in the inguinal canal following herniorraphy. Sterile bone wax pressed into bone ends prevents oozing.

Wound management

Care of the surgical wound is a responsibility of the entire surgical team. Chapter 1 discusses the homeostasis of wound healing. This chapter focuses on the clinical interventions and some of the perioperative factors that affect wound healing. Wound healing directly links to areas such as handling of tissues intraoperatively, wound closure materials and methods, and choice of dressings and drains.

Surgical technique

Traumatic tissue handling can affect its healing properties since bruised and damaged tissues take longer to heal. Careful handling and retraction of tissues is therefore essential intraoperatively. Close approximation of tissues and effective haemostasis both help to prevent blood clots collecting and encourage healing.

Complications of wound healing

Prevention of infection is essential if wound closure is to progress smoothly. Incisional infections can result in delayed healing times and unsightly scars, and may progress to systemic infection, further delaying the patient's discharge. Deep wound infections are serious conditions which occasionally may result in the removal of implants or the internal breakdown of tissues and surgical repairs. In vascular anastamoses, this can be fatal. The source of infection is often impossible to identify but may include contaminated instruments, poor sterile technique and environmental conditions, which stresses the need for a team approach to preventing contamination.

Wound disruption occurs in some patients because of wound closure materials failing, infection or mechanical stress on the wound. Dehiscence of wounds occurs when suture lines break down and the wound opens. Contents of body spaces, such as intestines, may erupt through the wound (evisceration). This is distressing and potentially fatal for the patient and needs urgent surgery. The dehiscence may be a sign of an underlying medical problem and so further careful wound management may be necessary.

Other common complications include:

- umbilical herniation following abdominal surgery because of weakening of abdominal wall muscles;
- hypertrophic scar formation (keloid scars);
- haemorrhage;
- sinus tract or fistula formation between areas of the body, e.g. the vagina and the colon;
- foreign body inclusion in the wound, e.g. grit or dirt in trauma procedures;
- adhesions to underlying body parts, e.g. adhesion of the anterior abdominal wall and colon.

Wound closure

The purpose of wound closure is to remove dead space, spread tension along suture lines, support the wound until tissue has repaired, and bring together and evert skin edges. Types of wound closure include staples, tape, adhesive and sutures. Each method has specific indications, advantages and disadvantages, and special considerations. This section mostly concerns sutures.

Suturing of tissue promotes primary wound healing by holding tissues together until enough healing occurs to withstand stress without mechanical support (Ethicon 2005).

Suture material is a foreign body which elicits a tissue reaction. During wound closure, a sterile field and meticulous aseptic technique are critical to reduce the risk of wound infection. Other complications of wound healing, such as hypertrophic scars, wide scars and wound dehiscence, may result from patient factors (e.g. nutritional status), incorrect suture selection or techniques that result in excessive tension across the wound.

Providing expert support during wound closure requires knowledge of surgical techniques and the physical characteristics and properties of the suture material and needle.

Synthetic sutures (Tables 9.5–9.7)

Natural collagen-based suture materials, made from collagen of mammal's intestines, are now banned in the European Union. Synthetic non-absorbable sutures produce little tissue reaction – these include synthetic substances such as polyamide and polypropelene polymers.

Coating sutures with agents to improve handling characteristics allows them to pass more easily through tissues and reduces tissue injury from their passage. Dyeing sutures also increases visibility.

Monofilament and multifilament sutures

Monofilament (single-stranded) sutures resist harbouring of micro-organisms, tie easily and provide less resistance to passage through tissue. Monofilament sutures become weakened if crushed or crimped by poor handling.

Table 9.5 Synthetic absorbable sutures (Ethicon 2005).

Type	Source	Uses and absorption
Coated Vicryl (polyglactin 910) suture	Braided multifilament suture coated with a copolymer of lactide and glycolide (polyglactin 370)	Tensile strength around 65% at 14 days post-implantation. Absorption completes in 56–70 days. These sutures cause only slight tissue reaction and may be used in the presence of infection. Used in general soft tissue approximation and vessel ligation
Monocryl (poliglecaprone 25) suture	Monofilament suture that is a copolymer of glycolide and E-caprolactone	Tensile strength is 50–60% at 7 days and nil at 21 days. Absorption is complete at 91–119 days. Used for subcuticular closure and soft tissue approximations and ligations
PDS II (polydioxanone) suture	Polyester monofilament suture made of poly (p-dioxanone).	Tensile strength is 70% at 14 days and 25% at 42 days. Used for soft tissue approximation, especially in paediatric, cardiovascular, gynaecological, ophthalmic, plastic and gastrointestinal surgery

Table 9.6 Natural non-absorbable sutures (Ethicon 2005).

Type	Source	Uses and absorption
Surgical silk	Raw silk spun by silkworms, often coated with beeswax or silicone	Tensile strength decreases and is lost over a period of 3–6 months
Surgical steel	Stainless steel (iron–chromium–nickel–molybdenum alloy) as a monofilament and twisted multifilament	High-tensile strength with little loss over time and low tissue reactivity. Used mainly in orthopaedic, neurosurgical and thoracic applications. This suture is also used in abdominal wall and sternum closure

Multifilament sutures are several monofilaments twisted or braided together, which increases tensile strength, pliability and flexibility, but unfortunately also increases friction through tissues. Absorbing fluid by capillary action may introduce pathogens into the wound. Both these features are reduced by coating the sutures with various substances, for example, Teflon.

Absorbable and non-absorbable sutures

Absorbable sutures provide temporary wound support, until the wound heals well enough to withstand stress. Absorption occurs by hydrolysis in synthetic materials.

The surgeon often uses non-absorbable sutures, such as nylon, for percutaneous skin closure, removing them after the wound has healed. Wound healing typically occurs in 6–8 days in healthy patients. When used internally, non-absorbable sutures become permanently encapsulated in tissue.

Suture selection often depends on surgeon training and preference since various suture materials are available for each surgical location and need. Normally, the surgeon uses the smallest diameter suture that adequately holds the healing wound edges.

Certain general principles apply to suture selection. For example, sutures are often no longer needed when a wound has

Table 9.7 Synthetic non-absorbable sutures (Ethicon 2005).

Type	Source	Uses and absorption
Nylon	Polyamide polymer suture material available in monofilament (Ethilon/ Dermalon suture) and braided (Nurolon/Surgilon suture) forms	Nylon has 81% tensile strength at 1 year, 72% at 2 years, and 66% at 11 years. Elasticity makes it useful in skin closure
Polyester fibre (Mersilene/Dacron suture (uncoated) and Ethibond/Ti-cron suture (coated))	Polyester, a polymer of polyethylene terephthalate. Sometimes coated with polybutilate (Ethibond suture) or silicone (Ti-cron)	Often used for vessel anastomosis and securing prosthetic materials, for example, heart valves
Polypropylene (Prolene suture)	Monofilament suture, an isomer of a propylene polymer	Prolene suture is not subject to degradation or weakening and preserves tensile strength for up to 2 years. The material does not adhere to tissues and is useful as a pull-out suture (e.g. subcuticular closure). Useful for contaminated and infected wounds, reduces sinus formation and suture extrusion. Often used in cardiovascular surgery

reached maximum strength therefore non-absorbable sutures are often used to close slowly healing tissues such as skin, fascia, and tendons. Absorbable sutures can close mucosal wounds, which are rapidly healing (Ethicon 2005).

Suture selection in contaminated tissues is important because of the risk of infection. For example, monofilament sutures are less likely to spread infection as they harbour fewer micro-organisms than multifilament sutures. Surgeons often select the smallest diameter monofilament suture materials, such as nylon or polypropylene, for repairing contaminated tissues.

Wound drains

The scrub practitioner should have a clear understanding of the features of surgical wound drainage to support the surgical team. This includes competence in the use of drains, methods of insertion, prevention of complications and safe securing of drains.

The purpose of a wound drain is to remove dead spaces, foreign objects or harmful materials that may lead to wound healing complications (Baxter 2003). Drains can also provide irrigation of wounds, relieve pressure within wounds (e.g. in the gastrointestinal tract) and hold open or stent hollow tubes (e.g. bile ducts). There are two basic categories of drains in use – open and closed.

Open drains (passive)

An open drain is open to the environment and can allow passage of air and fluid between the inside and outside environment. A Penrose drain is a soft tube of rubber which the surgeon places into the wound with the end sticking out and secured with a safety pin. Wound drainage occurs through this tube by the effects of body movements and gravity.

A sump drain is a double lumen tube which allows fluids to drain out of the wound through one channel, and filtered air to enter the wound through the other channel. This exchange of fluid with air encourages the flow of the fluid. A triple lumen tube allows the injecting of irrigations or medications into the wound site. Gentle suction is sometimes applied to sump drains to enable them to drain more effectively. A T-tube drain is a hollow tube in the shape of a T which is often used for drainage of bile fluid from the common bile duct.

Closed drains (active)

Vacuum drains are 'active' because they gently suck the exudates out of the wound. Vacuum drains only work in closed wounds as the negative pressure gradient must be maintained for them to work properly.

Although underwater seal drains are not active, they are closed because keeping the tubes under the water stops external air from entering the wound. The drainage bottle must remain below the level of the wound to ensure that water cannot syphon out of the jar and into the wound. These drains are often used in thoracic surgery as chest drains to drain air and fluid from the pleural cavity. As the patient breathes, the fluid in the submerged tube swings as the pressure in the pleural cavity changes. On removal of the air and fluid from the pleural cavity, the lung expands, the pleural cavity closes and the pressure stabilises. When this happens the water in the tube stops swinging and the drain can be removed.

Surgical dressings

The perioperative practitioner should understand the principles of surgical dressings and be able to apply them properly to provide the best environment for wound healing.

Purpose of wound dressing

Wound dressings have two main roles – to protect the wound from an unfavourable environment and to immobilise it. The ideal dressing is one which promotes the best environment for healing, provides a barrier to contamination, supports the wound and allows removal without further damage to the wound (Baxter 2003).

Wounds heal best under moist conditions, therefore a primary role of the dressing is to prevent excess drying out of the wound. The dressing also protects the wound from external contamination to prevent wound infection. Wounds can produce large amounts of exudates which can damage surrounding skin if allowed to collect. Therefore several dressings absorb and hold exudate, keeping it from damaging surrounding tissues.

Other features of dressings include helping with haemostasis, drainage and debridement of dead tissue, and acting as a carrier for therapeutic agents, such as antibiotics or antiseptics.

Types of dressing

Consideration of wound treatment must include a holistic assessment of the patient, since nutrition, illness and the patient's physical and psychological state can have an effect on wound healing. Wound healing has improved over the last 100 years, not only for medical reasons but also for social reasons such as better nutrition and housing and the arrival of the welfare state.

The choice of dressing, however, is still important to ensure ideal conditions for wound healing. The wound should remain moist but not macerated, free from infection, toxins and particles from the dressing itself, undisturbed by frequent dressing changes and kept at an optimum pH value (Baxter 2003).

Soft dressings are used for uncomplicated wounds which are closed by primary intention. Most surgical wounds fall into this category. These dressings normally consist of three layers. The first layer is a non-stick gauze which rests on the surface of the wound. It is important that this layer does not stick to the wound or new growth will be destroyed on its removal. The second layer is absorbent and can consist of relatively thicker padding which can absorb and remove the exudates from the immediate wound area. The third layer immobilises the wound area and so may be adhesive in many simple surgical dressings, or bulky and kept in position with bandages.

Single-layer dressings include semi-permeable membranes such as Opsite and Tegaderm. These are used for uncomplicated wounds and promote a moist, warm environment for best wound healing. Practitioners often use these for dressing cannulation sites. Spray dressings are also examples of single-layer dressings.

Wound packing is also a dressing which is used for deep wounds healing by secondary intention. The packing prevents the surface from closing up before healing of the deeper layers has completed. Packs can be made of various substances including plain gauze, impregnated gauze and hydrocolloids.

There is also a wide range of speciality dressings which are used for complex wounds and are therefore more common during longer episodes of patient care.

REFERENCES
Association for Perioperative Practitioners (AfPP) (2006) *Risk and Quality Management System*. AfPP, Harrogate.
Association for Perioperative Practitioners (AfPP) (2007) *Standards and recommendations for safe perioperative practice*. AfPP, Harrogate.
Baxter, H. (2003) Management of surgical wounds. *Nursing Times* **99** (13), 66.

Beesley, J. & Pirie, S. (2005) *Standards and Recommendations for Safe Perioperative Practice*. National Association of Theatre Nurses, Harrogate.

Davey, A., Ince, C. (2000) *Fundamentals of Operating Department Practice*. Greenwich Medical Media, London.

Department of Health (DH) (2009) *National Decontamination programme*. DH, London.

Doebbeling, B.N., Stanley, G.L., Sheetz, C.T., *et al.* (1992) Comparative efficacy of alternative hand-washing agents in reducing nosocomial infections in intensive care units. *New England Journal of Medicine* **327** (2), 88–93.

Clarke, P. & Jones, J. (1998) *Brigden's Operating Department Practice*. Churchill Livingstone, Edinburgh.

Ethicon (2005) *Wound Closure Manual*. Ethicon, Edinburgh.

Fell, C. (2000) Health and safety – Hand washing. *British Journal of Perioperative Nursing* **10** (9), 461–465.

Graff, L., Wigglesworth, N., Rose, D., *et al.* (2001) '*Surgical Drapes and Gowns in Today's NHS: Moving Forward From Traditional Textiles Report. Report from an Independent Multi-Disciplinary Working Group: May 2001*' Products http://www.molnlycke.com (accessed 19 August 2009).

Gruendemann, J.G. & Fernsebner, B. (1995) *Comprehensive Perioperative Nursing, Vol 1*. Jones and Bartlett, Boston.

Gruendemann, B.J. & Mangum, S.S. (2001) *Infection Prevention in Surgical Settings*. Saunders, New York.

Health Professional Council (HPC) (2008) *Standards of Conduct, Performance and Ethics*. HPC, London.

Hind, M. & Wicker, P. (2000) *Principles of Perioperative Practice*. Churchill Livingstone, Edinburgh.

Line, S. (2003) Decontamination and control of infection in theatre. *British Journal of Perioperative Nursing* **13** (2), 70–75.

Lipp, A. & Edwards, P. (2002) Disposable surgical face masks for preventing surgical wound infection in clean surgery. In: *The Cochrane Library*, Issue 1, Update Software, Oxford.

Medical and Healthcare Products Regulatory Agency (MHRA) (2003) *Surgical Gowns, Drapes and Coverings*. MHRA, London.

National Patient Safety Agency (2009) *WHO Surgical Checklist*. www.npsa.nhs.uk/advice (accessed 17 August 2009).

National Institute for Health and Clinical Excellence (2008) *Surgical Site Infection: Prevention and Treatment of Surgical Site Infection*. www.nice.org.uk (accessed 19 August 2009).

NHS Estates (2000) *Decontamination Review: Report on A Survey of Current Decontamination Practices in Healthcare Premises in England*. NHS Estates, London. www.decontamination.nhsestates.gov.uk/downloads/decontamination_review.pdf

Nursing and Midwifery Council (NMC) (2008) *Standards of Conduct, Performance and Ethics for Nurses and Midwives*. NMC, London.

Pearson, T. (2000) The wearing of facial protection in high risk environments. *British Journal of Perioperative Nursing* **10** (3), 163–166.

Pinney, E. (2000) Back to basics – hand washing. *British Journal of Perioperative Nursing* **10** (6), 328–331.

Surgical Tutor (2005a) *Sources of Surgical Infection.* www.surgical-tutor.org.uk/default-home.htm?principles/microbiology/surgical_infection.htm~right (accessed 01 February 2005).

Surgical Tutor (2005b) *Asepsis and Antisepsis.* www.surgical-tutor.org.uk/default-home.htm?core/preop1/asepsis.htm~right (accessed 01 February 2005).

Tanner, J., Woodings, D., & Moncaster, K. (2006) Preoperative hair removal to reduce surgical site infection. *Cochrane Database of Systematic Reviews.* The Cochrane Collaboration. John Wiley and Sons Ltd, Chichester.

Taylor, M. & Campbell, C. (1999a) Back to basics: The multidisciplinary team in the operating department. *British Journal of Theatre Nursing* **9** (4), 178–183.

Taylor, M. & Campbell, C. (1999b) Back to basics: Patient care in the operating department (1). *British Journal of Theatre Nursing* **9** (6), 272–275.

Wicker, P. (1991) Universal precautions: Infection control in a high risk environment. *British Journal of Theatre Nursing* **1** (9) 16–18.

Woodhead, K. (2005) Managing risk of swab and instrument retention. *Clinical Services Journal* **4** (1), 49–51.

World Health Organization (WHO) (2009) *WHO Guidelines for Safer Surgery 2009.* WHO, Geneva.

Patient Care During Recovery

10

Paul Wicker and Felicia Cox

LEARNING OUTCOMES

❏ Discuss the *role of the practitioner during postoperative recovery*.
❏ Identify the main *postoperative problems*.
❏ Discuss the *key clinical skills* and *underpinning knowledge* required of recovery practitioners.

ROLE OF THE RECOVERY PRACTITIONER

In 2002, NHS Education Scotland produced the document *A Route to Enhanced Competence in Perioperative Care* (NES 2002), which described the competencies displayed by perioperative practitioners working in anaesthetic, scrub and recovery roles. The section describing the recovery role covered areas such as patient assessment, airway maintenance, wound care and the skills to respond to developing postoperative problems. The working party also discovered that many of the skills and knowledge required by recovery practitioners are also displayed, albeit in a different context, in other perioperative roles. Therefore, the reader should refer to other chapters of this book to explore some of the areas not discussed in this chapter.

However, while practitioners in anaesthetic, scrub and circulating roles display many of the skills found in recovery, the unique environment of the recovery room lends a new aspect to the role. The lack of immediate medical support in the recovery room means that practitioners work in a more autonomous role than any other area of the operating department. Practitioners have to be able to make evidence-based decisions which support the postoperative patient at a stage of his or her treatment when he or she is highly vulnerable. Recovery practitioners must be able to recognise changes in the patient's condition, start suitable supportive therapies and oversee their effects, often with no immediate medical support.

Therefore, the recovery practitioner must efficiently and continually assess, plan, carry out and evaluate individual care and treatment for the postoperative patient to meet his or her individual needs. A major aim of the role is to aid in creating a calm therapeutic environment, using available resources in a safe and effective manner to reduce anxiety in postoperative patients.

The practitioner must also effectively communicate within a multidisciplinary team. This includes providing information to all healthcare workers interacting with the patient to aid continuity of care and cooperation between recovery and other departments.

Recovery room environment

One of the practitioner's main roles in the recovery room is to detect and prevent postoperative complications and to provide supportive interventions. Local policies often define the qualified staffing needed in recovery. The Association of Anaesthetists of Great Britain & Ireland (AAGBI 2002, 2005b) recommends this to be of the ratio of one qualified carer to one unconscious patient, with a minimum of two staff present when a patient is in the recovery area.

Arranging beds into individual bays promotes easy viewing of the patient and can provide easy access to the necessary equipment for patient care. Efficiency and effectiveness of movement are essential when time becomes critical for the safety of the patient. Therefore, the basic equipment for patient monitoring, airway maintenance, assisted ventilation and resuscitation must be available at the patient's head in each recovery bay (Box 10.1).

Under most circumstances patients are recovered on an operating department trolley, which is specifically designed for coping with patients whose airway might be compromised. In some units, patients are recovered on their own beds which have been brought from the ward. If this is the case, then it is important that the design of the bed facilitates safe postoperative care. For example, the bed should be able to tilt head-down

---

Box 10.1 Minimum equipment required for the recovery room

Fully equipped bed or trolley, for example:

- Oxygen supply.
- Apparatus tilt mechanism.
- Cot sides.
- Brakes.
- Suction.
- Attachments for IV stands.

Equipment to help maintain the patient's airway and normal respiration, for example:

- Oxygen supply (wall-mounted with tubing), face masks, Venturi masks and pocket masks (Figures 10.1 and 10.2).
- A T-piece system and a full range of oropharyngeal and nasopharyngeal airways.
- Suction with tubing.
- Yankauer oropharyngeal suckers and tracheobronchial suction catheters.
- Intubation equipment.
- Ambubag (self-inflating) and range of face masks.
- Monitoring equipment, such as oxygen saturation monitors, CO_2 monitor and other invasive monitors.

Monitors to assess the patient's haemodynamic state, for example:

- Sphygmomanometer and stethoscope or automatic blood pressure monitor.
- Central venous pressure.
- Electrocardiogram (ECG).

Cardiac arrest trolley with all the necessary equipment, for example:

- Defibrillator and ECG monitor.
- Intubation equipment.
- Emergency drugs.
- Sundry items (such as scissors, tape, pen and paper).

Patient heating device, for example:

- Electric heating blanket.
- Forced air warmer (e.g. Bair Hugger®).
- Ripple mattress.

---

to help increase cerebral blood flow during episodes of hypotension. It will also need cot sides, if appropriate, or other methods for preventing patients from falling out of bed, a suitable mattress to support the patient, especially if a cardiac arrest occurs, and fittings for suction and intravenous (IV) stands. The

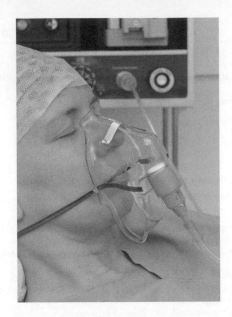

Fig. 10.1 Patient with a Venturi mask.

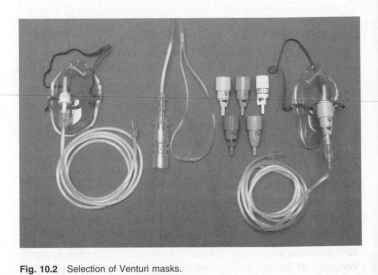

Fig. 10.2 Selection of Venturi masks.

practitioner should assess each patient's needs, and suitable means for patient support and transport should be provided.

Protection and support of the patient's airway is of primary importance during the immediate postoperative period. A developing airway obstruction may require the use of equipment such as face masks, airways and suction. The practitioner may also monitor the patient's haemodynamic state to identify conditions such as low blood pressure, slow pulse and postoperative bleeding, requiring the use of equipment such as central venous pressure monitors, pulse oximeter and electrocardiogram (ECG) monitor.

Various items of emergency equipment need to be readily available to help in the rapid and effective treatment of emergency conditions. For example, a fully stocked cardiac arrest trolley may have items such as a defibrillator, IV equipment and emergency medicines such as epinephrine (adrenaline) and atropine.

Recovery rooms will also need to stock equipment to warm the patient and help prevent postoperative shivering or accidental hypothermia, such as forced air warmers (e.g. the Bair Hugger®), electric blankets and fluid warmers.

All equipment should be checked daily and a record kept that this was undertaken.

Transfer of patient from the operating room to recovery

An anaesthetist and a qualified practitioner usually transfer the patient from the operating room to the recovery room. Patients may be on a bed or a trolley, accompanied by monitoring devices, IV equipment, wound drains, equipment for airway protection and so on.

Early assessment of the patient's condition is an important skill for the recovery practitioner to master. This includes receiving a full handover of the patient's care and treatment in the operating room, and a physical assessment of the patient's condition on admission to the recovery room. A full handover of information ensures the early identification of potential problems, effective treatment and prevention of complications. It is also essential for the practitioner to know anything relevant in the preoperative history that may be significant; for example, the patient may be hard of hearing, epileptic or allergic to certain medications.

A handover may include information such as:

- airway condition during surgery;
- vital signs;
- surgery performed and medical diagnosis;
- patient's general condition;
- anaesthetic and other medications used: non-steroidal anti-inflammatory drugs (NSAIDs) or opioid analgesics, muscle relaxants, antibiotics;
- any untoward problems that occurred in the operating room that might influence postoperative care (e.g. extensive haem-orrhage, cardiac arrest);
- abnormal pathology;
- any tubing, drains, catheters or other supportive aids;
- postoperative instructions from the anaesthetist, including, if required, specific information to report to the surgeon or anaesthetist (e.g. falling blood pressure or increasing loss from drains).

The practitioner carries out the preliminary assessment of patients on admission to the recovery room to ensure that their condition is stable and to provide a baseline for future observations (AAGBI 2005a). This may include an evaluation of:

- airway patency;
- depth and nature of respirations;
- skin colour;
- pulse volume and regularity;
- oxygen saturation;
- level of consciousness and the ability of the patient to respond to commands;
- evidence of haemorrhage or drainage from the operative site;
- temperature.

Care of the patient in recovery

The immediate care of the patient in recovery is a complex mix of many skills and a diverse range of knowledge. After early assessment a 'settling in' period follows where the practitioner commences observations, starts treatment and stabilises the patient's condition. Postoperative instructions from the anaesthetist and surgeon should be checked as soon as is practical. The practitioner may consider the following areas during this time.

The practitioner assesses the patency of the airway, gives oxygen as prescribed and positions the patient to maintain the airway. It is important to identify baseline recordings of respiration rate, depth and rhythm to assess the patient's condition before the anaesthetist hands over care (Younker 2008).

There is a high potential for rapid changes to the patient's haemodynamic state during the immediate postoperative period. Therefore, the practitioner should measure the pulse, recording the rate, rhythm and volume. As a general rule the patient has blood pressure recorded regularly (every 5–10 minutes). Normally, blood pressure should show a slow return to preoperative levels; however, the practitioner should not assess the reading by itself, but should assess it alongside other observations which form part of the overall assessment of the patient. For example, an anxious patient may have a raised blood pressure, despite excessive blood loss from a wound.

The practitioner should check wound sites, dressings and drains for signs of drainage, since excessive bleeding may need further investigation by the surgeon and possible return to the operating theatre.

Fluid balance is important in the immediate postoperative period because of blood loss during surgery and the hypotensive effects of several anaesthetic drugs. The practitioner should ensure that IV infusions are running at the prescribed rate via the correct route. All input and output from, for example, drains, catheters or IVs should be recorded. Various fluids may be given during the patient's recovery including, for example, crystalloids, blood and blood products and plasma expanders.

The postoperative patient may need various medicines during recovery, including antiemetics, analgesics (e.g. opioids and NSAIDs), antihypertensives and antibiotics. The anaesthetic chart usually lists any medications that the anaesthetist has prescribed for the immediate postoperative period. The practitioner should also check the patient's prescription chart for postoperative medicine regimes which the anaesthetist may have prescribed before surgery. Checking the intraoperative record before giving any medicines ensures that doses of the medicines will not be duplicated. Recording the effect of medicines given is essential to ensure that they produce the desired effect.

Postoperative pain can lead to further complications such as hypoxia, anxiety and restlessness. Good postoperative analgesia will encourage a rapid recovery (McMain 2008). The practitioner must carry out a formal pain assessment and give prescribed analgesia as required, noting the effect. Giving antiemetics helps reduce the emetic side effect of opioids.

A practitioner should remain with the conscious or semi-conscious patient since confused and disorientated patients may cause harm to themselves while awakening. The practitioner should assess the level of consciousness, observing for returning reflexes, for example swallowing, tear secretion, eyelash and eyelid reflexes, and response to stimuli both physical (not painful) and verbal. The patient should be oriented to time and place as often as is necessary since he or she is often disorientated and confused on waking. To reduce anxiety and increase cooperation, it is important to keep patients informed of all procedures, regardless of seeming unresponsiveness, as hearing returns before the ability to respond physically.

The patient should be positioned safely and comfortably. This is likely to be in the recovery position, which is a lateral position with the head on a pillow, and the upper leg resting on a pillow bent over the top of the lower leg. Keeping the patient's position comfortable may help relieve pain and help to prevent complications caused by abnormal positioning of limbs.

Postoperative hypothermia is a recognised complication of surgery and should be avoided as it may lead to other complications such as delayed wound healing, infection and, in extreme cases, organ failure. The patient must be kept warm and a space blanket or Bair Hugger® applied if needed. The recovery room environment should be kept at a warm temperature, above 21° C.

Assessment for discharge

The time that patients stay in the recovery room is dependent on the rate at which their condition returns to the physical, mental and emotional state where they can be left unattended between routine observations, and the absence of any postoperative problems which can be resolved during the immediate postoperative recovery (Swatton 2004, Smith & Hardy 2007). The practitioner should inform the anaesthetist of the patient's health status before the patient leaves the recovery area and follow the unit's discharge protocols to ensure efficient and safe patient care.

Common postoperative problems

Table 10.1 and Box 10.2 indicate some of the common postoperative problems and the patient's expected status on discharge. Under certain circumstances, for example during extended periods of ventilation, the patient's condition will vary from that described.

The main areas of concern for the recovery practitioner are neurological status, airway management, respiratory and cardiovascular function, pain relief and wound care

---

Box 10.2   Patient's expected state on discharge from the recovery area

- Conscious and oriented to a suitable level.
- All normal protective airway reflexes present.
- Acceptable respiratory function and normal oxygen saturation readings.
- Normal pulse and blood pressure readings for at least 30 minutes before discharge.
- No persistent or excessive bleeding from wound or drainage sites.
- Pain reduced to an individually acceptable level as assessed by formal pain intensity score.
- Postoperative nausea and vomiting absent.
- Body temperature within normal levels (a hypothermic patient's temperature must normally be above 36° C before discharge).

Table 10.1 Common postoperative problems.

Problem	Possible causes	Possible actions required (practitioner, surgeon or anaesthetist)
Airway obstruction	• Tongue occluding the airway because of poor positioning • Foreign material, e.g. blood, secretions, vomit, or swollen airway tissues • Laryngeal spasm • Bronchospasm	• Maintain recovery position supporting the jaw if unconscious or sit up if awake. Insert oral airway. Use suction to remove obstruction. Consider reintubation if required.
Hypoventilation	• Respiratory depression from anaesthetic agents such as opioids, volatile anaesthetics or barbiturates • Decreased respiratory drive caused by abnormal pCO_2 • Loss of hypoxic drive in patients with chronic pulmonary disease • Neuromuscular blockade from continued action of non-depolarising muscle relaxants caused by electrolyte imbalance, impaired excretion with renal or liver disease or hypothermia	• Ensure oxygen therapy is in place. Ventilate by hand if required using an Ambubag and mask. Ensure complete reversal of anaesthetic agents. Monitor SpO_2 and other blood gases
Hypotension	• Hypovolaemia caused by anaesthetic drugs (depression of the cardiovascular system or vasodilation), sympathetic block secondary to local anaesthetics or blood loss during surgery	• Lay the patient flat and raise legs to increase return blood flow to the heart and increase cerebral circulation if compromised • Wake patient up to stimulate the cardiovascular system • Check for blood loss from the wound site or drains in case of continuing bleeding • Increase rate of IV infusion to help replace fluids • Consider the need for blood transfusion

Hypertension	• Pain. • Carbon dioxide retention caused by poor ventilation • Distended bladder leading to pain or discomfort, caused by blocked or kinked catheters or obstruction caused by damage to tissues during surgery • Action of some anaesthetic drugs	• Assess the patient for pain and give prescribed analgesia. Check for bladder distension. Monitor respirations
Bradycardia	• May be the normal preoperative pulse rate in fit patients • Depression of the cardiovascular system caused by action of opioids • Anticholinesterases such as atropine • Pain stimuli	• Be aware of potential cardiac arrest and assess action required
Tachycardia	• Hypovolaemia causing the heart to compensate by beating faster • Pain stimuli • Fluid overload, e.g. caused by IV infusions • Fear or anxiety • Septicaemia • Actions of some anaesthetic drugs	• Be aware of possible cardiac arrest. Assess cause and act suitably according to local protocols. Check ECG and assess rhythm. Check blood pressure and central venous pressure

Cont.

389

Table 10.1 Continued.

Problem	Possible causes	Possible actions required (practitioner, surgeon or anaesthetist)
Nausea and vomiting	• Side effects of opioids • Hypotension • Abdominal surgery • Pain	• Prepare a vomit bowl and oral suction to protect the patient's airway. Place patient in suitable position for preserving or protecting the airway. Assess nausea score and give antiemetic as prescribed. Ensure the patient is not hypoxic
Pain	• Anxiety and restlessness causing increased pain from the operation site • Surgical trauma, e.g. at the wound site • Inadequate intraoperative or postoperative analgesia • Intraoperative harm to the patient not caused by surgery, e.g. inadequate positioning	• Speak to patient and assess cause of anxiety. Assess pain score, the nature and cause of pain and adjust pain relief. Give prescribed analgesia as required and record effectiveness
Hypothermia	• Vasodilatation or vasoconstriction • A recognised complication following surgery • Large infusions of blood and fluids	• Warm patient according to local protocols and with the equipment available. Be aware of the potential problems associated with heating patients too quickly
Wound haemorrhage	• Surgical issues such as inadequate wound closure, leaking vascular anastamosis, inadequate haemostasis • Blood disorders, e.g. sickle-cell anaemia or low platelet count • Transfusion reaction leading to abnormal clotting mechanisms	• Apply pressure to operative site and watch drains for signs of excessive leakage • Be aware of possible surgical complications and keep surgeon informed of developments • Ensure blood is available. Ensure availability of clip removers if wounds are closed by clips. Give fluids as needed • Prepare patient in case of return to the operating room

(Kehlet & Dahl 2003). Often, only the combined actions of the recovery practitioner, anaesthetist and surgeon provide the necessary care for the patient and resolve postoperative complications.

The patient must be awake, comfortable and physiologically stable before leaving the support of the recovery area (Box 10.2). The normal airway reflexes must be present to prevent problems with respiration, such as aspiration of stomach contents into the lungs, while returning to the ward or while under reduced postoperative supervision on the ward. Respiratory function must be satisfactory and oxygen saturation readings need to be within suitable levels to prevent hypoxia during the return to the ward. The patient should have also displayed normal pulse and blood pressure readings (AAGBI 2007) before discharge as this suggests a return to a normal preoperative state, reversal of anaesthetic and absence of bleeding or other postoperative complications.

Wound and drainage sites must be free from persistent or excessive bleeding since this may be a sign of postoperative complications which may need surgical intervention. This is especially important for surgery on or near the airway, for example thyroid surgery, since excessive bleeding may compromise breathing by causing obstruction.

The patient must have satisfactory pain relief before leaving the recovery area as this may be difficult to achieve on the ward or when pain has become established. Pain may also alter the patient's understanding of surgery and may influence future decisions about hospital treatment. Inadequate pain relief can also delay longer-term postoperative recovery by compromising respiration, reducing movement and exhausting the patient physically and emotionally.

It is important to reduce the risk of vomiting or airway problems during the patient's return to the ward since the conditions for airway control are likely to be less than ideal in the corridor or lift. The bed should contain all the necessary equipment including, for example, oxygen, suction, suitable monitoring and equipment for intubation or airway control.

To ensure continuity of care, the recovery practitioner must offer an accurate handover to the ward nurse collecting the patient (AAGBI 2005a). Clear, written documentation must support the handover by including, for example:

- operative procedure;
- anaesthetic administered;
- analgesia and pain assessment;
- antiemetics;
- oxygen therapy;
- IV therapy and fluid losses;
- drains;
- wound dressing;
- pressure ulcer risk assessment, including the Waterlow pressure ulcer assessment score (Waterlow 2005), a pressure sore severity score if a pressure sore is present and any measures taken.

A good handover of information helps to inform the ward staff about the patient's condition to:

- help plan postoperative care;
- improve communication between the patient, staff and relatives;
- help identify potential postoperative problems;
- assess the effect of analgesia;
- ensure that oxygen therapy continues in the ward;
- help identify future needs related to continuing recovery.

KEY CLINICAL SKILLS

The discussion in the previous paragraphs has highlighted the role of the recovery practitioner in helping the patient to full recovery. Many of the specific skills carried out by recovery practitioners have already been discussed in other chapters of the book. Therefore, the remainder of this chapter looks at the implication for postoperative recovery in four specific areas which are essential to good practice for the recovery practitioner:

- maintaining the airway;
- managing postoperative pain;
- maintaining fluid balance;
- monitoring haemodynamic status.

The reader should refer to previous chapters of this book for discussion of other skills practised by recovery practitioners.

Maintaining the airway

This section discusses the following areas:

- assessment of breathing and respiration;
- airway suction;
- extubation;
- insertion and removal of oral airways.

Assessment of breathing and respiration

The recovery practitioner must be skilled in assessing breathing and respiration, since there is an increased risk that the postoperative patient will have respiratory complications. Refer to Chapters 1 and 6 for discussion of respiratory assessment, physiology and respiratory conditions. Assessing the rate, depth and rhythm of breathing shows the patient's ability to manage his or her own airway and ventilation. This helps monitoring of the patient's return to a normal preoperative status, and aids diagnosis of respiratory conditions, initiation of treatment, monitoring of progress and evaluation of care.

Respiratory monitors are useful in the recovery area to assess respiratory function. For example, pulse oximetry is necessary to monitor SpO_2 (AAGBI 2007) and help avoid hypoxaemic incidents. Wright's respirometer or a peak flow meter can be used to assess respirations.

Airway suction

Competence in airway suction is an essential skill, since there are many possible causes of obstruction in the early postoperative period. Suction removes secretions or vomit from the pharynx in a safe and controlled manner for patients who are unable to cough effectively. Excessive mucus in the airways often produces a 'rattling' sound in the throat. Other sounds of obstruction include 'crowing', 'whooping' and 'stridor' caused by laryngeal spasm or obstruction of the vocal cords. Secretions are sometimes caused by irritation of the vocal cords and these secretions can be sucked out using suction catheters. Airway obstruction which progresses to complete obstruction becomes quiet or silent since the patient is not passing air through the vocal cords. In complete obstruction, the patient may also show signs of excessive effort as the body tries to breathe reflexively. Therefore, since 'no sound' suggests either perfect breathing or no breathing at all, other methods of assessing breathing should always be used in conjunction to hearing. These include, for example, the practitioner feeling for breaths on the reverse of his or her hand, watching for condensation coming and going on the inside wall of oxygen masks, observing for chest movements and intercostal in-drawing (accessory muscle use), and observing signs of excessive effort.

Oral or nasopharyngeal suction is the most common method of airway suction during recovery. Practitioners must be trained in the specific suctioning techniques prior to undertaking these procedures. Key points about suction include:

- oral suction is often carried out using rigid Yankauer suckers. Soft, Y-suction catheters passed through the nose are useful if the patient clenches their teeth;
- do not use contaminated or previously used suction catheters as these can increase the risk of respiratory infections (Pedersen *et al.* 2009);
- use the lowest possible suction pressure (Pedersen *et al.* 2009);
- do not occlude more than half the lumen of the endotracheal (ET) or tracheostomy tube if present (Pedersen *et al.* 2009);
- suction for no longer than 15 seconds (Pedersen *et al.* 2009);
- high flow, high capacity suction is required to cope with potentially large amounts of secretions or vomit;
- avoid traumatising the oral and respiratory mucosa, e.g. by forcing catheters past clenched teeth.

The patient may need tracheobronchial suction, using a soft Y-suction catheter, if there are secretions deep inside the lungs; for example, if still intubated or following tracheostomy. The practitioner must be aware that this procedure can be painful and distressing for both awake and semi-conscious, sedated patients (Puntillo 1994). A strict aseptic technique must be followed during this procedure because of the risk of deep respiratory infection. Only apply suction on withdrawal of the catheter, to avoid damaging the respiratory mucosa. Hypoxia is a risk because the suction draws out the patient's air supply, and the catheter itself causes a partial obstruction of the airway. The patient may therefore need preoxygenation and monitoring of SpO_2 is essential during the procedure.

Extubation

Extubation is normally an extended role and should only be carried out by practitioners who are specifically trained to undertake it. Patients often enter the recovery room still intubated. Semi-conscious patients may tolerate an ET tube for some time while awakening, and may remove it themselves as they wake up. This is a useful choice when managed properly and if there are no respiratory complications. Successful self-extubation suggests the patient is awake enough to maintain their own airway. During self-extubation, the practitioner should remain with the patient until extubated, cutting the ties and deflating the cuff at the right time, and performing oral suction if needed.

It may also be necessary to extubate the semi-conscious patient if the ET tube is irritating the airway and making the patient restless. The patient must be able to maintain his or her own airway and be able to breathe adequately before extubation. The key steps in extubation include:

- preoxygenate the patient if possible to help prevent hypoxia during extubation;
- remove any oral packs if present;
- apply suction to the mouth and pharynx;
- place the patient in the recovery position;
- remove the ties and deflate the cuff using a 20 ml syringe, ensuring the pilot balloon deflates;
- gently remove the tube, applying suction if necessary using a soft suction catheter;
- insert an oral airway if required (see Chapter 8 for measurement of oral airway).

The practitioner must watch the patient after the procedure for signs of hypoxia or respiratory distress and apply oxygen according to an assessment of the patient's condition (Hatfield & Tronson 2008). Equipment for re-intubation should be easily accessible in case the patient's condition deteriorates.

Insertion and removal of oral airways

Guedel airways are common in recovery because they are effective at keeping the upper airway clear of obstructions. These are curved, flattened tubes which are available in sizes including 4 for large patients, 2 or 3 for adults, 1 for young children and 0 or 00 for babies or neonates. They are normally clear plastic and disposable.

The Guedel airway is inserted upside-down to help passage over the tongue, and allowed to come to rest in the back of the mouth. If the patient gags, then either the airway is too big, or the patient is able to protect his or her own airway and so does not need an artificial airway. See Chapter 8 for a discussion on the measurement of oral airways.

The principles for removing oral airways are similar to those of extubation – patients should be breathing normally and protecting their own airway before removal. Similarly, the patient may need suction and should be watched for signs of hypoxia after the procedure.

Managing postoperative pain

This section discusses pain assessment, analgesic administration and treatment of complications. Most NHS trusts produce guidelines and protocols for managing postoperative pain and practitioners should be aware of how to apply these procedures to their own specific clinical setting.

Up to 70% of patients suffer acute pain in the recovery room (Hatfield & Tronson 2008). It is important to manage postoperative pain because it can interfere with ideal recovery by:

- increasing restlessness, leading to increased risk of cardiovascular problems and hypoxia;
- increasing the risk of postoperative nausea and vomiting;
- inhibiting normal respiration and increasing the risk of respiratory complications, such as obstruction from secretions, hypoxia and pneumonia;
- increasing the metabolic response (see Chapter 1) leading to increased risk of infection and delayed wound healing;
- causing the patient distress and anxiety.

The International Association for the Study of Pain defines pain as 'an unpleasant sensory or emotional experience associated with actual or potential tissue damage' (Merskey & Bogduk 1994). It is a subjective experience for which there are no objective measures. A mixture of pharmacological and non-pharmacological measures should be employed to reduce a patient's pain. Pharmacological therapy reduces pain by interfering with the receptor-mediated response (e.g. opioids such as morphine or fentanyl act as agonists at opioid receptors), reducing the transmission of pain signals along nerve fibres (e.g. local anaesthetics act at the sodium channels, inhibiting depolarisation and transmission of the pain signal) or by altering the perception of pain in the brain (Scott 2009). Because pain is not just a sensory or somatic experience, the patient's previous experiences of pain will influence their pain behaviours (Hagger-Holt 2009).

The analgesic regime should already have been discussed and agreed with the patient preoperatively (see Chapter 6). This is important so the patient is able to cooperate with medicine therapies and understands the choices available. Five steps in effective analgesia in the recovery area are:

- assessing the pain
- identifying the probable cause(s) of pain;
- educating and reassuring the patient;
- providing analgesia;
- identifying and treating complications.

Assessing the pain

A structured and regular pain assessment helps the practitioner to detect changes and assess pain even when the patient does not report it verbally. The practitioner must assess the patient's pain intensity competently and carry out any appropriate actions/interventions.

The subjective assessment of pain is simply a matter of asking the patient and believing what he or she says (Hatfield & Tronson 2008). This often points the way towards the analgesic therapy required and opens the way for the practitioner to offer emotional support.

An objective assessment of pain is difficult because there is only a general correlation between the actual damage caused to the body and the pain experienced by the patient. For example, there may be no obvious cause for a headache. Similarly, a patient with a leg wound may only complain of pain on respiration, while ignoring or not feeling pain from the leg wound. Severe pain also has systemic effects, such as tachycardia, bradycardia, hypertension or hypotension, nausea, vomiting, agitation and restlessness (McMain 2008). These signs and symptoms can mask the actual cause or presence of pain.

In semi-conscious patients, assessment of pain may be challenging – the patient cannot respond effectively to questions about the source, nature or intensity of his or her pain. Developing pain protocols, or defined courses of action according to specific criteria such as surgical procedure or patient condition, help to anticipate the patient's pain based on experiences of similar patients and researched evidence. Pain protocols can be useful because they ensure that all patients receive basic analgesic cover, therefore preventing pain developing. When the patient is awake and oriented, the protocol can be adjusted according to the objective assessment of his or her needs.

Therefore, several pain scoring methods have been produced which aid practitioners in the assessment of pain. Although there are several variations, the two main tools used in the recovery room are the numerical rating scale (NRS) and the verbal rating scale (VRS).

Numerical scales require patients to rate their pain on a scale of 0–10. For example, 0 = no pain whilst 10 is the worst pain imaginable. The accurate assessment of pain using a numerical scale depends on the patient's skills at self-awareness and self-assessment, as well as numerical understanding and ability. A verbal rating scale (Box 10.3) asks patients to rate their pain using descriptors of intensity.

Observation of the signs and symptoms of pain should supplement the objective assessment of a patient's pain, especially where the patient is unable to use the tools described above, for example when disorientated, confused, where he or she is

---

Box 10.3   Verbal pain rating scale

0   No pain
1   Mild pain
2   Moderate pain
3   Severe pain

---

unable to understand how to use the tool, or in babies or young children.

Pain behaviours vary from patient to patient. One patient in moderate to severe pain may be quiet, remain very still and be hypervigilant about the site of their pain, whilst another patient may be crying, anxious and restless.

Identifying the cause of pain
There are many causes of pain in the recovery area, coming from several sources, for example:

- preoperative medical conditions;
- poor positioning during surgery;
- cramps or muscle pain from depolarising muscle relaxants;
- headache or other 'hangover' effects from anaesthetic drugs;
- the surgical procedure including, for example, incisions, donor sites, infusion sites and catheters.

Most analgesic medicines have a systemic effect, and therefore act on pain from multiple sources. However, imagine a scenario where a patient, after an inguinal hernia repair, has a headache. The practitioner gives an opioid IV bolus, assuming that the patient is in pain from the wound (which may after all have been injected with a local anaesthetic and therefore may be pain free), which is not the most effective treatment for the patient's main problem. The practitioner must therefore develop skill at interviewing a potentially confused and disorientated postoperative patient to identify the source of pain. This includes having good communication skills, especially for identifying verbal and non-verbal clues about the source of the pain from the patient.

Educating and reassuring the patient

Anxiety can make pain worse; therefore, it makes sense to try to reduce anxiety to moderate the patient's pain experience. Interpreters, for non-English speaking patients, or family members may be useful for helping to reduce patient anxiety. Reducing anxiety about the cause of the pain may help the patient to relax tense muscles, adopt a positive attitude to the pain, relieve worry and cooperate with analgesic regimes. The practitioner needs to be skilled at assessing the patient's anxiety and be able to offer information, explanations or solutions to satisfy the patient. The practitioner must also be aware of cultural differences in relation to pain and pain relief.

Providing analgesia

Analgesia can be given by various routes to provide optimum relief from pain. Practitioners must be appropriately trained and experienced prior to administering analgesia, and IV injection is normally considered to be an extended role. Analgesic administration in the recovery room is normally either parenteral or by regional blockade (central and peripheral). The recovery practitioner should be familiar with all common methods of analgesic administration including IV, intramuscular (IM), subcutaneous, SC, oral, buccal, sublingual, rectal and epidural, as well as the principles of patient-controlled analgesia.

Opioids are widely used in the management of acute postoperative pain, and so the practitioner must have an understanding of the indications, effects and potential side effects, as well as complications of opioids. Opioids are often given intravenously in the recovery room. This is an ideal route because onset of action is rapid (less than 10 minutes), which is an advantage for patients in acute pain (Scott 2009). The IV route of administration is preferred as absorption of an IM dose may be erratic because of poor blood supply in a recovering postoperative patient. As well as opioids, paracetamol and the COX-2 inhibitor parecoxib may also be given by the IV route.

IV opioid patient-controlled analgesia (PCA) is popular in recovery since it allows the patients to titrate small doses of analgesia themselves, according to the pain that they feel, giving an accurate level of analgesia. Before commencing PCA, patients require a loading dose of opioid to ensure that pain is controlled with minimal side effects (Chumbley 2009). Patients should be educated preoperatively so that they are aware that only they must press the bolus request button, that addiction and overdose are very rare and that the device will make a noise when they request a dose – it is not an alarm to indicate malfunction.

Oral analgesia such as paracetamol may be given but the patient must be able to tolerate oral fluids. Consent must be sought prior to administration of rectal medicines such as diclofenac.

To safely care for patients who are receiving regional blockade staff are often required to undergo specialist training and education. Observation of practice and completion of a competency may be required depending on the employer.

Identifying and treating complications

The potential for side effects from opioid administration is high in recovery because the patient's surgery and anaesthesia already puts him or her at risk of the common side effects of opioids, namely cardiovascular and respiratory depression, sedation and postoperative nausea and vomiting.

A satisfactory dose of analgesia will make the patient's pain manageable, may make the patient drowsy and could result in a respiratory rate of around 8–10 breaths per minute. However, such patients may be at risk from hypoxia if the action of opioids continues to increase; for example, if an intramuscular dose is still being absorbed. The postoperative patient receiving opioids should therefore receive oxygen to help prevent the onset of hypoxia. Monitoring of blood pressure, pulse and SpO_2 is also essential to enable early identification of side effects.

Postoperative nausea and vomiting (PONV) can arise from several causes in the recovery room; for example, hypotension, anxiety, swallowed blood, abdominal procedures and opioid side effects (Royston & Cox 2003). Practitioners often underestimate patient distress caused by this condition, even though research suggests that patients would rather suffer pain than

PONV, and would be willing to pay a substantial amount of money for an effective antiemetic (Abraham 2008).

Conscious patients often give early signs of impending vomiting; for example, dry retching, nausea, pallor and increased salivation immediately before vomiting. Sitting patients up if awake can help them to vomit into a receptacle. Unconscious patients must be placed on their side, and suction used to remove the vomit. Tipping the bed so the patient is head down helps drainage out of the mouth and may prevent aspiration into the lungs. Antiemetics may be prescribed and their effectiveness should be monitored. The practitioner should also be aware of other possible complications of PONV, such as wound dehiscence, aspiration pneumonitis, oesophageal rupture and alveolar rupture leading to airway compromise. The lack of a universally effective antiemetic has led one author to believe that patient assessment is one of the key skills to preventing and treating PONV (Arnold 2002). See Chapter 3 for further discussion of pharmacology and administration of analgesics and antiemetics.

Opioids can also cause sedation because of their action on opioid receptors. Oversedation can lead to respiratory depression which may be reversed with incremental doses (100 μg which equates to 1.5 μg/kg) of the opioid antagonist naloxone. Naloxone is also used in smaller doses to reverse epidural opioid-induced itching.

Maintaining fluid balance

This section discusses postoperative fluid therapy, monitoring of fluid balance and inserting urinary catheters. See Chapter 1 for a discussion of fluid and electrolyte balance.

Postoperative fluid therapy

Normal homeostatic responses during surgery can mask postoperative hypovolaemia caused by blood loss in the operating room, but hypovolaemia can become obvious during the recovery period. This may be indicated by signs of tachycardia, reducing urine output and pallor. Many postoperative patients therefore have IV infusions in progression on return to recovery. Infusion solutions can include dextrose 5%, sodium chloride 0.9% (normal saline) or plasma volume expanders, such as dextran, voulven and gelofusin. Choice of IV solution is based on blood results, such as levels of serum sodium, urine osmolarity and interpretation of blood loss and normal fluid requirements by the body.

Fluid balance problems that the postoperative patient may face following surgery are:

- fluid depletion or overload;
- sodium depletion or overload;
- blood volume depletion or overload.

Fluid depletion or overload

An adult, under normal circumstances, needs a minimum of 2.5 litres of fluid intake per day. When the trauma of surgery and anaesthesia are added, this requirement normally increases. Therefore, the maintenance doses of fluids given intravenously are roughly 1 litre of sodium chloride and 2 litres of dextrose daily. Signs and symptoms that suggest water depletion include high serum sodium, concentrated urine and evidence of water loss through vomiting, diarrhoea and sweating (Hatfield & Tronson 2008).

Fluid overload is normally iatrogenic and a result of over-infusion of solutions such as dextrose. Acute overload of fluids can also be caused by bladder or prostate surgery because of absorption of irrigating solutions (Rao 1987). Signs and symptoms of fluid overload are wide and varied and may include, for example, feelings of dizziness, headache and nausea, restlessness and confusion progressing to hypertension, haematuria and bradycardia. Definitive diagnosis can be made by measuring serum sodium with results of less than 130 mmol/L. Medical management of serious fluid overload may include oxygen therapy, a diuretic such as furosemide and dopamine to support a failing cardiovascular system.

Saline depletion and overload

Saline depletion may be treated with saline infusions. Signs of saline depletion may include low urine output, tachycardia and low central venous pressure. Vomiting, gastric fluid loss or diarrhoea may cause saline depletion.

Saline overload can result in cardiac failure and the patient will present with such signs and symptoms as raised central venous pressure, pulmonary oedema and abnormal heart sounds. A diuretic such as furosemide can be used to treat this condition.

Blood volume depletion and overload

Blood volume depletion can present as surgical shock (see Chapter 1) if severe enough. Treatment of blood depletion in recovery is usually with crystalloid solutions, blood products or colloids. Blood or colloid overload in the operating room will present in recovery as left ventricular failure. Blood or colloid stays in the circulation and therefore puts undue strain on the heart. Treatment of overload is by diuretics or phlebotomy if required.

Fluid therapy

Fluid therapy should be recorded to avoid problems such as those mentioned above. All the usual vital signs, for example, anomalies in blood pressure, pulse, respiration or SpO_2, may indicate problems with fluid therapy. In particular the following methods may be specifically useful in suspected conditions:

- auscultation of the chest – can reveal pulmonary oedema (e.g. fine crackles) , abnormal heart sounds (e.g. gallop rhythm);
- central venous pressure – can show increased jugular venous pressure;
- chest x-ray – can show venous engorgement, lung oedema;
- blood results – identify serum sodium, potassium and other electrolyte disturbances;
- urinalysis – helps with diagnosis of saline overload or depletion.

Fluid therapy must be recorded accurately to help prevent errors in administration. This is especially important when drugs are added to infusions.

Urinary catheterisation

Many postoperative patients are catheterised to help in accurate fluid balance monitoring, and to help avoid postoperative complications. Indications for catheterisation include:

- postoperative conditions such as acute retention (e.g. as a result of opioid therapy);
- chronic retention with renal damage;
- to contribute to accurate fluid balance recording in at-risk patients;
- urinary incontinence caused by nerve damage, e.g. because of diabetes, spinal or neurological disease;
- to help with tissue viability during the intraoperative or postoperative periods.

Catheterisation is normally considered to be an extended role; therefore, practitioners should be appropriately trained and experienced before performing this procedure. Catheters are often inserted in the operating room, prior to the patient waking up; however, on occasion it may be necessary to catheterise a patient in recovery. Most catheters inserted for surgical reasons are intended for short-term use (1–6 weeks), and are made of plastic (if removed immediately on emptying the bladder) or latex with various coatings such as silver to reduce urethral trauma and infection. Catheters are usually of the Foley design, which have an eye at the distal end to promote drainage, and a balloon which prevents the catheter from falling out and reduces the chance of by-passing of urine. Specialty catheters include three-way catheters (for irrigating the bladder), double balloon (for controlling haemorrhage) and specialty tipped, for example Coude (olive) tip and whistle tip. The catheters come in lengths of 43 cm (male), 30 cm (female) and 26 cm (paediatric).

Catheter diameter is measured in Charrière (Ch) or French gauge (Fg), which are identical scales. Sizes range from 12 Ch/Fg to 24 Ch/Fg, where 12 Ch = 4 mm. Paediatric catheters are available from 6 Ch/Fg to 12 Ch/Fg. Balloon size varies from 3 ml to 30 ml and is printed on the pilot tube. The practitioner should always identify the correct balloon size and use the correct amount of sterile water to fill the balloon. All the relevant information should be recorded in the patient's notes.

It is important to use an aseptic technique and maintain good hygiene when managing catheters because of the risk of urinary tract infection (UTI). Between 1% and 4% of catheterised patients who develop a UTI go on to develop bacteraemia and septicaemia, of whom 13–30% die.

UTI associated with catheterisation can occur because of contamination during the catheterisation procedure, from contamination from the peri-urethral space, internal lumen of the catheter, drainage bag or a connection port. The recovery practitioner can help reduce the risk of UTIs by ensuring a satisfactory fluid intake, inserting the catheter aseptically and by teaching the patient catheter care (if appropriate, e.g. in day surgery). The catheter should be removed as soon as possible and prophylactic antibiotics should be considered in at-risk patients.

The practitioner should always use lubrication such as Instillagel, a water-based gel that contains 2% lidocaine for anaesthetic action and chlorhexidine for antiseptic cover. Instillagel provides analgesia within 3–5 minutes, reduces urethral trauma to a minimum and reduces contamination by bacteria. Use of Instillagel should be avoided in patients allergic to or sensitive to chlorhexidine as anaphylaxis has been reported (Parkes *et al.* 2009). Box 10.4 details the correct catherisation procedure.

There are many problems associated with catheterisation. Trauma caused by rough insertion of the catheter can cause bleeding. This can lead to pain and discomfort, anxiety and blockage of the catheter. The practitioner should always insert catheters gently to help prevent damage to the urethra. Catheters can become blocked by encrustations (biofilm) or by bleeding, especially following surgery on the renal and urinary systems. Pain can be caused by spasm of the urethra, trauma, irritation, allergy and so on. The cause of the pain must always be assessed and suitable measures taken. The catheter may be pulled out by semi-conscious or confused patients, or when transferring the patient from bed to table. This is especially painful and dangerous when the balloon is still inflated. A non-deflating balloon is also dangerous and may need surgery to remove the catheter. The balloon may also burst, leading to the

---

Box 10.4   Catheterisation procedure

The procedure should be carried out aseptically and the patient should be socially clean before starting.

Initiating male catheterisation
- Place patient supine with legs straight.
- Retract foreskin and clean with saline 0.9%, clean from tip of penis towards glans.
- Change sterile gloves if necessary.
- Insert 11 ml of Instillagel, hold glans firmly between thumb and forefinger to prevent reflux and wait 2–3 minutes.

Initiating female catheterisation
- Place patient supine, legs abducted and bent at the knees, heels together.
- Spread the labia and find the urethral opening.
- Clean area from front to back with sodium chloride 0.9%.
- Be aware of possibility of false placement of the catheter into the vagina. Folds of skin may also be mistaken for the urethra.

Catheterisation procedure
- Select correct size and catheter.
- Gently insert a size 12–14 Fg catheter into the urethra.
- Gently feed the catheter along the urethra only touching the outside plastic covering and not the catheter itself, until urine drains.
- Attach bag or spigot.
- Gently advance the catheter and ensure all the balloon is in the bladder.
- If resistance is felt do not force catheter, remove it and send for help.
- Take a urine sample for microbiology at this point if needed.
- Inflate the balloon with the correct amount of sterile water, watching the patient for verbal and non-verbal signs of pain.
- Aseptically connect the catheter to drainage bag and secure to the patient's leg.
- In males, retract the foreskin and ensure area is clean and dry, then replace foreskin in normal position. Be aware of risk of paraphimosis.

---

risk of retained latex fragments and painful removal of the catheter.

Monitoring haemodynamic status

This section discusses the use of monitoring in recovery, in particular, blood gases, blood pressure, central venous pressure and pulse oximetry.

Much of the recovery practitioner's time involves assessing, interpreting and recording patients' physiological measurements. Monitors can supplement the visual and verbal signs and symptoms of developing complications by providing objective evidence of particular measurements. Chapter 2 discusses the use of equipment, and Chapter 1 considers several of the physiological parameters, including ECG. This section focuses on the practical use of monitors in the recovery environment.

Monitoring blood gases

Recovery practitioners are increasingly becoming involved in this procedure, which is now seen as an extended role. Arterial blood gases can be taken from an arterial cannula, or from the radial, femoral, brachial or dorsalis pedis arteries, in order of preference. Care should be taken to assess the suitability of the artery chosen and the practitioner must consider systemic factors such as diabetes or vascular disease. The practitioner must be able to undertake an Allen's test before cannulation of the radial artery. This test involves occluding the radial and ulnar arteries in turn and observing for flushing of the hand when one is released. If either is occluded, then neither can be used for blood gases because of the danger of damage to the blood supply to the hand.

Arterial monitoring kits are available to help obtain the sample. The blood must be stored in a cool container and sent to the lab as soon as possible. The form accompanying the sample must be fully and carefully completed, because of the importance of the readings. Applying a pressure pad should help to stop bleeding over the puncture site and the practitioner should watch the site carefully for bleeding over the next few minutes.

Various physiological measurements can be made from blood gases; for example, pH, pO_2, pCO_2 and bicarbonate among others. The practitioner must be familiar with normal levels and be able to respond quickly to abnormal results. Blood gases are often taken to the intensive care unit for testing.

Monitoring blood pressure

Most recovery areas now have automatic blood pressure monitors; however, it is a useful skill to be able to monitor blood pressure using a manual sphygmanometer. In brief, the following procedure may be used to take manual blood pressure:

- explain to the patient what you are doing as you attach the cuff to the upper arm;
- place your fingers on the radial pulse;
- inflate the cuff to about 30 mmHg above the point at which the pulse disappears;
- take your finger off the radial pulse and listen with a stethoscope to the blood flow returning to the brachial artery in the cubital fossa.

The point where the first sound is heard is the systolic pressure; the diastolic pressure is when the sound disappears completely.

Manual blood pressure measurements are prone to errors because of factors such as the patient moving, agitation and excessive movement, wrong size of cuff used, inaccurate readings being taken and so on. An alternative is to use an oscillometric blood pressure monitor which automatically inflates and deflates the cuff at intervals. This device is now widely used in the recovery areas and has largely superseded manual methods of blood pressure monitoring. It helpfully alerts the user to kinks in the tube or errors in cuff placement. Again, errors are possible in these readings, although the automatic function makes it a useful monitor for busy practitioners (Burton 2000).

A potentially more accurate way of measuring blood pressure is to use an arterial catheter connected to a transducer. Arterial lines are often connected in the operating room prior to admission into the recovery unit. Errors can occur using this method because of false calibration or faulty set-up; however, it is generally accepted to be the most accurate way of assessing blood pressure. The practitioner should remember that it is not individual readings that are important during patient recovery, but the trend, which can show an improving or worsening condition. Readings from blood pressure monitors should also be supplemented by a holistic assessment of the patient. For example, a patient sitting up in bed, conversing with a practitioner, is unlikely to have a blood pressure of 60/40 mmHg, regardless of what the equipment records.

Central venous pressure

Central venous pressure (CVP) monitors are used to measure filling of the right side of the heart and can point out signs of fluid imbalance. These monitors also help to guide fluid replacement, to infuse medicines and to provide venous access when peripheral cannulation is difficult. The normal reading for CVP is between 0 and 5 cmH$_2$O. Although the measurement of CVP is undertaken in most recovery units using sophisticated monitors that can also transduce arterial pressure, measurements may also be made manually using a manometer. The measurement is taken by measuring the distance a column of water is pushed up a measuring tube by the central venous pressure. The practitioner should refer to manufacturer's manuals or trust procedures to ensure the correct setting up of the equipment, since various errors in setting up can lead to false readings. In brief:

- medical staff insert the central venous catheter;
- identify a zero reference point – the zero of the measuring tube should be level with the right side of the heart, which is roughly midway between the anterior and posterior of the chest (mid-axillary line). Mark the point for future reference with a permanent pen;
- ensure there is a continuously flowing infusion to prevent occlusion of the catheter;
- open the tap in both directions – this shuts off the infusion and opens a direct pathway between the measuring tube and the patient;
- measure and record the distance the water is pushed up the tube;
- close the tap to the tube, opening it to the infusion.

The CVP is especially useful in a bleeding patient since venous pressure alters before arterial pressure. As blood volume falls, the CVP also falls, sometimes rapidly, and before arterial pressure is affected. Comparison of CVP readings to arterial blood pressure can help with the diagnosis of conditions such as hypovolaemia, shock, cardiac failure and abnormalities in fluid balance. Complications of CVP include infection, pneumothorax, arterial puncture and air embolism caused by disconnection in the system.

Pulse oximeters

Pulse oximeters are useful in the postoperative patient since they are non-invasive, quick and easy to apply, give an accurate indication of SpO_2 and are a good guide to whether the patient is hypoxic (Pedersen *et al.*, 2002, Wright 2003). The pulse oximeter reads the absorption of light by haemoglobin, which is affected by oxygen saturation. This produces a visual and auditory signal which gives an indication of SpO_2. The readings can be affected by shivering, hypothermia, hypovolaemia and cardiac function.

Readings should be approaching 100% when on oxygen, or greater than 90% when breathing room air, in an otherwise healthy patient, before discharge from the recovery room. In most circumstances haemoglobin saturation greater than 90% means the patient is not hypoxic. However, SpO_2 also depends on the pH of the blood and if the patient is acidotic, saturation can remain high, but SpO_2 may be low. Therefore, again the practitioner should not rely on this monitor by itself, but must use it as part of the holistic patient assessment. In all situations, a falling reading of less than 90% should be investigated because of the increasing danger of hypoxia as saturation decreases.

REFERENCES

Abraham, J. (2008) Acupressure and acupuncture in preventing and managing postoperative nausea and vomiting in adults. *Journal of Perioperative Practice* **18** (12), 543–551.

Arnold, A. (2002) Postoperative nausea and vomiting in the perioperative setting. *British Journal of Perioperative Nursing* **12** (1), 24–30.

Association of Anaesthetists of Great Britain & Ireland (AAGBI) (2002) *Immediate Postanaesthetic Recovery*. AAGBI, London.

Association of Anaesthetists of Great Britain & Ireland (AAGBI) (2005a) *Day Surgery 2* (revised edn). AAGBI, London.

Association of Anaesthetists of Great Britain & Ireland (AAGBI) (2005b) *The Anaesthesia Team* (revised edn). AAGBI, London.

Association of Anaesthetists of Great Britain & Ireland (AAGBI) (2007) *Recommendations for Standards of Monitoring During Anaesthesia and Recovery*, 4th edn. AAGBI, London.

Burton, J. (2000) Oscillometric blood pressure monitors. *British Journal of Perioperative Nursing* **10** (12), 624–626.

Chumbley, G. (2009) Patient-controlled analgesia. In Cox, F. (ed) *Perioperative Pain Management*. Wiley-Blackwell, Oxford.

Hagger-Holt, R. (2009) Psychosocial perspectives of acute pain. In: Cox, F. (ed) *Perioperative Pain Management*. Wiley-Blackwell, Oxford.

Hatfield, A. & Tronson, M. (2008) *The Complete Recovery Book*. Oxford University Press, Oxford.

Kehlet, H. & Dahl, J. (2003) Anaesthesia, surgery, and challenges in postoperative recovery. *The Lancet* **362**, 1921–1928.

McMain, L. (2008) Principles of acute pain management. *Journal of Perioperative Practice* **18** (11), 472–478

Merskey, H., Bogduk, N. (1994) *Classification of Chronic Pain*, 2nd edn. IASP Press, Seattle, 209-214.

National Health Service Education Scotland (NES) (2002) *A Route to Enhanced Competence in Perioperative Practice*. NES, Scotland.

Parkes, A.W., Harper, N., Herwadkar, A., & Pumphrey, R. (2009) Anaphyslaxis to the chlorhexidine component of Instillagel: a case series. *British Journal of Anaesthesia* **102** (1), 65–68.

Pedersen, T., Dyrlund Pedersen, B., & Møller, A.M. (2002) Pulse oximetry for perioperative monitoring (Cochrane Review). In: *The Cochrane Library*, Issue 1. Update Software, Oxford.

Pedersen, C.M., Rosendahl-Nielsen, M., Hjermind, J., & Egerod, I. (2009) Endotracheal suctioning of the adult intubated patient – what is the evidence? *Intensive and Critical Nursing* **25** (1), 21–30.

Puntillo, K.A. (1994) Dimensions of procedural pain and its analgesic management in critically ill surgical patients. *American Journal of Critical Care* **3** (2), 116–122.

Rao, P.N. (1987) Fluid absorption during urological endoscopy. *British Journal of Urology* **60**, 93–99.

Royston, D. & Cox, F. (2003) Anaesthesia: the patient's point of view. *The Lancet* **362** (9396), 1648–1658.

Scott, K. (2009) How analgesics work. In: Cox, F. (ed) *Perioperative Pain Management*. Wiley-Blackwell, Oxford.

Smith, B. & Hardy, D. (2007) Discharge criteria in recovery – 'just in case'. *Journal of Perioperative Practice* **17** (3), 102–107.

Swatton, S. (2004) A discharge protocol for the postanaesthesia recovery unit. *British Journal of Perioperative Nursing* **14** (2), 74–80.

Younker, J. (2008) Care of the intubated patient in the PACU: The ABCDE approach. *Journal of Perioperative Practice* **18** (3), 116–120.

Waterlow, J. (2005) From costly treatment to cost-effective prevention: using Waterlow. *British Journal of Community Nursing* **10** (9) S25–6, S28, S30.

Wright, J. (2003) Introduction to pulse oximetry. *British Journal of Perioperative Nursing* **13** (11), 456–460.

Index

accidental hazards 183–7

accountability 51, 134, 143–6, 172–4, 364

AcH (acetylcholine) 28, 113, 118, 129

acid–base balance 4, 9–11

acidosis 10–11, 13, 38, 44, 199

ACTH (adrenocorticotrophic hormone) 43

ADH (antidiuretic hormone) 7, 8, 12, 26, 43–4

adrenaline (epinephrine) 12, 18, 25, 28, 43, 125, 127, 129–31, 293–5, 325, 383

adrenergic (adrenoceptor) agonists 129, 130–1

adrenergic (adrenoceptor) antagonists 129, 130, 132

advanced scrub practitioner / first assistant to the surgeon 158–9, 233–4

AFC (Agenda for Change) 164–5

AIDS (acquired immunodeficiency syndrome) 184

airway management 34, 65, 261, 278–9, 383–5, 387–92

 ARDS (acute respiratory distress syndrome) 294

 bronchospasm 293

 in recovery 393–6

 mechanical ventilation/ intubation 280–94

 paediatric 330–1

 see also tracheal intubation

airway suction 393–5

aldosterone 7, 8, 26, 43–4

alfentanil 65, 123

alkaloids 113

alkalosis 10–11, 12, 38, 44

allergic reactions, respiratory system 40

alveoli 35–7, 40–1, 64–5, 294

anaemia 112, 258, 390

anaesthesia

 drugs to support body systems 112–3, 115–6, 122, 126–32

 drugs which may be administered during anaesthesia 313

 elderly patient 333–5

 electrolyte balance 11–13

 epidural 124, 317–21, 322, 323–4

 general anaesthesia 115–124, 277–95, 333

 historical development 111–2

 hypothermia 200–3, 331–2, 334–5

 impact on the body 41–46

 induction, general anaesthesia 277–84

 induction complications, general anaesthesia 284–95

 local anaesthesia 124–6, 131, 234, 271–2, 325–8

 maintenance and emergence, general anaesthesia 313–5

 metabolic response 41–6

anaesthesia (*cont'd*)
  monitoring 68–77, 115, 393,
    407–9
  neuromuscular block 76
  paediatric patient 63, 116, 119,
    282, 304–5, 307–9, 327,
    328–32
  pregnant patient (caesarean
    section) 332–3
  regional 313–25, 334–5
  reversal agents 114–5
  sedation 271–2, 313, 327–9
  spinal 316–7, 318, 319, 321,
    323–4, 332
  temperature control 75–6,
    200–3, 295–6, 297, 313–5,
    334–5
  TIVA (total intravenous
    anaesthesia) 65–67,122–3,
    313
  triad of 112, 277–8
anaesthetic assistant 230–1, 234,
  236–43
anaesthetic chart 104, 385
anaesthetic equipment 54–76,
  271–3, 295–312
  airway filter/humidifier
    296–7, 302
  anaesthetic machine 54–68
  catheter mount 297, 302
  ET (endotracheal tube) 280,
    282, 304–8, 331
  face masks 295–6
  laryngoscope 302–4, 310, see
    also tracheal intubation
  LMA (laryngeal mask airway)
    280–1, 297–302
  Magill forceps 309–10
  nasal cannula 312, 316, 324
  nasopharyngeal airway
    279–80, 308–9
  oropharyngeal airway 279–80,
    290, 308–9

  oxygen mask 311–12, 325
  pulse oximeter 73, 393, 411
  Ryles (nasogastric) tube
    309–10
  ventilators 63–5
anaesthetic gases
  gas supply 55–61
  scavenging systems 61
  vaporisers 61–3, 64
  ventilators 63–5
anaesthetic practitioner
  airway management 272,
    278–80, 287–8, 330–1
  anaesthesia 271–7
  anaesthetic machine 54–65
  anaesthetic monitoring
    equipment 68–76
  anaphylaxis 295
  consent 141–2
  cricoid pressure (Sellick's
    manoeuvre) 284–7, 333
  cricothyroidotomy 291
  elderly patient 334–5
  laryngoscopy 302, 303–4
  LMA (laryngeal mask airway)
    281–2, 298
  local nerve block 327–8
  maintenance/emergence from
    anaesthesia 313–5
  malignant hyperpyrexia 296
  pacemakers 83
  paediatric patient 141, 329–32
  pregnant patient 332–3
  pressure sores 197, 219
  regional anaesthesia 316,
    324–5
  roles and responsibilities
    159–60, 313–5
  Ryles tube 309–10
  sedation 329
  spinal anaesthesia/epidural
    318–23
  temperature, patient 202

TIVA (total intravenous
anaesthesia) 68
tracheal intubation 280–4,
287–9, 209–1, 302–5, 306,
309–10
analgesia, postoperative 122–4,
267, 321, 386, 396–7, 400–1,
406
anaphylaxis 30, 207, 273, 293,
294–5, 406
ANF (atrial natriuretic factor) 7, 8
angiotensin 26
anoxia 44, 196
antibiotics 40, 111–3, 261, 313,
341, 345, 348, 375, 384–5, 406
anticholinergic agents 126, 129,
313
anticoagulants 265
antiemetics 12, 122, 126, 128,
265–6, 313, 385, 386, 392, 402
see also PONV
antiplatelet drugs 265
ARDS (acute (adult) respiratory
distress syndrome) 41, 293–4
arteries and veins, structure and
functions 15–16
arteriogram 259
aspiration of stomach contents
11, 241, 265, 276, 284, 292–3,
300, 305, 333, 341, 391, 402
aspirin 265
asthma 40, 131, 293
atenolol 28
atracurium 120–1
atria see heart
atropine 28, 113–4, 126, 128–30,
277, 383, 389
autonomic nervous system 18,
113, 126, 129

barbiturates 388
barium swallow or enema 259
baroreceptors 25, 43

bicarbonate (HCO_3^-) electrolyte
balance 7–8, 10
biological hazards 183, 209–11
bleeding see surgical haemostasis
blood based pH buffers 9–11
blood clotting
deep vein thrombosis 263
disorders 323, 390
positive feedback mechanism
4
preoperative treatment 112
role of calcium 9
wound healing 47
blood disorders
preoperative treatments 112
postoperative problems 390
blood gases 32, 35– 39, 388,
407–8
blood glucose 4, 44–6
blood infection (septicaemia)
215, 340, 389, 406
blood osmolarity 7, 8, 26–7
blood pressure
effects of drugs 28, 115, 119,
121, 126, 129–132
homeostasis 2–3, 24–7, 195
in shock 27–31
monitoring 73–4, 116, 258,
383–5, 407–9
blood sugar see blood glucose
blood tests 258
body-weight, and drug dosage
calculations 106–7
bougie 282, 284, 290, 307–8, 329
bradycardia see heart
breathing, assessment of 32,
38–9, 393–4
see also airway management;
respiratory system
bronchitis 40, 131
bronchospasm 122, 131, 132, 207,
293–4, 388
buffer systems (pH) 4, 9–11

burns 7, 41, 82–3, 91
bupivacaine 123–4, 127, 322, 326

caesarean section 332–3
calcium (Ca^{2+}) electrolyte 7–9
cancer, of the lung 41
cannulation, intravenous 111
capnography 72, 74
carbon dioxide laser 88–9
carbon dioxide levels 14, 32–36, 37–9, 74
cardiac output 20, 24, 27, 30, 31
cardiac rhythms 16–24
cardiogenic shock 29–31, 132
cardiovascular homeostasis 14–32
care pathways 257–8
care planning 253–4
catheterisation 341, 405–7
catheters, types of 405
cell membrane 5–6, 8
cerebral embolism 217
change management 134, 163–5
chemical hazards 92, 183, 203–6
chest infection 260–1
children see paediatric patient
chlorhexidine 108, 347, 406
chloride electrolyte 9
chloroform 111
cholinergic agents 129
cholinergic blocking agents 113, 126, 129–30, 313
circulating practitioner 79, 157–8, 317, 340, 363–4
circulatory system see cardiovascular homeostasis
CJD (Creutzfeldt–Jacob disease) 251
clinical governance 134, 149, 165–74, 235,
    Care Quality Commission 167
    Clinical Negligence Scheme for Trusts 166–7
    Healthcare Commission 167–8
    National Clinical Audit 167
    National Institute for Clinical Excellence NICE 166, 169
    NHS Constitution 168
    NHS Litigation Authority 168–9
    NHS Modernisation Agency 169
    National Patient Safety Agency 166, 170
    National Clinical Assessment Service 171
    Patient Advice and Liaison Service 166, 171
    performance indicators 166, 171–2
clinical leadership competencies 235–6
clinical supervision 134, 148–50, 172–3
cocaine
    local anaesthetic 124, 127
    drug abuse 184
cold viruses 40
colloids (plasma expanders) 13, 31, 404
communication, and patient care 134–8, 139, 140, 146–7, 159, 191, 209, 235, 249–50, 273, 392
complaints 137, 146–7, 171
computers, electronic health records 150–2
consent 141–3, 186, 252
Control of Substances Hazardous to Health Regulations see COSHH
cortisol release 43
COSHH (Control of Substances Hazardous to Health Regulations) 2002 203–6, 349
count board 363

cricoid pressure (Sellick's manoeuvre) 284–7
cricothyroidotomy 291
crystalloid infusates 13–4, 31, 385
CT (computerised tomography) 259
CVP (central venous pressure)
  in hypovolaemic shock 31–2
  postoperative monitoring 410–1
cyclizine (Valoid) 12, 113, 128, 266

day surgery 249–50, 252, 257, 259, 406
deep vein thrombosis see DVT
dehydration 7, 11, 12, 26, 41, 264
dextran 13, 265, 403
diagnostic imaging 259
diagnostic screening 249, 258–9
diarrhoea, loss of fluid and electrolytes 7, 12–13, 26, 403–4
diathermy see electrosurgery
diazepam 113
diclofenac 109, 401
digoxin 28, 106, 109
discharge planning 251, 252–3
distributive shock 29–30
diuretics 7, 403–4
dobutamine, to treat cardiogenic shock 32
documentation of care 146–8, 199
dopamine 28, 130–1, 403
doxapram 124
drugs see pharmacology
DVT (deep vein thrombosis) 97, 217–21, 263–5, 313

EBME (electrical and biomedical) department 52–3, 80, 89
ECF (extracellular fluid) 5, 8, 9, 11, 44

ECG (electrocardiogram, electrocardiograph) 18–24, 74, 116, 234
elderly patient 11, 107, 202, 251, 260, 262, 333–5
electrolyte and water homeostasis 2, 3–14
electrolyte metabolism 8–9
electrolyte replacement therapy 13
electronic health records 150–2, 180, 364
electrosurgery (diathermy) 68–83, 210–1
  bipolar 79–80
  hazards 82–4, 92, 210–11, 344
  monopolar 78–9
emergency equipment, recovery room 383
emphysema 41, 131, 291
endoscopic retrograde cholangiopancreatography 259
endoscopic retrograde pyelogram 259
endotracheal intubation see tracheal intubation
enflurane 61
ephedrine 28, 131
epidural anaesthesia 124, 317 21, 322, 323–4
epinephrine see adrenaline
equipment, care and competent use 52–4
  see also anaesthetic equipment; surgical equipment
ET (endotracheal) tubes, types and sizes 74, 282, 304–8, 331
  see also tracheal intubation
ether 111, 277
European driving licence 150
extubation 395–6

face masks
  general anaesthesia 295–7,
    381–3
  recovery 382–3
  see also oxygen masks;
    surgical face masks
fasting, preoperative 11, 241, 266
FBC (full blood count) 258
fentanyl 113, 122–3, 322, 326, 397
first assistant to the surgeon see
    advanced scrub practitioner
fluid balance 2, 4, 6–7, 11–14,
    385, 392, 402–4
fluid compartments of the body
    5–6
fluid replacement therapy 13–4,
    31–2, 42–6, 410

gastric aspiration 11, 265, 284,
    292–3, 305, 333, 391
GCS (graduated compression
    stockings) 218–9, 264–5
general anaesthesia 115–124,
    277–95, 333
glucagon release, response to
    trauma 43
glucose intolerance, following
    surgery 44–5
glyceryl trinitrate 108
glycopyrronium bromide
    (glycopyrrolate) 130

HACI (hospital acquired
    infection, nosocomial
    infection) 212–6, 340–2
haemorrhage 7, 25–6, 112, 130,
    384, 390
haemostasis (surgical) 365–9
hair removal see shaving
haloperidol 266
halothane 61, 295
hand washing 98, 185, 187, 213,
    216, 340, 344

Hartmann's solution 14
hay fever 40
hazards
  accidental 183, 184–7
  biological 209–11
  chemical hazards 92, 183,
    203–6
  deep vein thrombosis 217–21,
    263–5
  definition 180
  electrosurgery 82–4
  infection control 212–7
  lasers 90–3
  needlestick injuries 186–7
  radiation 199
  stress 212
  see also risk management
Health and Safety at Work Etc.
    Act 1974 52, 187, 208
health and safety see risk
    management
Health Professions Council see
    HPC
heart 16–24
  abnormal rates and rhythms
    20–24, 30, 44, 200, 207
  normal sinus rhythm (NSR)
    18–20
  rate 19–24
  structure and functions
    16–19
heparin 264–5
hepatitis B, infection control
    184–7, 207
hepatitis C, infection control
    184–7
herpes whitlow infection 183,
    209–10
high block (or total spinal block)
    321, 324
HIV (human immunodeficiency
    virus), infection control
    184–7, 207, 209

homeostasis 2–4
  blood pressure 2, 3, 24–7
  cardiovascular 14–32
  respiratory system 32–9
  support using fluid
    replacement therapies 11–14
  surgical haemostasis 365–9
  water and electrolytes 5–14
hospital acquired infection see
  HACI
humour, in patient
  communications 250
hydrogen (H⁺) electrolyte balance
  7, 10–11
hyoscine 113, 114, 126, 130
hypercapnia 38, 294
hyperglycaemia 44–5
hypertonic solutions 13
hypnotic drugs 113
hypocapnia 38
hyponatremia 43
hypotension 12, 29, 43, 74, 126,
  207, 294, 323, 324, 327, 358,
  401
hypothalamus 7, 26–7, 43, 201
hypothermia 107, 200–3, 331–2,
  334, 386, 411
hypotonic solutions 13
hypovolaemia 4, 7, 12, 42–46,
  321, 402, 410, 411
hypovolaemic shock 31–32
hypoxia 29, 41, 46, 66, 112, 262,
  284, 292, 294, 386, 391–6, 401,
  411

ICF (intracellular fluid) 5, 8, 14
IM (intramuscular) injection 110
immune system 40
infection control 98, 212–7,
  340–52
  cost 212–3
  HACI (hospital acquired
    infections) 212–6, 340–2

MRSA (methicillin resistant
  Staphylococcus aureus) 98,
  215–6
sources of contamination
  343–52
standard precautions 340–3
surgical scrub procedure
  343–5
surgical site infections 201,
  212–6
virus transmission 184–7
wound healing 369
inflammation wound healing 46
inflammatory response (phase of
  metabolic response) 42–4
information technology within
  the NHS 150–2
informed consent see consent
infusates 13–14
injections, routes of 109–11
instrument reprocessing, local
  350
insufflator machine 95, 96, 98
insulin release, response to
  trauma 4, 44–5
insulin resistance, following
  surgery 45
intraperitoneal drug
  administration 111
intravenous cannulation 111
introducer (to aid intubation)
  282, 290, 300, 307
intubation see tracheal intubation
investigations, preoperative 241,
  259–60
iodine 108, 347
IRDS (infant respiratory distress
  syndrome) 36–7, 41
isoprenaline 28, 130–1
isotonic solutions 13–4
IV (intravenous) injection/
  infusion 13, 65, 111, 116,
  161, 400

joint stiffness 261

ketoacidosis 11

laboratory tests (diagnostic
    screening) 258–9
lactic acidosis 11, 42
laparoscope 93–4
laparoscopy 80, 94–8
laryngitis 34, 40
laryngoscope 280, 290, 302–4,
    310
laryngospasm 291–2
laser
    hazards 90–3
    in surgery 85–90
    plume 83, 92, 344
latex allergy (practitioners and
    patients) 206–9
lidocaine (lignocaine) 108, 124–7,
    406
LMA (laryngeal mask airway)
    280–1, 297–302
local anaesthesia 108, 124–6, 131,
    234, 271–2, 325–8
local anaesthetics 108, 114,
    124–6, 127, 141, 287, 316, 317,
    321, 323, 324, 325–7, 388, 397
local field block 325–7
local infiltration 327
local nerve block 327
lung cancer 41
lymphatic system 14, 33

Magill forceps 309–10
malignant hyperthermia/
    hyperpyrexia 66, 74, 200,
    273, 295–6
manual handling 187–92
    see also patient – correct
    positioning
manual handling operations,
    legislation 187

medical gases see anaesthetic
    gases
Medicines Act 1968 102
Mental Capacity Act 2005 142
metabolic acidosis see acidosis
metabolic alkalosis see alkalosis
metabolic response to trauma
    41–6
metoclopramide (Maxolon) 12,
    128, 266
Misuse of Drugs Act 1971 102
Misuse of Drugs Regulations
    2001 102
monitoring the patient 68–76, 77,
    407–11
morphine 12, 102, 113–4, 122–3,
    128, 277, 397
MRI (magnetic resonance
    imaging) 259
MRSA (methicillin resistant
    Staphylococcus aureus) 98,
    215–6
mucous membranes, drug
    administration via 108–9
muscle cells 8
muscle contraction 6, 9
muscle relaxants 76, 118–20, 121
muscle wasting, following
    surgery 45
muscles, intramuscular (IM)
    injection 110

naloxone 124, 402
nasal cannula 312, 316, 324
nasogastric tube (Ryles tube)
    309–10
nasopharyngeal airway 279–80,
    308–9
nausea and vomiting see
    antiemetics; PONV
ND:YAG laser 88–9
needle phobia 135, 248, 327
needle-stick injuries 186–7

negative feedback mechanisms 4
negligence 146, 166–7, 168–9, 194, 362
neonates 106, 331, 396
neostigmine 115, 120, 129–30
nerve cells, action potential 6
NES perioperative working parties 230–42
neuromuscular block 76, 118, 388
nitrous oxide 56, 58–61, 69–71, 115–6, 277
NMC (Nursing and Midwifery Council) 144, 146, 197, 237
non-invasive blood pressure monitoring 73–4
non-medical anaesthetist (nurse anaesthetist) 161–2, 234
noradrenaline (norepinephrine) 25, 32, 43, 129–132
NSR (normal sinus rhythm) see heart
nurses, training in perioperative care 233
Nursing and Midwifery Council see NMC

ODP (operating department practitioner) 102, 140, 146, 155–6, 160, 232–3, 329
oliguria 31, 44
ondansetron 12, 113, 266
operating department practitioner see ODP
operating room, hazards within 180–3
opiate antagonists 115, 124
opiates 43, 115, 120–3, 267, 390, 400–2
oral airways, insertion and removal 393, 396
organisational hazards 212
oropharyngeal airway 279–80, 290, 308–9

osmolarity 5, 7–9, 14, 26–7
osmosis 5–6
osmotic diuresis 45
osmotic pressure 5, 7, 13, 14
overhydration 12
oxygen
    cardiovascular system 14–18
    homeostasis 2–3
    100% oxygen administration 200, 278, 290, 292, 293, 294, 295
    oxygen mask 311–2, 394
    oxygen saturation 32, 73, 282, 384, 391, 411
    preoxygenation of patient 115, 284, 395
    respiratory system 32–7
oxygen analyser (anaesthetic machine) 55, 57, 67
oxygen mask 311–12, 325

pacemakers (and electrosurgery) 22, 30, 82, 83
paediatric patient
    anaesthesia 328–32
    anaesthetic room 139
    catheterisation 405
    consent 141
    drug dosage 106
    inhalational anaesthetics 116, 119
    intubation 282, 304–5, 307, 308, 309
    suction 84
    sutures 371
    topical anaesthesia 327
    ventilators 63
pain assessment systems 386, 396–9
pain management 120, 161, 267, 396–402
    see also analgesia
pancuronium 120–1

paracetamol 400, 401
parasympathetic depressants
    113–4, 115
parasympathetic nervous system
    24–5, 43, 126, 129–30
patient
    consent 141–3, 186, 252, 262,
        401
    correct positioning 353–61
    dignity 139, 140, 353
    effective communication with
        134–9
    family and friends 256, 257,
        328, 400
    fears and worries 135–9, 154,
        248–9, 250, 257, 266, 330, 400
    patient roles 256
    physiological assessment
        254–5
    preoperative preparation
        247–51, 353–4
    psychosocial assessment 255–7
    religious or spiritual needs 256
    see also elderly patient;
        paediatric patient; trauma
        patient
patient advocacy 139–41
PCA (patient-controlled
    analgesia) 161, 267, 400–1
performance indicators 167,
    171–2
perioperative practitioner
    accountability 51, 143–6, 172
    attitude 271, 400
    communication skills 135–9,
        249–50, 399
    continuing professional
        development 149, 235
    developing role 231–5
    preoperative preparation
        247–51
    professional bodies 232, 235
    roles 154–163

route to enhanced
    competencies 235–6
training 231–9
see also perioperative team
perioperative team 154–63
    advanced scrub practitioner/
        first assistant to the surgeon
        158–9, 234
    anaesthetic assistant 230–1,
        234, 236–43
    anaesthetic practitioner 160,
        271–7, 277–95, 295–312,
        313–35 see also anaesthetic
        practitioner
    circulating practitioner 157–8,
        317, 340, 363–4
    non-medical anaesthetist
        (nurse anaesthetist) 161–3,
        234–5
    operating department
        practitioner 102, 140, 146,
        155–6, 160, 232–3, 329
    operating room orderly/
        support staff 154–6
    operating room support
        worker 58, 95–6, 97–8, 154,
        277, 286, 293
    reception practitioner 159–60
    recovery practitioner 160–1,
        202, 379–411 see also
        recovery practitioner
    scrub practitioner 95, 97–8,
        143, 156–8, 234, 339, 342, 361,
        363–4, 367
    surgeon's assistant 234
    surgical care practitioner 159,
        234
    teamwork 152–4
personal protective equipment/
    clothing 184–6, 188, 203–4,
    214, 342
pethidine 102, 122–3
pH buffering systems 4, 9–11

pharmacodynamics (actions and effects of drugs) 106–7
pharmacokinetics (how the body manages drugs) 105
pharmacology
  absorption of drugs 105, 108–111, 116–7, 125, 400
  anaesthetic chart 104, 385
  blood pressure homeostasis 24–7
  cardiovascular system 14–32
  controlled drugs 102–3
  dose calculation 106–7
  drug administration routes 107–11
  drug errors 101–3
  drug interactions 105, 107, 110
  drugs administered during general anaesthesia 115–24
  elderly patients 107
  half-life of drugs 105
  legislation 102–3
  local anaesthetic agents see local anaesthetics; local anaesthesia
  metabolism of drugs 105
  paediatric patients 106
  preoperative drugs 112–4
  safe practice during administration 103–4
  therapeutic level of drugs 106–7
  therapeutic margin/ratio of drugs 106
  see also specific drugs
phenoperidine 123
phenothiazine group (antiemetics) 126, 128
phentolamine 28, 132
phosphate electrolyte 9, 10, 11
pneumonia 40, 333, 396

PONV (postoperative nausea and vomiting) 7, 11–2, 113, 265–6, 287, 324, 391, 401–2, 403, 404
  see also antiemetics
positioning the patient 353–61
  see also manual handling
positive feedback mechanisms 4
postoperative complications 260–8, 387–91
postoperative nausea and vomiting see PONV
postoperative pain 396–401
postoperative patient, care in recovery 384–7
potassium
  (K⁺) electrolyte 5, 7–8
  infusates 14
  serum 44, 121, 404
preassessment clinics 249–50
  see also preoperative assessment
pregnancy (patient)
  anaesthesia (caesarean section) 332–3
  hypotension 358
pregnancy (practitioner), occupational hazards 205–6
preoperative assessment 190, 197, 249, 253–7, 263–4, 266–7, 333, 355
preoperative checklist 197, 274–7
preoperative drugs 112–4
preoperative equipment check 53–4
preoperative fasting 11, 266
preoperative investigations 241, 259–60
preoperative preparation and planning 247–51, 353–4
preoperative visiting 231, 248–51, 255

pressure sore risk assessment scales 198–9, 263

pressure sores and ulcers 191, 192–99, 262–3, 334

prions 299

prochlorperazine (Stemetil) 128

professional development (perioperative) 149, 235

propofol 65, 66, 117

propranolol 28, 132

protein depletion, following surgery 45

pulmonary embolism 217, 263

pulse lavage 84–5, 86, 342

pulse oximetry 73, 393, 411

pulse pressure 29, 44

pyrexia, postoperative 12

radiation hazards 199

radio-opaque dyes, use in investigations 259

RDS (respiratory distress syndrome) 41

see also ARDS; IRDS

reception area, communication with patient 137–8

record keeping see documentation of care

recordable items, counting and checking 361–5

recovery practitioner 379–411

airway management 383–5, 387–90, 393–6

assessment of patient condition 383–4

care in recovery 384–7

catheterisation 405–7

fluid balance maintenance 385, 402–4

haemodynamic status monitoring 385, 407–11

pain management 385–6, 389–1, 396–401

postoperative complications 387–91

transfer of patient 383–4, 387, 391–2

recovery room 380–3

reflective practice 148–9, 150, 236

regional anaesthesia 313–25, 334–5

religious needs of the patient 142, 256

remifentanil 65, 123

renal depression, effects on water and electrolyte balance 7, 11, 12

renin/angiotensin mechanism 26

renin release, response to trauma 43

respiratory depression 116, 118, 122–3, 124, 324, 401, 402

respiratory system 32–41, 260–1

RIDDOR (Reporting of Injuries, Diseases and Dangerous Occurrences Regulations 1995) 147–8

risk assessment 52, 179–84, 342–3, 352–3

risk management

accidental hazards 183–7

biological hazards 183, 209–11

chemical hazards 92, 183, 203–6

deep vein thrombosis 217–18, 219, 263–5

latex allergy 206–9

maintenance of equipment 187

manual handling 187–92

organisational hazards 212

pressure ulcers 192–9

radiation hazards 199

standard precautions 188, 340–2, 343

temperature control 62, 75–6, 200–3, 386–7

see also infection control

RSI (rapid sequence induction) 284, 292–3
Ryles (nasogastric) tube 309–10

salbutamol 108, 130–1, 293
SC (subcutaneous) injection 109–10
scavenging system 61
scrub practitioner
  managing recordable items 361–5
  roles and responsibilities 79–80, 91, 95, 97–8, 143, 156–8, 339
  surgical homeostasis 365–9
  wound management 369–76
sedation 271–2, 335
  antiemetic induced 126, 128
  opioid induced 401, 402
  regional/local anaesthesia 313, 327–9
Sellick's manoeuvre (cricoid pressure) 284–7, 333
sepsis 34, 42, 45, 293, 334
septicaemia 215, 340, 389, 406
sharps, safe practices 185–6, 364
shaving 346–7
shock
  blood pressure 27–31
  cardiogenic shock 29–31, 32, 132
  central venous pressure (CVP) 31–2, 410
  distributive shock 29–30
  hypovolaemic shock 31–32
  surgical shock 41–6, 404
sinusitis 40
skin, drug administration via 108
skin preparation, for surgery 91, 108, 234, 268, 345–8
smoke inhalation, risk from electrosurgical plume 83–84, 92, 210–11, 344

smoking, risks associated 196, 260, 263, 293
sodium (Na⁺)
  depletion/overload 403
  electrolyte 7, 8
  hypovolaemia 14
  reabsorption 26
  retention/loss 12, 44
  serum sodium 403–4
spinal anaesthesia (intrathecal block) 316–7, 318, 319, 321, 323–4
spiritual needs of the patient 142, 256
SSIs (surgical site infections) 201, 212–6
standard precautions (infection control) 340–3
stomach contents, risk of aspiration 11, 265, 284, 292–3, 305, 333, 391
stress, in the operating room 212
suction equipment 67, 84, 85, 393–5
supraventricular tachycardia see heart
surfactant (respiratory system) 36–7
surgery, effects on the body 11–13, 41–6
surgical dressings 375–6
surgical equipment 51–4, 76–98, 187, 348–50, 366–8
surgical face masks 85, 92, 138, 185, 211, 342, 344–5
surgical gowns and drapes 350–2
surgical haemostasis 365–9
surgical safety checklist 217, 248, 275–6, 364
surgical scrub procedure 216, 343–4
  see also infection control

surgical shock 41–6, 404
    see also shock
surgical smoke inhalation risk
    83–4, 92, 210–11, 344
surgical technique, and wound
    healing 369
sutures, types and selection
    370–3
suxamethonium 118–21, 200,
    295
suxamethonium apnoea 120
swab board see count board
sympathetic nervous system
    24–5, 29, 43, 126, 129
sympatholytics see adrenergic
    antagonists
sympathomimetics see
    adrenergic agonists

tachycardia see heart
teamwork 134, 152–4
temazepam 113
temperature control 62, 75–6,
    200–3, 386–7
temperature monitoring 75–6
tissue repair, wound healing
    stages 46–9
TIVA (total intravenous
    anaesthesia) 65–8, 121–3
tracheal extubation 395–6
tracheal intubation
    awake 287–8
    complications 288–94
    difficult 288–90, 307–8
    equipment 302–312
    failed 290–1, 332
trauma patient 251
trauma, the metabolic response
    41–6
tuberculosis 40
TV and camera monitoring,
    surgical procedures 93–95

U&Es (urea and electrolytes) 259
ultrasound investigations 259
urinalysis 258, 404
urinary catheterisation 262, 324,
    405–7
UTI urinary tract infection
    261–2, 340, 406

vaporisers 54, 61–3
vapour analyser 74–5
vasopressin, to treat cardiogenic
    shock 32
VDU (visual display unit), for
    surgical procedures 93–5
veins and arteries, structure and
    functions 15–16
venogram 259
ventilation systems (operating
    room) 348
ventilators (aid to breathing)
    63–6
ventricle see heart
vicarious liability 145, 155
virus transmission, infection
    control 184–7
visitors perioperative 180, 181
vomiting see PONV; antiemetics

warfarin 265
water and electrolyte
    homeostasis 5–14
    see also fluid balance
water retention 8, 12
wound closure 370–3
    drains 374–5
    dressings 375–6
    healing 46–9, 369–70
    infections 201, 214–5, 268,
        345–7, 348, 369–70, 375–6
    management 369–76

X-rays 199, 259